NMR in Living Systems

NATO ASI Series

Advanced Science Institutes Series

A series presenting the results of activities sponsored by the NATO Science Committee, which aims at the dissemination of advanced scientific and technological knowledge, with a view to strengthening links between scientific communities.

The series is published by an international board of publishers in conjunction with the NATO Scientific Affairs Division

A	Life Sciences	Plenum Publishing Corporation
B	Physics	London and New York
C	Mathematical and Physical Sciences	D. Reidel Publishing Company Dordrecht, Boston, Lancaster and Tokyo
D	Behavioural and Social Sciences	Martinus Nijhoff Publishers
E	Engineering and Materials Sciences	The Hague, Boston and Lancaster
F	Computer and Systems Sciences	Springer-Verlag
G	Ecological Sciences	Berlin, Heidelberg, New York and Tokyo

Series C: Mathematical and Physical Sciences Vol. 164

NMR in Living Systems

edited by

T. Axenrod

Department of Chemistry,
City College of the City University of New York, U.S.A.

and

G. Ceccarelli

Institute of Physical Chemistry,
University of Pisa, Italy

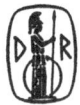

D. Reidel Publishing Company

Dordrecht / Boston / Lancaster / Tokyo

Published in cooperation with NATO Scientific Affairs Division

Proceedings of the NATO Advanced Study Institute on
NMR in Living Systems
Altavilla Milicia (Sicily), Italy
August 26-September 7, 1984

Library of Congress Cataloging in Publication Data

NATO Advanced Study Institute on NMR in Living Systems
    (1984) : Altavilla Milicia, Italy)
    NMR in living systems.

    (NATO ASI series. Series C, Mathematical and physical sciences ; vol. 164)
    "Proceedings of the NATO Advanced Study Institute on NMR in Living Systems, Altavilla
Milicia, Sicily, Italy, August–September 1984" – T.p. verso.
    "Published in cooperation with NATO Scientific Affairs Division."
    Includes index.
    1. Nuclear magnetic resonance – Congresses. 2. Biology – Technique – Congresses.
I. Axenrod, T. II. Ceccarelli, G. (Giulio) III. Title. IV. Series: NATO ASI series. C,
Mathematical and physical sciences ; no. 164.
QH324.9.N8N38 1984   574'.028   85–30044
ISBN-13: 978-94-010-8535-9   e-ISBN-13: 978-94-009-4580-7
DOI: 10.1007/978-94-009-4580-7

Published by D. Reidel Publishing Company
P.O. Box 17, 3300 AA Dordrecht, Holland

Sold and distributed in the U.S.A. and Canada
by Kluwer Academic Publishers,
190 Old Derby Street, Hingham, MA 02043, U.S.A.

In all other countries, sold and distributed
by Kluwer Academic Publishers Group,
P.O. Box 322, 3300 AH Dordrecht, Holland

D. Reidel Publishing Company is a member of the Kluwer Academic Publishers Group

TABLE OF CONTENTS

PREFACE

PREFACE

In the four decades since its discovery nuclear magnetic resonance (NMR) has become an indispensable tool for obtaining chemical information often inaccessible by other methods. With the development of instruments of increasingly higher magnetic field strengths, the integration of powerful computers and the availability of an expanding array of flexible software new applications and developments have proliferated rapidly. Among the more exciting new advances is the use of NMR spectroscopy to probe biological systems.

The last ten years have witnessed tremendous progress in the development of new NMR imaging and spectroscopic techniques for research and diagnostic applications. The ability to investigate metabolic processes and anatomical structure of intact biological systems under conditions that are totally non-destructive and non-invasive clearly provides much of the impetus for the intense activity that has been generated in the fields of medicine, radiology and the allied basic sciences. Significant advances have been made in this brief period: Whole-body proton NMR imaging today provides anatomical definition of normal and abnormal tissue with a contrast and detection sensitivity often superior to those of X-ray computed tomography and other competing imaging methods. Biochemical pathways, using NMR spectroscopy of protons, carbon-13 and phosphorus-31 nuclei in live animals and man can readily be followed by surface-coil methods to detect metabolites in localized regions. Indicative of the importance and widespread acceptance of these techniques is the explosive growth that the NMR literature is experiencing. This augers well for the future.

NMR as a probe in biological systems is by its very nature an interdisciplinary effort and its continued advancement depends on a combination of expertise drawn from many areas. These range from the basic physical and biomedical sciences through engineering and computer technology. The contents of this volume are taken in large part from the lectures presented at the NATO Advanced Study Institute on "NMR in Living Systems" held in Altavilla Milicia (Sicily), Italy during September 1984. One of the objectives of the Institute, and of this volume, was to bring together individuals from the different fields who could contribute to an authoritative over-all review of the present state-of-the-art.

In view of the range of interests and levels of NMR experience brought to the Institute by the participants, the program was designed to impart an in-depth knowledge of basic theory essential to the later treatment of more advanced techniques and specialized applications which are at the frontiers of the field today. The basic concepts including the resonance phenomenon, Fourier transform methods, relaxation mechanisms, spin-spin coupling, chemical shift spectroscopy, two dimensional NMR, computer data processing and instrument design were presented in the introductory phases of the program. With this as fundamental background, the various methods of obtaining and interpreting images, measuring cation concentrations in cells and following metabolic processes by topical NMR methods were then examined. The power, versatility and limitations of each of these methods were considered in relation to complementary methods presently available. Future research needs were explored and strategies for coping with the burgeoning literature were outlined.

Grateful acknowledgment is made to the NATO Scientific Affairs Division for the generous support of the Advanced Study Institute.   Special thanks are due to Professor Mariella Brai and Dr. Mario Valenza whose handling of many of the organizational details greatly facilitated the smooth operation of the Institute. Finally , we take this opportunity to express our appreciation to the lecturers for their advice and assistance in planning the program and for their cooperation and contributions in producing this volume.

Theodore Axenrod
Giulio Ceccarelli

New York, N.Y. (USA)
Pisa (Italy)
December 1984

AN OVERVIEW OF BIOLOGICAL APPLICATIONS OF NMR

Cherie L. Fisk and Edwin D. Becker
National Institutes of Health
Bethesda, Maryland 20205, USA

ABSTRACT. Since its discovery in 1946, NMR has developed to one of
the most widely used tools in chemistry and is rapidly becoming an
essential technique in biology and medicine. In this introductory
chapter the use of NMR in biology and biochemistry is traced from
early studies of small molecules of biological interest, through the
study in vitro of biopolymers and cell constituents, to the current
applications of in vivo spectroscopy and imaging. The development of
improved instruments and introduction of new methods that are essential to current uses are emphasized.

1. INTRODUCTION

The last few years have seen an explosive growth in the application
of nuclear magnetic resonance (NMR) to the study of living systems,
ranging from cells in tissue culture, through perfused organs to
intact animals and human beings. Increasingly, NMR data provide
detailed insights into metabolic processes, and the use of NMR
imaging already rivals or surpasses other imaging modalities, such as
x-ray, in its capacity to define anatomical features in humans and to
serve as a leading diagnostic tool. Some biologists and medical
practitioners view NMR as a new technique since it has only recently
made an impact in their fields. But NMR was discovered nearly 40
years ago (1), and in these four decades has moved gradually from a
phenomenon of interest to physicists to an essential tool in chemistry, biochemistry and now biology and medicine.
    To put the current uses of NMR in perspective, we first review
briefly the origins of the method and its early applications to
chemistry and biochemistry, then trace the extensions of its use as
instruments were improved and new techniques developed. Finally, we
comment on the present status and probable future developments in the
field.

1

T. Axenrod and G. Ceccarelli (eds.), NMR in Living Systems, 1–17.

2. PHYSICAL BASIS OF NMR

NMR arises from the interactions between the magnetic moments of
atomic nuclei and strong magnetic fields imposed in the laboratory.
We shall not provide a detailed account of NMR theory here, since
such developments are available in a number of textbooks ($\underline{2}$), but we
shall summarize the important results and equations. Some features
of NMR spectra can be understood only by the use of quantum mechan-
ics, while others can equally well be explained in classical terms.
Both classical and quantum mechanical approaches lead to the fundamental equation of NMR (first derived classically by Larmor in
another connection):

$$\nu_o = \left[\frac{\gamma}{2\pi} \right] B_o \tag{1}$$

where ν_o is the resonance frequency; γ, the magnetogyric ratio, is a
property of the particular nuclide being studied (H-1, P-31, etc.);
and B_o is the magnetic field applied to the sample. In the classical
picture of NMR the nuclear magnetic moment can be pictured as precessing, like a spinning top, about the magnetic field at the frequency ν_o as illustrated in Figure 1.

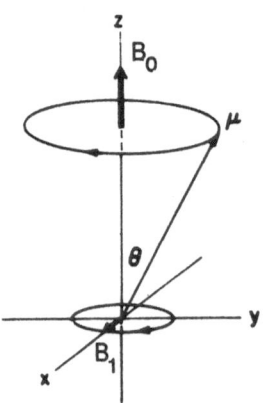

Figure 1. Precession
(at the Larmor frequen-
cy, ν_o) of a magnetic
moment, μ, about a fixed
magnetic field, B_o. For
detection of the NMR
signal, a radio-
frequency field, B_1,
(rotating in the xy
plane also at the Larmor
frequency) is intro-
duced. Interaction
between B_1 and μ (resonance) produces a signal
in the spectrometer.

In the first few years after the discovery of NMR in 1946 major
attention was focussed on obtaining accurate values of γ for various
nuclei, in understanding the interactions between the nuclear magnets
and the radio-frequency waves used to study their resonance properties, and in elucidating the mechanisms by which nuclei relax back to

equilibrium after being disturbed in an NMR experiment. As the
stability of NMR spectrometers and the homogeneity of magnets improved, physicists studying NMR were surprised to find that the
resonance frequencies of nuclei depended on the chemical compounds in
which the nuclei resided. This "chemical shift," initially a source
of annoyance in limiting the precision of the measurement of γ, soon
became the cornerstone for the development of NMR as a chemical tool,
as it was realized that nuclei could serve as probes of electronic
structure in molecules. The Larmor equation was thus modified to
take into account the electronic shielding, σ, around each nucleus:

$$\nu_0 = \left[\frac{\gamma}{2\pi}\right] B_0 \, (1 - \sigma). \qquad (2)$$

In particular, the observation in 1951 of three lines in the proton
NMR spectrum of ethanol (Figure 2) demonstrated the utility of NMR in
the structure elucidation of organic molecules.

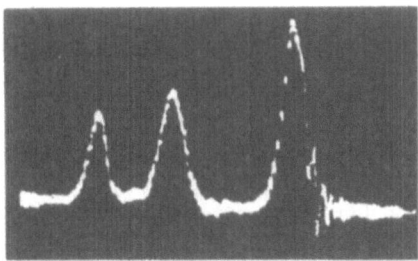

Figure 2. Oscillograph trace of the 32-MHz NMR signal from
ethanol obtained in 1951. The peaks from left to right
represent OH, CH_2, and CH_3. [Reprinted by permission from
J.T. Arnold, S.S. Dharmatti and M.E. Packard, _J. Chem.
Phys._ 19: 507 (1951). Copyright © 1951, American Institute
of Physics.]

     Soon after the discovery of the chemical shift, the continued
improvement in NMR instruments permitted the discovery of electron
coupled spin-spin interactions that cause splittings of chemically
shifted NMR lines into multiplets. The rapid development of theory
to account for the details of the sometimes complex NMR spectra and
the resultant correlation of NMR properties with features of molecular structure led to widespread use of NMR in chemistry by the
mid-1950's. Because H-1 has a large magnetic moment, hence gives
higher sensitivity than any other stable nuclide, proton NMR became

most popular and was used almost exclusively for organic chemical
applications.

3. EARLY BIOCHEMICAL APPLICATIONS

Most of the early NMR investigations devoted to biological and
biochemical problems were really just the study of organic molecules
which happened to have biological functions, but these studies
provided the basic data needed for the applications to complex
biological systems that were to come much later. Among the early
studies of proton NMR at 40 or 60 MHz were many structural and
conformational studies. For example, porphyrins were studied extensively by proton NMR beginning in the late 1950's and early 1960's.
Early observations centered on ring current effects and substituent
effects on chemical shifts (3), and thus laid the groundwork for
later studies of heme proteins. Around the same time, one of the
first examples appeared where proton NMR was used to establish a
complete alkaloid structure (4). In this study the new "high field"
60-MHz spectrometer was essential for accurate spin-spin coupling
analysis, and permitted the identification of non-equivalence due to
molecular asymmetry in the alkaloids lunacrine and lunine. The
characterization of a multitude of alkaloid structures followed,
aided by higher fields and introduction of double resonance techniques including nuclear Overhauser enhancement experiments. By
1972, a review of the previous three years' research in the alkaloid
field discussed over 400 structures (5).

Initial studies of steroids at 40 MHz focussed on points of
unsaturation and on the angular methyl groups which appeared as
sharp, intense signals superimposed upon a broad, unresolved spectrum
from the steroid backbone (6). This broad absorption was useful as a
finger-print, sensitive to minor changes in substitution. By 1970,
measurements of steroids had been reported at 220 MHz (7), and
nuclear Overhauser and solvent effects were used to aid structure
determination. A reviewer wrote that year in assessing the NMR of
steroids over the previous decade (8): "It is standard practice to
record the NMR spectra of all new steroids and it is unusual to read
a paper describing original work in the steroid field, which does not
cite NMR measurements as evidence for chemical structure."

Nucleic acid bases, nucleosides and nucleotides have been
fruitfully studied ever since pioneering work in the late 1950's at
40 MHz (9). The unambiguous determination of the predominant tautomeric form (amino or imino) in certain nucleic acid bases was a
problem solved by proton NMR in the early 1960's (10). Likewise
hydrogen bonding leading to base-pair interactions could easily be
observed even at low field as downfield shifts in amino proton
resonances (11). Research examining the association of bases and
nucleosides in aqueous solution (base stacking) began in 1964 with
observations of concentration and temperature dependent chemical
shifts (12). Numerous studies of mononucleosides and mononucleotides

centered around efforts to elucidate their conformations and intermolecular interactions in solution (13). Higher field instruments
clearly contributed to success in this field, allowing for complete
analysis of complex ribose spin-spin coupling patterns.

A large body of literature developed on structural, configura-
tional and conformational studies of carbohydrates building upon the
first extensive studies at 40 MHz (14). Empirical rules were developed for chemical shift calculations which depended upon the axial
or equatorial positioning of substituents. Along with the application
of double resonance techniques, improvements in sensitivity and
resolution permitted detection of long-range couplings and increasingly sophisticated analyses. The study of conformational equilibria
was also emphasized in early studies of sugars. At low temperatures,
anomeric species could be frozen out, and individual resonances
observed for different anomers (15).

The NMR history of amino acids and peptides began in 1957 with a
40-MHz proton NMR study of simple amino acids and dipeptides in
aqueous solution (16). The authors focussed on sensitivity of the
chemical shift to ionic form. At the somewhat higher fields of 60 MHz
and 100 MHz the spectra of all common amino acids were subsequently
obtained, and further studies yielded information about the relative
populations of different conformations in amino acids from analyses
of proton spin-spin coupling patterns. Spectral analysis played a
large role in conformational studies of larger, particularly cyclic
peptides. Focussing on the NH proton resonances in order to study
backbone conformation, authors deduced dihedral angles from coupling
to the alpha protons, and identified hydrogen-bonded protons from
deuterium exchange rates and the temperature dependence of their
chemical shifts (17).

The first spectrum of a protein obtained in 1957 at 40 MHz
(Figure 3) left much to the imagination, with only 4 broad bands
resolved. In subsequent studies, protein spectra were often recorded
under denaturing conditions (high temperature, urea or TFA). Also,
high concentrations were needed (for example, 20% solutions) leading
to further degradation in spectral resolution from molecular association effects and high solution viscosities. By the mid-1960's higher
fields and time-averaging techniques (discussed later) contributed to
significantly improved protein spectra in which aromatic protons
arising from histidine, phenylalanine and tyrosine could be readily
resolved. This observation led to numerous subsequent studies where a
protein's histidine chemical shifts were recorded as a function of
the solution pH, and thus the microscopic pKa values determined (18).

Some of the very first spectra of biological materials were in
fact spectra of water of hydration on biopolymers. As early as 1950,
spectra were obtained for proteins, carbohydrates and vegetable
tissue, where water was the only signal observed (19). In another
early study, broadening of the water line due to interaction with
solute DNA was detected, whereas proteins such as egg albumin caused
no measurable effect (20). In 1961 the technique proton relaxation
enhancement (PRE) was introduced (21). This technique still involved

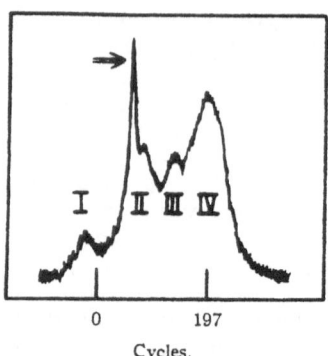

Cycles.

Figure 3. 40-MHz NMR spectrum of ribonuclease. [Reprinted by permission from M. Saunders, A. Wishnia, and J.G. Kirkwood, J. Am. Chem. Soc. 79: 3289 (1957). Copyright © 1957, American Chemical Society.]

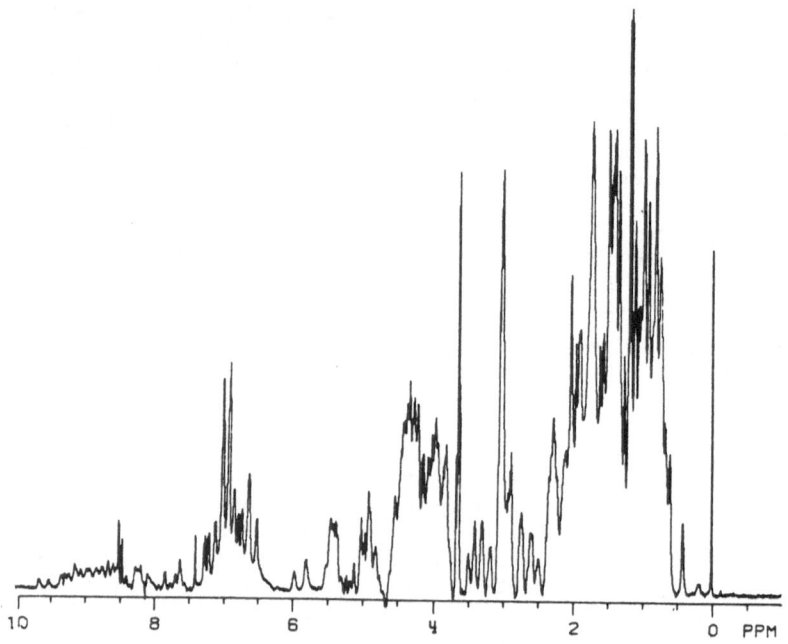

Figure 4. 500-MHz NMR spectrum of ribonuclease. [Reprinted by permission from J.S. Cohen, L.J. Hughes, and J.B. Wooten in Magnetic Resonance in Biology (J.S. Cohen, ed.), 2: 130 (1983). Copyright © 1983, John Wiley & Sons, Inc.]

measurement of the relaxation properties of water in the presence of biopolymers. But rather than being limited to a study of the water-biopolymer interaction itself, the water served as a probe for paramagnetic ion-biopolymer interactions. The first system studied was the binding of transition metal ions to DNA. Subsequent work established the PRE technique as a probe for the investigation of active sites in enzymes.

The experiments discussed above report early observations of proton NMR. Although sensitivity was obviously a limitation with other nuclei, substantial contributions using C-13 and P-31 NMR were made on molecules of biological interest. By 1960, the P-31 NMR spectra of ADP and ATP had been obtained (22). The P-31 chemical shifts were shown to be sensitive to the pH and ionic environment, an observation that foreshadowed current intense research activity monitoring metabolic changes in in vivo systems. Carbon-13 NMR was extremely difficult with early spectrometers, and yet a large body of useful data was collected in several laboratories. The first studies of C-13 chemical shifts and coupling constants in organic compounds in 1957 were carried out with neat liquids or in saturated solutions (23). Extreme sensitivity problems prevented studies at lower concentrations. Thus, it was not until more than a decade later that the the first molecules of biochemical interest began to be studied by C-13 NMR. Comprehensive surveys of natural abundance C-13 data for nucleosides and nucleotides were published, and C-13 enrichment was used to develop relationships between C-H vicinal coupling constants and conformation. Initial C-13 observations of amino acids were accomplished with double resonance techniques (INDOR) or with en-riched samples (24). Later studies designed to determine character-istic chemical shifts of amino acids in peptides largely relied upon pulse Fourier transform techniques discussed below.

4. DEVELOPMENTS IN INSTRUMENTS AND TECHNIQUES

The exploitation of NMR in biology and biochemistry has depended markedly on the phenomenal improvements over the years in NMR instru-mentation. As higher magnetic fields of excellent homogeneity have become available, it has been possible to unravel features of complex molecules that could scarcely be envisioned at lower fields. For example, the spectrum of ribonuclease at 40 MHz of Figure 3 has improved today to that shown in Figure 4 at 500 MHz. It is often not appreciated that along with an order of magnitude improvement in spectrometer frequency over the last 20 years has come an improvement in instrumental sensitivity of about a factor of 400, as illustrated in Table I. This arises both from the higher field and observation frequency (including a more favorable Boltzmann distribution) and from improved electronics and better probe design.

Table I. Signal/Noise for Various Spectrometers

Year	Spectrometer Frequency (MHz)	S/N *
1961	60	6
1965	100	30
1969	220	80
1978	200	300
1978	360	800
1984	500	2500

Strongest peak in methylene proton signal of ethylbenzene,
1% by volume. Single scan or single pulse.

Three other developments in NMR technique have also played a
vital role in permitting the application of NMR to the typical low
concentrations of molecules and to the insensitive nuclei found in
biological systems. The first is the principle of time-averaging,
first utilized in NMR about 1963. Figure 5 reproduces one of the
first published NMR spectra obtained by extensive time-averaging.

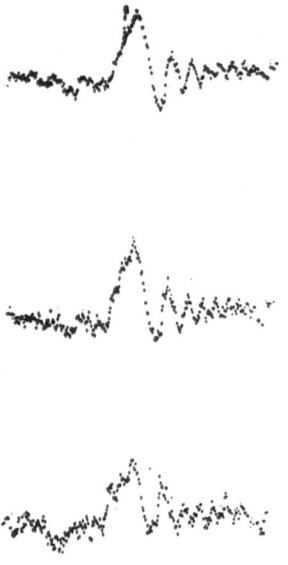

Figure 5. 6.5-MHz
natural abundance
deuterium NMR spectrum
of tap water obtained by
time averaging. The
lower curve is the
result of 1000 scans,
the center of 3000 scans
and the upper curve of
4000 scans. Each scan
occupied 0.4 seconds.
[Reprinted by permission
from M.P. Klein and G.W.
Barton, Jr., Rev. Sci.
Instr. 34: 754 (1963).
Copyright © 1963,
American Institute of
Physics.)

The concept of accumulating signal so as to average out random
noise had long been known in physics and engineering, but the application of the principle to a broad spectral range depended on the

availability of suitable digital computers. With time-averaging methods it was now possible to study NMR spectra at lower concentrations than heretofore and thus investigate molecules, especially biopolymers, of limited solubility. Since the signal/noise improves only as the square root of the number of repetitions, there is a practical limit to the sensitivity improvement that can be obtained.

The real value of time-averaging became apparent only with the next major advance in NMR methods--the introduction of pulse Fourier transform (FT) techniques. The use of short, high power radio-frequency (RF) pulses to excite NMR signals had been used since the early days of NMR, but only for samples with a single resonance line. As discussed in more detail in the following chapter, an ensemble of identical nuclei precessing at a given frequency can be represented by a "magnetization" vector, M, depicted in Figure 6. The effect of the RF pulse (which introduces the radio-frequency field B_1 shown in Figure 6a) is to cause the magnetization to tip from its equilibrium position along the z' axis to a new position with a component in the x'y' plane. With the proper choice of RF power and pulse width, the magnetization can be made to go through $90°$ (a $90°$ pulse) and end entirely in the x'y' plane. The interaction of the magnetization with the RF coil, located in the x'y' plane, induces a signal, the magnitude of which decreases with time as the individual nuclei go out of phase due to relaxation processes and magnetic field inhomogeneities.

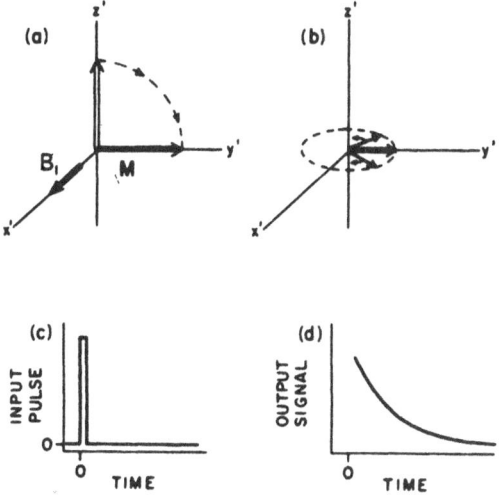

Figure 6. Application of a radio-frequency pulse to a single type of nucleus. (a) A $90°$ pulse along x' rotates M from the equilibrium position to the y' axis. (b) M decreases as the individual nuclear magnetic moments dephase. (c) Input signal, a $90°$ pulse, corresponding to (a). (d) Exponential free induction decay (FID) corresponding to (b). The output signal is proportional to:

$$e^{-t/T_2^*}$$

The resulting signal--the free induction decay (FID)--is simple in form for a single resonance, as shown in Figure 6d, but the presence of NMR signals at several frequencies leads to a complex FID. It had been known since 1957 that for any NMR signal, however complex, the FID and the true spectrum are related by the mathematical process of Fourier transformation. The seminal paper by Ernst and Anderson in 1966 (25) first developed the concept of pulse FT NMR in a practical way, and as mini-computers became available for use with NMR spectrometers, FT NMR became the method of choice because of its versatility and its ability to provide at least an order of magnitude further enhancement in sensitivity.

The virtue of FT NMR, as compared with older continuous wave (cw) methods, is that all spectral information is obtained in the FID in a period of about one second (sometimes less). Thus in the time that it would take to scan one spectrum by cw methods the FIDs from many pulse repetitions can be coherently added in computer memory and in a few seconds (sometimes less) can be Fourier transformed to produce a spectrum with much improved signal/noise (again in proportion to the square root of the number of FIDs accumulated). Relaxation effects (to be discussed in a later chapter) provide some limitations on the use of FT methods, but the versatility of pulse techniques permits pulse FT methods to be used for measurement of relaxation times and in some instances to overcome what might appear to be fundamental limitations.

The third major advance in techniques stems from the development of a theoretical framework to exploit the versatility of pulse methods in obtaining narrow line spectra from solids and in correlating spectral features as an aid to interpretation. Because of magnetic dipolar, and in some cases electric quadrupolar, interactions, NMR spectra of solids are often extremely broad, thus masking information on chemical shifts. Methods largely developed by Waugh and his co-workers beginning around 1968 (26) now permit crystalline and amorphous solids and solid-like materials such as membranes to be studied by high resolution NMR. Meanwhile, the expansion of FT NMR techniques into two dimensions has increased our ability to correlate proton and C-13 chemical shifts in the spectra of biopolymers, to examine chemical exchange processes and to exploit much of the high resolution NMR information available in solids. A later chapter provides a detailed discussion of two-dimensional NMR.

With the advent of FT NMR have come new data handling procedures, such as mathematical filtering (resolution enhancement) and difference spectroscopy. Spectral editing pulse techniques can both suppress specific types of resonances for spectral simplification and can select resonances of interest for detailed analysis. Also, effective pulse sequences have been developed to permit studies of exchangeable protons in spectra once dominated by an overpowering water signal.

Nuclear Overhauser Effect (NOE) measurements, and particularly 2D NOE techniques, are now available to the spectroscopist interested in defining spatial relationships in primary, secondary and tertiary

biopolymer structure. With 2D-J-connectivity and 2D-NOE sequential
assignment techniques (27), comprehensive proton resonance assignments in small proteins and polynucleotides of known sequence are now
possible. Inter-proton distances derived from these experiments can
then be utilized as constraints in conformational studies aimed at
defining macromolecular conformations in solution. Two-dimensional
techniques are also applicable to carbon-13 NMR spectroscopy of
biopolymers for heteronuclear correlation experiments in which
enrichment is often employed to increase sensitivity.

The study of nuclei other than hydrogen and carbon has also
blossomed with the advance in NMR technology, permitting, for example, detailed studies of the internal dynamics of deuterated biopolymers and membrane systems using deuterium NMR. The sensitivity
of the solid state line shape to molecular motion provides data for
the testing of various models of internal motion. The good signal to
noise ratios which can now be obtained in single scans of specifically deuterated membrane preparations (Figure 7) demonstrate the
increased potential of these techniques for the study of the internal
motion of individual membrane constituents.

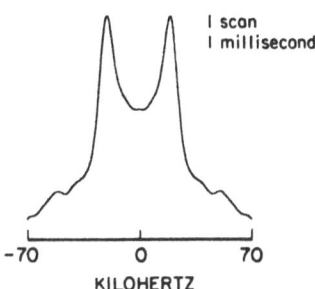

Figure 7. Deuterium quadrupole echo Fourier transform NMR
spectrum of [γ-d$_6$]valine biosynthetically incorporated into
the purple membrane of H. halobium R$_1$ in excess water at
-100 °C. The spectrum arises from the 21 valines in the
purple membrane protein (approximately 126 deuterons).
[Reprinted by permission from M.A. Keniry, A. Kintanar,
R.L. Smith, H.S. Gutowsky, and E. Oldfield, Biochemistry
23: 288 (1984). Copyright © 1984, American Chemical
Society.]

5. NMR IN LIVING SYSTEMS

Thus far we have discussed the development of essential NMR instruments and techniques and the application of NMR methods to the study
of important biological systems in vitro. Some of the current areas
of excitement are summarized in the first part of Table II. The main
focus of this book, however, is on NMR studies in living systems,
ranging from cells to intact animals and humans, as summarized also
in Table II.

Table II. Biological Systems Studied by NMR

IN VITRO STUDIES

- Small inorganic and organic molecules of biochemical
  significance

- Isolated, purified macromolecules such as proteins,
  polynucleotides, polysaccharides, and lipid bilayer
  assemblies

- Intact cellular organelles and membranes

IN VIVO STUDIES

- Intact organisms, single cells, and cultured cell
  populations maintained alive by various perfusion
  media and techniques

- Excised intact organs and tissue maintained viable
  by perfusion

- Surgically exposed organs and tissue (in live animals)
  placed within NMR receiver coils

- Organs and tissue using externally mounted coils on
  live animals and humans

- Organs and tissue in intact, unperturbed individuals
  (animal or human) using imaging techniques

The interest in studying living cells with NMR techniques stems
from experiments performed nearly 30 years ago. As early as 1956, it
was reported that most of the NMR signal from the water in human red
blood cells appeared as a broad resonance showing a slow exchange
with D_2O (28). Relaxation times for water in cells and excised
tissues were estimated in other early experiments, and found to be

substantially less than in distilled water. In addition, studies performed during the mid-1960's detected changes in T_1 and T_2 values of muscle tissue depending upon the hormonal state of the animal before tissue excision (29). Continued interest in defining and explaining the properties of water in biological tissue led to the report that the relaxation times of cancerous tissues were significantly longer than those from normal tissues (30). Differences in the NMR responses of various tissues are, in fact, a basis for the success of NMR imaging which will be discussed below.

The high resolution study of living mammalian cells began in 1973 with the observation that the P-31 chemical shifts of intracellular phosphates such as orthophosphate and 2,3-diphosphoglycerate are sensitive to intracellular pH (31). Since that time, numerous studies have concentrated on the quantitation of soluble (mobile) cell constituents including ions and metabolites in order to elucidate biosynthetic pathways, cellular metabolic activity, and transport phenomena in vivo. The technical challenge has been to develop methods for adequate oxygenation and nutrient supply to cells maintained in the dense populations necessary for NMR experiments. Creative methods for perfusion and cell growth on hollow fibers, beads, and in agar threads have been developed to meet these needs. The P-31 NMR research on cells, particularly that directed toward the characterization of intracellular ionic conditions and quantitation of the products of phosphate metabolism, provides a strong background for the interpretation of the spectra of intact tissue and for tests of tissue viability. In 1974, the first such report appeared showing P-31 spectra from intact excised rat hind-leg muscle packed in an NMR tube containing ringer solution (32). The P-31 signals from the high energy phosphates (creatine phosphate and ATP) were indeed observable and intracellular ionic conditions could be inferred from the chemical shifts of inorganic phosphate and ATP. This opened up possibilities for monitoring phosphate metabolism during muscle contraction and recovery (33). Recent studies have demonstrated the capability of current instrumentation to obtain proton spectra of tissues from a single transient that are of sufficient quality for the estimation of tissue metabolite concentrations and intracellular pH (34). This increase in sensitivity should provide additional impetus for the use of NMR as a non-invasive probe of physiological processes.

It is also possible to study metabolism in whole perfused organs and, with appropriate probe design, to study organs exposed surgically and then placed within the NMR receiver coil. Thus, for example, cardiac high-energy phosphate metabolic responses to physiological stresses such as cardiac arrest may be followed with NMR.

Methods that permit spectra to be obtained from living, unperturbed individuals, both animal and human, have resulted from two parallel developments: (1) surface coils (often coupled with magnetic field profiling); and (2) NMR imaging. Surface coils were first utilized around 1980 to monitor the metabolic state of skeletal muscle and brain in rats (35). The intensity of a surface coil radio-frequency field decreases with distance from the plane of the coil, thus detecting signals from a sensitive volume that extends to a depth equal to approximately the diameter of the coil. These coils have been used to obtain _in vivo_ spectra both by placing them on the surface of an individual adjacent to the organ or tissue of interest, and by actually surgically implanting the coil within an animal for studies over extended periods of time. Spatial localization of the NMR signal detected by surface coils has been aided by developments in static magnetic field profiling (sometimes called "topical NMR") and more recently in the design of "depth pulse sequences" (<u>36</u>). Surface coils were used in 1981 for one of the first reported applications of NMR to a clinical use, a diagnosis of McArdle's syndrome by observing the P-31 spectrum of the patient's arm muscle at rest and during aerobic exercise (<u>37</u>). Applications of _in vivo_ spectroscopy using several different nuclei will be presented in several later chapters.

The use of NMR to obtain two-dimensional or three-dimensional images analogous to those obtained with x-rays and computed axial tomography (CAT scan) has developed rapidly from its inception in the laboratory in 1973 (<u>38</u>) to current commercialization of clinical instruments for whole-body human imaging. The principle of NMR imaging is simple and is illustrated in Figure 8.

Sample cross-section

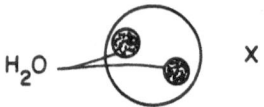

Field gradient

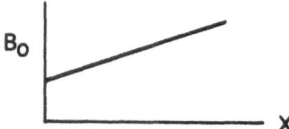

Spectral response

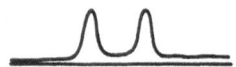

Figure 8. The principle of NMR imaging

From Equation (2) it is clear that a given substance (such as water) has an NMR frequency that is proportional to the applied magnetic field. If a known linear gradient is introduced into the magnetic field in one dimension, the observed frequency becomes a marker for location of the observed material, and a non-uniform distribution in the direction of the gradient provides a profile such as shown in Figure 8. By applying gradients sequentially in several directions and back-projecting, one can obtain two-dimensional images, a process identical to that used in CAT scans. Much more efficient and sophisticated methods are available for NMR and are discussed in detail in subsequent chapters.

Most NMR images of humans and animals represent primarily water, since it is the dominant proton-containing substance in the body. To the extent that other substances, such as lipids, with different chemical shifts have sufficient intensity to be observed, the images can be distorted since a given frequency now arises from more than one magnetic field, hence from more than one location. However, with suitable methods to disentangle the effects, "chemical shift imaging" potentially provides a great deal of additional information. Even a single chemical species such as water gives rise to a signal that depends on both the concentration of the substance and its local environment. The value of NMR in anatomical imaging stems largely from variations in water content in different tissues and on relaxation parameters. Indeed, as will be shown in later chapters, specific pulse sequences are employed to maximize the contrast between different tissues.

6. THE FUTURE

The future of NMR studies in living systems is very bright indeed. Magnets have now progressed to the point that high homogeneity can be obtained at field strengths up to about 1.5 teslas (about 60 MHz for proton NMR) with magnet bores of about 1 meter. Meanwhile, spectrometer sensitivity has improved so that low concentrations of nuclei such as P-31 and C-13 can be observed in highly localized volumes. As techniques for chemical shift imaging improve, studies of anatomical imaging and spectroscopy will merge. In vivo NMR applications rest on a solid base of molecular data, which itself is rapidly growing. Likewise, new developments in the physics of NMR such as two-dimensional and multi-quantum techniques, will doubtless have substantial spin-offs in the study of living systems. Finally, the complementary nature of x-ray CAT scans and NMR imaging in providing anatomical information on hard and soft tissue, and the complementary contributions from NMR and positron emission tomography (PET) in the study of physiology augur well for an explosion in our understanding of biological processes and in the diagnosis of many diseases. The remaining chapters in this book address many of these points in detail and present a picture of the current state of the art.

REFERENCES

(1)(a) F. Bloch, <u>Phys. Rev.</u> 70: 460 (1946); F. Bloch, W.W. Hansen and
       M. Packard, <u>Phys. Rev.</u> 70: 474 (1946).
   (b) E.M. Purcell, H.C. Torrey and R.V. Pound, <u>Phys. Rev.</u> 69: 37
       (1946).
(2)(a) E.D. Becker, <u>High Resolution N.M.R.</u>, Second Edition, (Academic
       Press, New York, 1980).
   (b) D.G. Gadian, <u>Nuclear Magnetic Resonance and its Applications
       to Living Systems</u>. (Oxford University Press, New York,
       1982).
   (c) R.K. Harris, <u>Nuclear Magnetic Resonance Spectroscopy. A
       Physicochemical View</u>. (Pitman, London, 1983).
(3) E.D. Becker, R.B. Bradley and C.J. Watson, <u>J. Am. Chem. Soc.</u> 83:
    3743 (1961).
(4) S. Goodwin, J.N. Shoolery and L.F. Johnson, <u>J. Am. Chem. Soc.</u> 81:
    3065 (1959).
(5) T.A. Crabb, in <u>Annual Reports on NMR Spectroscopy</u>, (E.F. Mooney,
    ed.), (Academic Press, New York, 1975), 6A: 249.
(6) J.N. Shoolery and M.T. Rogers, <u>J. Am. Chem. Soc.</u> 80, 5121 (1958).
(7) N.S. Bhacca, A.I. Meyers and A.H. Reine, <u>Tetrahedron Letters</u>,
    2293 (1968).
(8) J.E. Page, in <u>Annual Reports on NMR Spectroscopy</u>, (E.F. Mooney,
    ed.), (Academic Press, New York, 1970), 3: 149.
(9) O. Jardetzky and C.D. Jardetzky, <u>J. Biol. Chem.</u> 233: 383 (1958);
    O. Jardetzky and C.D. Jardetzky, <u>J. Am. Chem. Soc.</u> 82: 222
    (1960).
(10) H.T. Miles, R.B. Bradley and E.D. Becker, <u>Science</u> 142: 1569
     (1963).
(11) R.R. Shoup, H.T. Miles and E.D. Becker, <u>Biochem. Biophys. Res.
     Commun.</u> 23: 194 (1966).
(12) S.I. Chan, M.P. Schweizer, P.O.P. T'so and G.K. Helmkamp,
     <u>J. Am. Chem. Soc.</u> 86: 4182 (1964).
(13) P.O.P. T'so, M.P. Schweizer, and D.P. Hollis, <u>Ann. N.Y. Acad.
     Sci.</u> 158:256 (1969).
(14) R.U. Lemieux, R.K. Kullnig, H.J. Bernstein, and W.G. Schneider,
     <u>J. Am. Chem. Soc.</u> 80: 6098 (1958).
(15) P.L. Durrette, D. Horton and N.S. Bhacca, <u>Carbohydrate Res.</u> 10:
     565 (1969).
(16) M. Takeda and O. Jardetzky, <u>J. Chem. Phys.</u> 26: 1346 (1957).
(17) (a) D.W. Urry and M. Ohnishi, in <u>Spectroscopic Approaches to
         Biomolecular Conformation</u>, (D.W. Urry, ed.), (American
         Medical Association, Chicago, 1970), 263.
     (b) V.F. Bystrov, in <u>Progress in NMR Spectroscopy</u>, (J.W. Emsley
         et al., ed.), (Pergamon Press, Oxford, 1978.)
(18) J.S. Cohen, in <u>Experimental Methods in Biophysical Chemistry</u>,
     (C. Nicolau, ed.), (Wiley, London, 1973), 521.
(19) T.M. Shaw and R.H. Elksen, <u>J. Chem. Phys.</u> 18: 1113 (1950).
(20) B. Jacobson, W.A. Anderson and J.T. Arnold, <u>Nature</u> 173: 772
     (1954).

(21) J. Eisinger, R.G. Shulman and W.E. Blumberg, Nature 192: 963
     (1961); J. Eisinger, R.G. Shulman, and B.M. Szymanski, J. Chem.
     Phys. 36: 1721 (1962).
(22) M. Cohen and T.R. Hughes, J. Biol. Chem. 235: 3250 (1960); M.
     Cohen and T.R. Hughes, J. Biol. Chem. 237: 176 (1962).
(23) P.C. Lauterbur, J. Chem. Phys. 26: 217 (1957).
(24) W.J. Horsley and H. Sternlicht, J. Am. Chem. Soc. 90: 3738
     (1968); W. Horsley, H. Sternlicht, and J.S. Cohen, J. Am. Chem.
     Soc. 92: 680 (1970).
(25) R.R. Ernst and W.A. Anderson, Rev. Sci. Instrum. 37: 93 (1966).
(26) (a) J.S. Waugh, L.M. Huber and U. Haeberlen, Phys. Rev. Lett.
         20: 180 (1968).
     (b) A. Pines, M.G. Gibby, and J.S. Waugh, J. Chem. Phys. 59: 569
         (1973).
(27) (a) G. Wagner and K. Wuthrich, J. Mol. Biol. 155: 347 (1982).
     (b) J. Feigon, W. Leupin, W.A. Denny, and D.R. Kearns,
         Biochemistry 22: 5943 (1983).
(28) E. Odeblad, B.N. Bhar and G. Lindstrom, Arch. Biochem. Biophys.
     63: 221 (1956).
(29) E. Odeblad and A. Ingelman-Sundberg, Acta Obst. et Gynec.
     Scandinav. 44: 117 (1965).
(30) R. Damadian, Science 171: 1151 (1971).
(31) R.B. Moon and J.H. Richards, J. Biol. Chem. 248: 7276 (1973).
(32) D.I. Hoult, S.J.W. Busby, D.G. Gadian, G.K. Radda, R.E. Richards
     and P.J. Seeley, Nature 252: 285 (1974).
(33) M.J. Dawson, D.G. Gadian and D.R. Wilkie, J. Physiol. 267: 703
     (1977).
(34) C. Arus, M. Barany, W.M. Westler and J.L. Markley, J. Magn.
     Reson. 57: 519 (1984).
(35) (a) J.J.H. Ackerman, T. H. Grove, G.G. Wond, D.G. Gadian and
         G.K. Radda, Nature 283: 167 (1980).
     (b) J.J.H. Ackerman, P.J. Bore, D.G. Gadian, T.H. Grove and G.K.
         Radda, Phil Trans. R. Soc. Lond. B. 289: 425 (1980).
(36) (a) P.E. Hanley and R.E. Gordon, J. Magn. Reson. 45: 520 (1981).
     (b) M.R. Bendall and R.E. Gordon, J. Magn. Reson. 53: 365
         (1983).
(37) B.D. Ross, G.K. Radda, D.G. Gadian, G. Rocker, M. Esiri and J.
     Falconer-Smith, New Engl. J. Med. 304: 1338 (1981).
(38) P.C. Lauterbur, Nature 242: 190 (1973).

THEORETICAL BACKGROUND TO HIGH RESOLUTION NMR PARAMETERS AND NUCLEAR
SHIELDING CALCULATIONS

G. A. Webb
Department of Chemistry
University of Surrey
Guildford, Surrey
England

"...What people have learnt before reaching a certain, critical, age
they are inclined to regard as factual, or ordinary; and what they
hear later, as theoretical ... The critical age seems to depend on the
psychological type."
    K. R. Popper, "The Logic of Scientific Discovery", Hutchison,
    London, 1975, p.425.

ABSTRACT.   An attempt is made to provide the quantum mechanical basis
used in an interpretation of nuclear shielding data.   The various
models in common use are discussed and emphasis is laid on their
ability to provide some chemical detail of the molecular factors
causing nuclear shielding and shielding variations.   Most calculations
relate to nuclei from the first e.g. ^{13}C, $^{14,15}N$, ^{17}O, or second, e.g.
^{29}Si, ^{31}P, rows of the periodic table.   Recently interest has moved
towards the shieldings of heavier nuclei.   Thus an account is given of
the possible importance of relativistic effects in discussions of the
NMR parameters of heavy nuclei.   The possible shielding influences
arising from both specific and non specific solute-solvent interactions
are considered.   Finally, mention is made of ring current effects on
the shielding of protons in the neighbourhood of conjugated ring
systems.

INTRODUCTION

    NMR is a non-invasive technique for the detection and characteri-
sation of specific compounds in intact biological tissues.   From the
standpoint of living systems NMR applications fall into two principal
categories.
    The first being NMR imaging which seeks to map nuclear spin-
density, usually that of mobile protons, or relaxation times.   The
initial reports of work in this area appeared in 1973.   Over the
intervening years the development of this technique has been very
rapid, as witnessed by the appearance of three books dealing with this

19

T. Axenrod and G. Ceccarelli (eds.), NMR in Living Systems, 19–37.

topic during the past three years (1-3).

NMR imaging has tended to be mainly concentrated in the field of medical applications. Prototype systems became available for clinical use in 1980 and commercial systems are now available from various sources. Other commonly encountered names for this branch of NMR are zeugmatography and tomography.

The second principal category of NMR applications is that of high resolution NMR, which forms the basis of the present discourse. High resolution NMR permits the identification and measurement of metabolites, metabolic analogues, drugs, pH etc. The first reports of applications of this kind appeared in 1974 and progress over the intervening decade has been very rapid.

High resolution clinical NMR systems are now available for human limb or whole body studies. The observation of a high resolution NMR spectrum from a small part of a large body gives rise to the field of topical magnetic resonance (TMR).

In common with other forms of molecular spectroscopy, high resolution NMR provides spectra consisting of a number of lines and bands, whose relative position, relative intensity and shape may be analysed to yield molecular parameters.

I see it as my present remit to attempt to provide the groundwork for an understanding of some of these NMR parameters in terms of molecular structure (4).

The NMR parameters in question are σ, which describes the shielding experienced by the resonating nucleus due to its molecular electronic environment; J, which relates to nuclear spin-spin coupling via intervening electrons and thus depends upon relative nuclear and electronic dispositions; and the times, T_1 and T_2, which concern the relaxation processes encountered by the nuclei which became excited in the NMR experiment. Relaxation rates can provide information, inter alia, on molecular dynamics (5).

The theoretical background to all of these NMR parameters lies in mathematical models, an understanding of which can provide useful molecular information.

The theoretical aspects of the interpretation of relaxation data require methods which are fundamentally different from those required for an understanding of σ and J. A discussion of the basis of T_1 and T_2 requires some knowledge of the thermodynamics of irreversible processes, or a semi-classical description of the time evolution of expectation values or a quantum mechanical account of large ensembles. The present account does not deal with relaxation processes but further details may be found elsewhere (6).

In contrast to this the molecular interpretation of values of σ and J relies on theoretical models which are used to describe isolated molecules. These models are presented within a quantum mechanical framework.

Background to Nuclear Shielding Calculations

The molecular shielding of a nucleus in an NMR experiment, from the applied magnetic field, is due to the electrons and nuclei present in the vicinity of the nucleus in question. In practice one measures the chemical shift, δ, which is the shielding difference between two nuclei of the same species in different environments, e.g. those found in reference and sample molecules, σ_{Ref} and σ_{Sample}.

$$\delta = \sigma_{Ref} - \sigma_{Sample} \qquad (1)$$

Hence a high frequency NMR line shift, denoted by an increase in δ, corresponds to a decrease in nuclear shielding. A basic description of the various factors, responsible for producing nuclear shielding variations, requires a knowledge of the changes occurring in the electronic environment of the nucleus concerned (4,7).

Perhaps the three most important requirements of a reliable theory of nuclear shielding are;

A   It should be capable of producing quantitatively satisfactory results,

B   An interpretation should be available which provides some chemical detail of the molecular factors causing nuclear shielding, and, perhaps more importantly, shielding variations

C   It should be possible to apply the theory to moderately sized molecules without the requirement of excessive computational effort.

In spite of the many approximations involved, molecular orbital (MO) theory (8) is generally accepted to provide the most satisfactory description of molecular electronic structure at the present time.

Small molecules, with only light atoms, can be dealt with by rather sophisticated ab initio MO techniques, whereas semi empirical MO descriptions are available for larger molecules and for those containing nuclei up to, and including, the first transition series of elements.

In general the most time consuming step in MO calculations is the evaluation of two-electron integrals. For a basis set of size n there are approximately n^4 of these integrals to be evaluated for a given ab initio calculation. Whereas, for a semi empirical calculation the corresponding number of integrals is n^2. In addition, the use of truncated basis sets, in semi empirical calculations, reduces the size of n for a given molecule. Thus semi empirical MO calculations are less demanding on computer time and, although their results may be less satisfactory than those from ab initio calculations, they are the most widely used for calculations on larger molecules, e.g. those containing in excess of about fifty valence electrons.

In recent years multinuclear FT NMR instrumentation has led to the study of a wide variety of nuclei (9). It is perhaps salutary to realise that, of the eighty two elements in the periodic table, up to and including lead, all but four have one or more stable NMR active isotopes. The exceptions being Tc and Pm which have no stable isotopes at all, Ar and Ce. None of these four are particularly important from the point of view of living systems.

However, a number of heavy nuclei are of importance in bioinorganic chemistry, e.g. metalloproteins and enzymes. Thus an understanding of the factors controlling the NMR parameters of heavier nuclei is of some importance.

Before turning to a more detailed description of the models available for nuclear shielding calculations let us consider the approximate shielding ranges found for some NMR nuclei.

TABLE I

Some Approximate Nuclear Shielding Ranges in p.p.m.

Nucleus	Shielding Range	Nucleus	Shielding Range
H	20	Cr	1800
Li	10	Mn	3000
B	200	Fe	1300
C	650	Co	18000
N	1000	Cu	800
O	1500	Zn	100
F	800	As	650
Na	20	Se	1800
Mg	15	Ag	900
Al	500	Cd	800
Si	400	Sn	2300
P	700	Sb	3500
S	700	Xe	7400
Cl	1000	Pt	13000
K	50	Hg	3600
Ca	20	Tl	7000
Ti	1700	Pb	10000
V	7600		

As shown in Table I the shielding range experienced by a given nucleus depends, to some extent, upon its position in the periodic table. Thus the range appears to be related to electronic structure which, in turn, controls the chemistry of the element concerned. Thus the shielding ranges for the elements of the first two groups of the periodic table tend to be much smaller than those for nuclei from the later groups.

In general, heavier nuclei have much larger shielding ranges, e.g. cobalt and rhodium have the largest ranges known to date at about 18000 p.p.m. Additionally many nuclei, such as thallium, have a very solvent dependent nuclear shielding range (10).

As first pointed out by Jameson and Gutowsky twenty years ago (11) the range of shielding for a given element tends to increase with atomic number, and the periodicity of the shielding range largely follows that in $<r^{-3}>np$, where $<r^{-3}>np$ refers to the expectation value of the inverse cube of the separation of the valence p electrons from the nucleus in question. This function increases as one passes across the periodic table, due to incomplete screening of the nuclear charge by the valence electrons. In addition, an increase in $<r^{-3}>np$ is found upon descending a periodic group as the valence p electrons become more penetrating. Thus the factor $<r^{-3}>$, for the valence electrons concerned, appears to play an important role in any theoretical model of nuclear shielding. However, as we shall see later, the nuclear shielding range is more satisfactorily attributed to the differential of $<r^{-3}>$, with respect to the change in nuclear environment, rather than to $<r^{-3}>$ itself.

Thus there are a number of problems to be overcome in the production of a satisfactory account of nuclear shielding. These may be summarised as first, the choice of the most appropriate M.O. procedure. Second, the formulation of a suitable quantum mechanical model relating to $<r^{-3}>$, and its evaluation for light and heavy nuclei. Third, since such models are based upon the concept of a molecule in a vacuum some allowance must be made for medium effects in comparing the calculated and observed results. These effects can include those due to specific interactions, such as hydrogen bonding, and non-specific effects arising from the bulk electric and magnetic properties of the solvent employed.

The remainder of this discourse is devoted to giving some indication of the current state of play in relation to these problems.

Nuclear Shielding Models

Quantum mechanical calculations of the nuclear shielding tensor are usually furnished in the formalism due to Ramsey (12). This leads to the shielding tensor being described by a sum of diamagnetic, σ^d, and paramagnetic, σ^p, components:

$$\sigma = \sigma^d + \sigma^p \qquad (2)$$

where σ^d relates to the concept of the free electron rotation about the nucleus and σ^p relates to the hindrance to this rotation produced by the other electrons and nuclei in the molecule. It cannot be too strongly stressed that the terms "diamagnetic" and "paramagnetic" do not refer to the magnetic properties of the molecule under consideration but are due to the mathematical shapes of the expressions for σ^d and σ^p.

There are a number of drawbacks to Ramsey's shielding model in discussions of molecular problems (4,7). Amongst the difficulties encountered are that, as molecular size increases, σ becomes the relatively small difference between the two large and variable terms, σ^d and σ^p, which are of opposite sign. Consequently the value obtained for σ may be in considerable error.

A second problem is that the evaluation of σ^p requires a knowledge of all the excited molecular electronic states. Finally, the values obtained for σ^d and σ^p depend upon the origin chosen for the calculation. This can clearly lead to difficulties when comparing results from different sources.

A more suitable model for dealing with problems of molecular interest is one in which a number of localised shielding contributions are considered. Such an approach permits nuclear shielding to be considered as a sum of expressions, each of which can be related to particular atoms and bonds in a molecule (13).

A development along these lines has been made by Pople (14,15)

using a MO theory within the framework of an independent electron model.
The resulting expression for the shielding tensor may be written as:

$$\sigma = \sigma^d(\text{loc}) + \sigma^d(\text{nonloc}) + \sigma^d(\text{inter})$$

$$+ \sigma^p(\text{loc}) + \sigma^p(\text{nonloc}) + \sigma^p(\text{inter}) \tag{3}$$

The various diamagnetic and paramagnetic terms in equation (3) bear no
direct relationship to their counterparts bearing these names in
Ramsey's approach.

The local terms, $\sigma^d(\text{loc})$ and $\sigma^p(\text{loc})$ arise from electronic
currents localised on the atom containing the nucleus of interest;
$\sigma^d(\text{nonloc})$ and $\sigma^p(\text{nonloc})$ are due to currents on neighbouring atoms
while $\sigma^d(\text{inter})$ and $\sigma^p(\text{inter})$ are derived from shielding currents not
localised on any atom in the molecule, e.g. ring currents.   The two
interatomic terms in equation (3) produce a shielding contribution of a
few parts per million at most.   The data given in Table I reveal that
most nuclei have shielding ranges of several hundred parts per million;
consequently shielding effects due to ring currents are normally neglected when discussing chemical shift trends of most nuclei;   an exception
being that of the hydrogen nuclei as discussed later.

The difficulties noted above, with respect to the evaluation of
the shielding terms resulting from Ramsey's model, are absent when
Pople's sum-over-states (SOS) approach is used together with gauge-
invariant atomic orbitals (GIAO's) to evaluate the terms given in
equation (3).   However, inclusion of the molecular electronic excited
states is usually the least satisfactory aspect of SOS nuclear shielding
calculations.

A means of obviating the requirement of excited state information
is to use finite perturbation theory (FPT) rather than the SOS procedure.   Ditchfield (16,17) has successfully adopted this approach, at
the ab initio level with GIAO's, in a discussion of the nuclear
shielding of small molecules containing light atoms.   Some molecules
of biological interest have also been studied by means of the shielding
model developed by Ditchfield.   Promising shielding data have been
presented for the various nuclei in N-methylformamide (18), imidazole
(19) and cytosine (20) as a result of small basis set ab initio calculations.

An extension of this model to larger molecules is, at present, only
feasible by the employment of semi empirical CNDO/INDO parameters (21,
22).   By this means satisfactory [11]B and ^{13}C shielding results have
been reported which show that multicentre terms play an important role
in determining σ, particularly when multiple bonding occurs.

A different, but related, approach is that due to Schindler and
Kutzelnigg who use localised MO's with individual gauge origins in order
to describe the nuclear shielding in terms of localised (chemically
interesting) quantities (23).   This is known as the IGLO, (individual
gauge origin for localised MO's), procedure.   The IGLO's tend to be
approximately spherical in shape which results in the paramagnetic
shielding contributions being rather smaller than those produced by
means of GIAO's.   Consequently any error in the calculation of the

paramagnetic contribution to the shielding is likely to be of less importance when IGLO's are employed. _Ab initio_ IGLO shielding calculations have been reported for the ^{1}H and ^{13}C nuclei in about one hundred compounds (24). In most cases the agreement with experimental data appears to represent an improvement over that found by earlier _ab initio_ shielding calculations.

TABLE II (24)

^{13}C Shieldings (ppm) Relative to CH_4

Molecule	Nucleus	IGLO (a) Dz	I	II	IGLO Increment	Experiment
C_2H_6		-5.7	-11.9	-13.2	-15.4	-14.3
C_3H_8	CH_3	-12.6			-17.6	-24.3
	CH_2	-7.6			-22.4	-25.8
C_2H_4		-129.6	-134.2	-135.1	-134.6	-129.8
CH_2=CH	CH_2	-127.1	-125.4		-120.7	-119.8
CH=CH_2	CH	-139.2	-147.9		-134.0	-140.4
CH_3 C CH_3	CH_3				-20.2	-20.0
CH_3 C CH_3 CH_3	C				-140.6	-123.9

(a) Dz is a double zeta basis set, I is a contracted triple zeta set plus one set of polarisation functions for d orbitals on carbon and p orbitals on hydrogen, II differs from I only in the contraction of the p groups.

As shown in Table II, a particularly interesting aspect of IGLO calculations is that orbital contributions to nuclear shielding appear to be transferable. Thus it is possible to assign specific shielding contributions to particular molecular regions and, consequently, to develop an _ab initio_ incremental system for nuclear shielding which should be of particular interest to workers dealing with large molecules.

In spite of its various limitations Pople's SOS model with CNDO/INDO parameters is the most widely adopted one for the calculation of nuclear shielding.

Within the confines of the approximations inherent to CNDO/INDO type calculations, the rotationally averaged values of the local shielding terms for nucleus A, which is assumed to have only s and p valence electrons, are given by equations (4) and (5)

$$\sigma_A^d(\text{loc}) = \frac{\mu_o e^2}{12\pi m} \sum_\nu^A P\nu\nu <|\Gamma_{A\nu}^{-1}|\nu> \tag{4}$$

$$\sigma_A^p(\text{loc}) = \frac{-\mu_o e^2 h^2}{6\pi m^2} <r^{-3}>_{np} \sum_j^{occ} \sum_k^{unocc} (E_k - E_j)^{-1}$$

$$\times \left[(C_{jAj}C_{zAk} - C_{zAj}C_{yAk}) \sum_B (C_{yBj}C_{zBk} - C_{zBj}C_{yBk}) \right.$$

$$+ (C_{zAj}C_{xAk} - C_{xAj}C_{zAk}) \sum_B (C_{zBj}C_{xBk} - C_{xBj}C_{zBk})$$

$$+ \left. (C_{xAj}C_{yAk} - C_{yAj}C_{xAk}) \sum_B (C_{xBj}C_{yBk} - C_{yBj}C_{xBk}) \right] \tag{5}$$

Where $P\nu\nu$ is the charge density in the atomic orbital ν that is at an average distance $\Gamma_{A\nu}$ from nucleus A, C_{xAj} is the LCAO coefficient of the P_x orbital on atom A in the MO j etc. The summation over neighbouring atoms B includes A. In Equation (5) E_k and E_j refer to the energies of MO's k and j that are unoccupied and occupied, respectively, in the ground state. The excitation energies, E_k-E_j are for the excited singlet states which are mixed with the ground state by the applied magnetic field.

From the ordering of the LCAO coefficients in equation (5) it is apparent that $\sigma\to\sigma^*$, $\sigma\to\pi^*$, $n\to\sigma^*$ and $n\to\pi^*$ singlet transitions may be expected to contribute to $\sigma_A^p(\text{loc})$. It is also clear that both atoms A and B must possess valence p electrons for $\sigma_A^p(\text{loc})$ to be non zero.

Hence, within the SOS description at the semi empirical MO level, the nuclear shielding of the elements of groups I and II of the periodic table has no contribution from $\sigma_A^p(\text{loc})$. The restricted nuclear shielding ranges of these elements are thus understandable in terms of small variations in the other contributions to equation (3). In general, such changes are markedly smaller than those normally observed in $\sigma_A^p(\text{loc})$.

Expressions analogous to equations (4) and (5) are available for the nonlocal shielding terms (4). Calculations on first-row nuclei show that $\sigma_A^d(\text{nonloc})$ contributes less than 1 p.p.m. to the total shielding whereas the magnitude of $\sigma_A^p(\text{nonloc})$ depends on the multiplicity of the bonding involved (25). The largest value of $\sigma_A^p(\text{nonloc})$ found for first-row nuclei is about -12 p.p.m. for the central atom in the azide anion, and the corresponding value of $\sigma_A^p(\text{loc})$ is -261 p.p.m. (26).

Thus within the framework of Pople's SOS model, nuclear shielding is largely described by $\sigma_A^d(\text{loc})$ and $\sigma_A^p(\text{loc})$, with $\sigma_A^p(\text{nonloc})$ being of marginal importance for multiply bonded light nuclei. Consequently the small shielding range of hydrogen, and other atoms with only s valence electrons, is ascribed to variations in $\sigma_A^d(\text{loc})$ at least in part.

Equations (4) and (5) have been evaluated by means of various semi-empirical MO parameter sets. These calculations reveal that $\sigma_A^d(loc)$ usually varies by less than 5% for a given nucleus in a range of molecular environments (27). Hence, for the majority of nuclei, shielding variations are primarily due to a change in the value of $\sigma_A^p(loc)$.

The restricted shielding range of the hydrogen nuclei is not accounted for by a change of less than 5% in $\sigma_A^d(loc)$. There are additional influences to be considered such as ring current effects which are mentioned later.

Closer inspection of equation (5) reveals three potential sources of variation for $\sigma_A^p(loc)$, namely $<r^{-3}>np$, the excitation energy E_k-E_j, and the MO coefficients of the p orbitals.

TABLE III

Some SCF Dirac-Fock values of $<r^{-3}>np$ [28] (a)

Element (n=2)		Element (n=3)		Element (n=4)		Element (n=5)	
B	0.775	Al	1.089	As	7.026	Sn	7.274
C	1.661	Si	2.030	Se	9.518	Sb	9.977
N	3.020	P	3.273	Br	12.339	Te	12.929
O	4.948	S	4.849			I	16.152
F	7.544	Cl	6.799			Hg	194.732

(a)   Values are in (atomic units)$^{-3}$

As shown in Table III, the value of $<r^{-3}>np$ depends critically on the position of the nucleus in question within the periodic table. In general, the larger values of $<r^{-3}>np$ are those which are more susceptible to change giving rise to larger nuclear shielding ranges.

An expression analogous to equation (7) has been derived for d orbital shielding contributions (11). Since the d orbital contribution to $\sigma_A^p(loc)$ also has a $<r^{-3}>$ dependence it shows a periodic variation analogous to that of the p orbitals.

We now appear to have some understanding of the relationship between nuclear shielding and $<r^{-3}>$. In practice it is usually not feasible to separate changes in $<r^{-3}>$, for the valence electrons, from those in the relevant excitation energies and MO coefficients.

In closing this section we note that equation (5) is often simplified by means of the closure approximation and the replacement of E_k-E_j by ΔE. This is usually referred to as the average excitation energy (AEE) approximation. Because ΔE corresponds to some unknown weighted average of singlet transition energies it is usually not calculated a priori but treated as an empirical parameter.

Within the AEE approximation equation (5) becomes

$$\sigma_A^p(loc) = \frac{-U_o e^2 h^2}{8\pi m^2} \frac{<r^{-3}>np}{\Delta E} \sum_B Q_{AB} \qquad (6)$$

where $Q_{AB} = \frac{4}{3} \delta_{AB} (P_{xAxB} + P_{yAyB} + P_{zAzB})$

$$- \frac{2}{3} (P_{xAxB}P_{yAyB} + P_{xAxB}P_{zAzB} + P_{yAyB}P_{zAzB})$$

$$+ \frac{2}{3} (P_{xAyB}P_{xByA} + P_{xAzB}P_{xBzA} + P_{yAzB}P_{yBzA}) \tag{7}$$

and δ_{AB} is the Kronecker delta and the P's are the elements of the charge density bond order matrix. Thus the first set of terms on the right-hand side of equation (7) is a charge density expression, while the remaining two sets correspond to bond orders.

Relativistic Effects for Heavy Nuclei

The electronic properties of heavy atoms are influenced by relativistic effects. Essentially two such effects need to be considered in dealing with NMR parameters. The first of these arises from changes in the radial parts of the wavefunctions of heavier nuclei. Such changes may be contemplated in the following manner. In order for electrons to resist the enhanced positive change of a heavy nucleus they must move at greater velocities in their Bohr orbits. The increase in velocity eventually leads to a relativistic mass increase which results in the electrons closest to the nucleus being attracted more to it. Consequently the radii of the innermost orbits tend to contract. This contraction may lead to a greater screening of the nuclear charge for the outer electrons such that the radii of their orbitals may expand. As can be seen from equations (4) and (5) changes in the separation between a given nucleus and the surrounding electrons are expected to significantly alter both the diamagnetic and paramagnetic shielding contributions. That this is the case for σ^d is shown clearly for the heavy nuclei featured in Table (IV) (29) while Table V gives the ratio of the calculated relativistic to non-relativistic values of $<r^{-3}>$ for a number of electrons in various atoms. The data in Table V show the general contraction of inner orbitals and the expansion of the outermost ones which will influence the value calculated for σ^p.

TABLE IV (29)

Some Atomic Values of σ^d in ppm

Element	Non-Relativistic Value	Relativistic Value
He	59.9	59.9
Ne	553	559
Ar	1130	1159
Kr	2472	2727
Xe	3949	4947
Hg	6595	11290

TABLE V (28)

Ratio of Relativistic to Non-Relativistic Values of $\langle r^{-3} \rangle$

Element	Orbital	Ratio	Element	Orbital	Ratio
C	2p	0.999	Cd	2p	1.055
N	2p	0.999		3p	1.076
O	2p	0.999		3d	0.996
F	2p	0.999		4p	1.079
				4d	0.978
Cl	2p	1.004			
	3p	1.003	Hg	2p	1.181
				3p	1.263
As	2p	1.023		3d	1.022
	3p	1.032		4p	1.286
	3d	0.988		4d	1.033
	4p	1.025		4f	1.278
				5p	1.293
Br	2p	1.026		5d	0.964
	3p	1.036			
	3d	0.989			
	4p	1.028			

The second relativistic effect which must be taken into account arises from the breakdown of Russell Saunders coupling in favour of j-j coupling of electronic angular momenta (30). This breakdown is the the result of an increase in the magnitude of the electronic spin-orbit coupling parameter. The result being that some spin triplet character is mixed into the ground spin singlet state, of a diamagnetic molecule, by mechanisms which are comparable to the contact and dipolar inter- actions found in the theory of nuclear spin-spin couplings. The resulting spin triplet character of the ground state produces a local magnetic field at a given nucleus thus giving rise to a change in nuclear shielding.

Such shielding influences are often known as heavy atom effects. For example, compared to methane the ^{13}C nuclei of CH_3I, CH_2I_2, CHI_3 and CI_4 are shielded by 18.5, 51.7, 137.6 and 290.2 ppm respectively. INDO parameterised calculations show that spin-orbit coupling effects on ^{13}C shieldings of the halomethanes are small for chlorine substitution, essential for bromine substitution and predominant when iodine substi- tution occurs (31). In the case of HI, spin-orbit coupling appears to contribute 51% of the total proton shielding (32).

Recently, expressions have been reported for the relativistic formulation of the paramagnetic part of the Ramsey shielding expression (33,34) and of that of the Pople shielding theory (35). However, evaluation of these terms for molecules is still awaited. Nonetheless it does seem very likely that relativistic influences will play a major role in the determination of the shieldings of heavier nuclei.

TABLE VI   Comparison of some INDO/S–SOS calculated nitrogen shieldings
of some N-heterocycles with experimental data

System	Shielding source	N-1	N-2	Average
	Calc. Expt.	172.42	111.89	142.16 172.6
	Calc. Expt.	177.40	114.78	146.09 177.2
	Calc. Expt.	158.91 206.0	158.91 206.0	
	Calc. Expt.	174.83 221.3	117.73 125.5	
	Calc. Expt.	172.96 217.7	128.45 134.7	
	Calc. Expt.	170.76 217.0	166.45 196.0	
	Calc. Expt.	165.40 204.5	165.40 204.5	
	Calc. Expt.	166.31 180.8	114.15 76.5	
	Calc. Expt.	169.05 182.2	124.64 94.4	
	Calc. Expt.	177.90 186.4	168.93 146.4	
	Calc. Expt.	192.13 200.6	80.58 65.1	
	Calc. Expt.	195.04 207.2	102.68 90.8	

Medium Effects on Nuclear Shielding

Interactions between solute and solvent molecules in a given solution may be treated as belonging to either of two categories; namely specific and nonspecific interactions. Specific effects include those arising from hydrogen bonding, complex formation and those that take place when shift or relaxation reagents are added to a solution to be studied by NMR. In general, such interactions are predictable from a knowledge of the chemistry of the system concerned. Calculations of nuclear shielding in the presence of specific interactions may be performed by using the supermolecule approach (36,37).

Nitrogen atoms are often potential molecular sites for hydrogen bond formation. Thus nitrogen NMR can be a very satisfactory means of investigating hydrogen bonding. Supermolecule calculations of the minimum basis set ab initio variety, within the FPT framework, have been employed to study the effects of hydrogen bonding on the nitrogen shielding of formamide (18) and imidazole (19). The experimental shielding trends are qualitatively reproduced by these calculations. However, in the case of imidazole better agreement with experiment is obtained from some INDO/S SOS shielding calculations (38).

The results of some INDO/S SOS supermolecule calculations of nitrogen shielding changes, due to hydrogen bond formation and protonation, in some heterocyclic systems are shown in Table VI (38).

The rather poorer agreement between the ab initio and experimental nitrogen shielding changes, upon hydrogen bond formation, most probably arises from the necessity of using a minimum basis set in the calculations. For the present it seems that semi empirical MO calculations of nitrogen shielding effects, arising from hydrogen bonding in N heterocyclic systems, must suffice.

Nonspecific solvent effects on NMR parameters may be discussed on the basis of two types of model. In one the solvent is taken as a continuum, characterised by its macroscopic dielectric constant, ε. The electrostatic interactions between the solute and solvent molecules are accounted for in terms of the reaction field theory (39). The second type of model permits the shielding changes to be interpreted in terms of interactions between pairs of molecules. A general pair interaction model includes terms due to van der Waals forces, bulk susceptibility effects, electric moment effects and the magnetic anisotropy of nonspherical solute molecules (40).

Precise mathematical expressions are not available for many non-bonded interactions. Consequently continuum models tend to be more popular for investigating solvent effects on NMR parameters. The most widely used of these, to date, seems to be the solvaton model (41). By means of this model the solvent induced shift is proportional to $(\varepsilon - 1)/2\varepsilon$. Some INDO/S SOS shielding calculations, incorporating the solvaton model, predict that the nitrogen shielding of nitromethane will decrease by ～10 ppm as ε increases from ～2 to ～46 (42). This is in good agreement with observation and suggests that the solvaton model may be suitable for determining the solvent induced changes in nitrogen nuclear shielding that may occur in biomolecules. At present nitrogen shielding variations in such molecules are frequently attributed to a

Table VII Some CNDO/S calculated contributions to the ^{31}P shielding
        tensor[a] and charge,[b] Q, on the phosphorus atom, as a function
        of the dielectric constant (ε) of the medium

Molecule	ε	$\sigma^P(3p)$	$\sigma^P(3d)$	σ^P_{Total}	σ_{Total}	$(r^{-3})_{3p}^c$	$(r^{-3})_{3d}^c$	Q^b
PH_3	1	-293.57	-6.44	-300.01	652.39	1.452	0.290	4.716
	2	-301.55	-6.45	-307.98	644.32	1.467	0.293	4.668
	4	-302.37	-6.46	-308.81	643.49	1.473	0.295	4.643
	10	-303.88	-6.45	-310.31	641.99	1.479	0.296	4.628
	20	-305.41	-6.44	-311.72	640.58	1.481	0.296	4.623
	40	-306.05	-6.43	-312.49	639.81	1.482	0.296	4.621
	80	-306.82	-6.43	-313.26	639.04	1.482	0.296	4.619
$PH_2(CH_3)$	1	-310.69	-5.53	-316.22	636.56	1.434	0.287	4.774
	2	-314.55	-5.46	-320.01	632.77	1.444	0.289	4.742
	4	-316.48	-5.42	-371.90	630.88	1.449	0.290	4.727
	10	-317.63	-5.39	-323.02	629.76	1.452	0.290	4.717
	20	-318.00	-5.40	-323.40	629.38	1.453	0.291	4.717
	40	-318.09	-5.40	-323.48	629.30	1.453	0.291	4.712
	80	-318.13	-5.39	-323.52	629.26	1.453	0.291	4.711
$PH(CH_3)_2$	1	-352.16	-4.20	-356.71	596.47	1.418	0.284	4.827
	2	-355.87	-4.14	-360.01	593.17	1.424	0.285	4.806
	4	-357.51	-4.11	-361.62	591.56	1.427	0.285	4.795
	10	-358.58	-4.10	-362.68	590.50	1.429	0.286	4.789
	20	-359.02	-4.10	-363.11	590.07	1.430	0.286	4.787
	40	-359.10	-4.09	-363.19	589.99	1.430	0.286	4.786
	80	-359.15	-4.09	-363.24	589.94	1.430	0.286	4.785
PF_3	1	-347.27	-8.30	-355.56	595.72	1.503	0.301	4.553
	2	-354.90	-8.17	-363.06	588.22	1.516	0.303	4.512
	4	-358.85	-8.13	-366.98	584.30	1.523	0.305	4.491
	10	-361.18	-8.09	-369.26	582.02	1.527	0.306	4.478
	20	-361.80	-8.09	-369.88	581.40	1.528	0.306	4.474
	40	-362.28	-8.08	-370.36	580.92	1.529	0.306	4.472
	80	-362.54	-8.07	-370.61	580.67	1.529	0.306	4.471
POF_3	1	-110.31	-25.84	-136.14	812.59	1.597	0.319	4.263
	2	-110.56	-24.51	-135.07	813.66	1.637	0.327	4.150
	4	-110.54	-23.87	-134.40	814.33	1.657	0.331	4.086
	10	-110.49	-23.53	-134.02	814.71	1.669	0.334	4.051
	20	-110.45	-23.41	-133.87	814.86	1.673	0.335	4.039
	40	-110.43	-23.33	-133.76	814.97	1.675	0.335	4.034
	80	-110.43	-23.78	-133.71	815.02	1.675	0.335	4.031

[a] The shielding tensor contributions are given in ppm.
[b] The charge on the phosphorus is given in terms of the electronic
   charge density.
[c] Values given in au^{-3}, where 1 au = 5.2918 x 10^{-11} m.

conformational change upon change of solvent (43). Shielding calculations employing the solvaton model may reveal just how realistic such an interpretation is.

The results of some CNDO/S SOS solvaton calculations of ^{31}P shielding are shown in Table VII (44).

The shielding of the trivalent phosphorus compounds is predicted to decrease by up to 15 ppm as ε increases from 1 to 80. A much smaller shielding variation, in the opposite direction, is expected for pentavalent phosphorus compounds. The shielding decrease of the trivalent phosphorus nucleus, as ε increases, is explained in terms of a contraction of the phosphus p orbitals, i.e. an increase in $<r^{-3}>_{sp}$, which leads to an enhanced paramagnetic shielding term. The difference in the solvent sensitivity between the tri and penta-valent phosphorus compounds is accounted for by means of lone pair effects on nuclear shielding.

Ring Current Effects on Nuclear Shielding

The interatomic terms included in equation (3) incorporate the hypothetical ring currents. Since hydrogen nuclei have a rather small nuclear shielding range the shielding changes, of a few ppm, attributed to ring currents can be of significance in hydrogen NMR. In general ring current effects are ignored for other nuclei.

Normally the ^1H nuclei directly bonded to a conjugated ring system are deshielded by 3-4 ppm. For example the CH signals of Phe, Tyr, Trp and His appear in the region of 6.8 to 8.1 δ thus they are well separated from all other amino acid CH resonances of proteins (45). In contrast, ^1H nuclei from other amino acid residues may be found in positions above or below a conjugated ring due to protein folding. The NMR signals from such protons are usually highly shielded; perhaps by 1 ppm or so, greater than the shielding of methyl protons. This enhanced shielding is also considered to be due to ring current effects.

If one assumes that specific solute-solvent interactions and paramagnetic species are absent, then conformation dependent shieldings of aliphatic protons, in a protein, can be related to the proton micro-environment by means of ring current effects.

Traditionally, it has been assumed that ring current shielding variations are attributable to the delocalized π electrons of conjugated ring systems. Large basis set ab initio calculations of proton shielding purport to show that σ, rather than π, electrons are responsible for ring current effects (46,47). Thus one may be lead to the conclusion that a ring current can arise from a summation over all natural orbitals of those lines of currents which encircle the axis of a molecule (48).

Putting the question of ring current origins to one side there are three main approaches to the problem of calculating ring current effects on proton shieldings (4, 45). These are the classical dipole model (D) of Pople (49), the semiclassical current loop model of Johnson and Bovey (JB)(50) and the quantum mechanical model of Haigh and Mallion (HM)(51). The delocalised electrons are represented by an equivalent point dipole at the centre of the ring in the D model. In the JB

scheme, a local magnetic field is considered to be produced by two
current loops parallel to the plane of a conjugated ring and at a given
distance above and below this plane.   The HM approach incorporates
London's theory of diamagnetic ring currents and compares the shielding
of a given proton with that of a benzene proton.

Comparison of the predictions obtained from these three models
shows that they are significantly different for protons in the plane of
the ring, and close to it.   In biological applications the interest
tends to reside in ring current effects on protons beyond the van der
Waals dimensions of the conjugated ring.   In these circumstances the
three models provide very similar shielding predictions.   An analogous
situation occurs when the shielding of out-of-plane protons is considered.   Ring stacking produces a ring plane and proton separation of
0.33-0.34 nm.   Estimates from the three shielding models are very comparable for protons separated from a ring plane by 0.3 nm or more.

In practice tables of predicted ring current shielding effects are
available for both the HM and JB models as a function of the proton
position with respect to the conjugated ring.   Thus graphical displays
of contour maps of shieldings can be produced for a given ring position.
A good example of the use of ring current calculations in making proton
NMR assignments is to be found in the case of hen egg white lysozyme
(52).   A total of 45 experimental shifts are available for analysis,
comprising 25 from aliphatic protons and 20 from aromatic protons.
Fig. 1 shows a plot of these shifts versus those calculated by the D,
JB and HM ring current models.   Thus ring current effects appear to
provide the dominant explanation for the 45 observed proton shifts in
lysozyme.   Further examples are to be found in the application of the
JB model to the ^{1}H spectra of nucleic acid bases (53,54), and the use
of a double dipole model for the porphyrin ring current (55) in the
analysis of the ^{1}H NMR spectra of some chlorophyll derivatives (56).

Conclusions

I hope that the foregoing discourse has presented the view that
Ramsey's shielding model is not too interesting from the chemical point
of view.   The approaches of Pople, Ditchfield and Schindler and
Kutzelnigg are potentially more rewarding.

For molecules of a reasonable size semiempirical methods, e.g.
INDO/S SOS, are still the workhorse.

In calculating nuclear shielding data an isolated molecule is not,
in general, a good representation of reality.   Both specific and non-
specific solvation effects can be important.

For molecules containing heavy nuclei relativistic influences will
almost certainly be of significance in estimations of nuclear shielding.

Finally, various models are available for the calculation of the
effects of ring currents on proton shieldings.   Such effects can play
a significant role in the analysis of the complicated proton spectra of
large systems such as proteins and chlorophyll derivatives.

Figure 1

Plots of the experimental proton shieldings of lysozyme against those
calculated by various ring current models. The methyl and coupled
protons are represented by ●, while the conjugated ring protons are
denoted by O. The lines represent least-squares regressions.

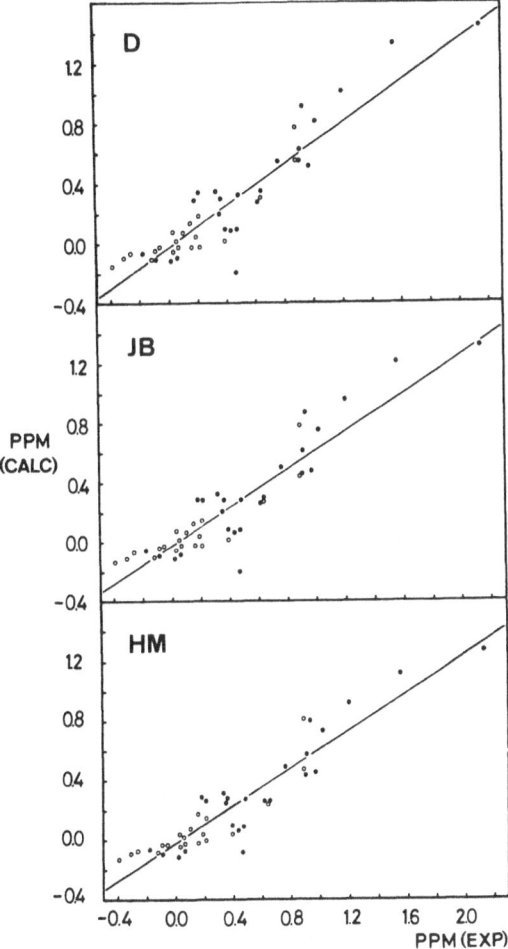

References

(1)   'NMR in Medicine', L. Kaufman, L.E. Crooks and A.D. Margulis,
        Eds., *Iagku-Shoin, New York*, 1981.
(2)   P. Marsfield and P. Morris, *Adv. Magn. Reson.*, 1982, Supplement
        2.
(3)   'NMR Imaging', C.L. Portain, A.E. James, F.D. Rollo and R.R.
        Price, Eds., *W.B. Saunders, Philadelphia*, 1983.
(4)   I. Ando and G.A. Webb, 'Theory of NMR Parameters', *Academic
        Press, London*, 1983.
(5)   R.T. Boeré and R.G. Kidd in 'Annual Reports on NMR Spectroscopy',
        G.A. Webb, Ed., *Academic Press, London*, Vol. 13, p.320 (1982).
(6)   J. Reisse in 'The Multinuclear Approach to NMR Spectroscopy',
        J.B. Lambert and F.G. Riddell, Eds., *Reidel*, p.63 (1982).
(7)   K.A.K. Ebraheem and G.A. Webb, *Prog. NMR Spectrosc.*, 11, 149
        (1977)
(8)   J.A. Pople and D.L. Beveridge 'Approximate Molecular Orbital
        Theory', *Mc-Graw Hill, New York*, 1970.
(9)   'NMR of Newly Accessible Nuclei', ed. P. Laszlo, *Academic Press,
        New York*, Volumes 1 and 2, 1983.
(10)   J.F. Hinton, K.R. Metz and R.W. Briggs in 'Annual Reports on
        NMR Spectroscopy', G.A. Webb, Ed., *Academic Press, London*, Vol.
        13, p.211 (1982).
(11)   C.J. Jameson and H.S. Gutowsky, *J. Chem. Phys.*, 40, 1714 (1964)
(12)   N.F. Ramsey, *Phys. Rev.*, 78, 689 (1950).
(13)   A. Saika and C.P. Slichter, *J. Chem. Phys.*, 22, 26 (1954).
(14)   J.A. Pople, *J. Chem. Phys.*, 37, 53 (1962).
(15)   J.A. Pople, *J. Chem. Phys.*, 37, 60 (1962).
(16)   R. Ditchfield, *J. Chem. Phys.*, 56, 5688 (1972).
(17)   R. Ditchfield, *Mol. Phys.*, 27, 789 (1974).
(18)   F. Ribas Prado, C. Giessner-Prettre, A. Pullman, J.F. Hinton,
        D. Harpool and K.R. Metz, *Theoret. Chim. Acta*, 59, 55 (1981).
(19)   F. Ribas Prado, C. Giessner-Prettre and B. Pullman, *Org. Magn.
        Reson.*, 16, 103 (1981).
(20)   C. Giessner-Prettre and B. Pullman, *J. Amer. Chem. Soc.*, 104,
        70 (1982).
(21)   A.R. Garber, P.D. Ellis, K. Seidman and K. Schade, *J. Magn.
        Reson.*, 34, 1 (1979).
(22)   P.D. Ellis, Y.C. Chou and P.A. Dobosh, *J. Magn. Reson.*, 39, 529
        (1980).
(23)   M. Schindler and W. Kutzelnigg, *J. Chem. Phys.*, 76, 1919 (1982).
(24)   M. Schindler and W. Kutzelnigg, *J. Amer. Chem. Soc.*, 105, 1360
        (1983).
(25)   G.A. Webb in 'NMR and The Periodic Table', R.K. Harris and B.E.
        Mann, Eds., *Academic Press, London*, 1978, p.49.
(26)   M. Jallali-Heravi and G.A. Webb, *J. Magn. Reson.*, 32, 429 (1978).
(27)   K.A.K. Ebraheem, G.A. Webb and M. Witanowski, *Org. Magn. Reson.*,
        8, 317 (1976).
(28)   J.P. Desclaux, Atomic data and Nuclear data tables, 12, 311
        (1972).
(29)   D. Kolb, W.R. Johnson and P. Shorer, *Phys. Rev.*, 26A, 19 (1982).

(30)   J.C. Slater, 'Quantum Theory of Atomic Structure', *Mc-Graw Hill, New York*, 1960, Chapter 25.

(31)   A.A. Cheremisin and P.V. Schastnev, *J. Magn. Reson.*, $\underline{\underline{40}}$, 459 (1980).

(32)   I. Morishima, K. Endo and T. Yorezawa, *J. Chem. Phys.*, $\underline{\underline{59}}$, 3356 (1973).

(33)   P. Pyykkö, *Chem. Phys.*, $\underline{74}$, 1 (1983).

(34)   N.C. Pyper, *Chem. Phys. Letters*, $\underline{96}$, 204 (1983).

(35)   Z.C. Zhang and G.A. Webb, *J. Mol. Struct.*, $\underline{\underline{104}}$, 439 (1983).

(36)   D.L. Beveridge and G.W. Schnuelle, *J. Phys. Chem.*, $\underline{\underline{78}}$, 2064 (1974).

(37)   G.A. Webb and M. Witanowski, Molecular Interactions, $\underline{5}$ (1984) in the press, Wiley, New York.

(38)   B. Na Lamphun, G.A. Webb and M. Witanowski, *Org. Magn. Reson.*, $\underline{21}$, 501 (1983).

(39)   C. Böttcher, 'Theory of Electric Polarisation', *Elsevier, Amsterdam*, Vol. $\underline{1}$, (1973).

(40)   W.T. Raynes, A.D. Buckingham and H.J. Bernstein, *J. Chem. Phys.*, $\underline{\underline{36}}$, 3481 (1961).

(41)   I. Ando and G.A. Webb, *Org. Magn. Reson.*, $\underline{\underline{15}}$, 111 (1981).

(42)   M. Witanowski, L. Stefaniak, B. Na Lamphun and G.A. Webb, *Org. Magn. Reson.*, $\underline{\underline{16}}$, 57 (1981).

(43)   M. Witanowski, L. Stefaniak and G.A. Webb in 'Annual Reports on NMR Spectroscopy', G.A. Webb, Ed., *Academic Press, London*, $\underline{\underline{11B}}$, (1981).

(44)   B. Na Lamphun and G.A. Webb, *Org. Magn. Reson.*, $\underline{\underline{21}}$, 399 (1983).

(45)   S.J. Perkins, *Biol. Magn. Reson.*, $\underline{4}$, 193 (1982).

(46)   P. Lazzeretti, E. Rossi and R. Zanasi, *J. Chem. Phys.*, $\underline{\underline{77}}$, 3129 (1982).

(47)   P. Lazzeretti, E. Rossi and R. Zanasi, *J. Amer. Chem. Soc.*, $\underline{\underline{105}}$, 12 (1983).

(48)   J.A.N.F. Gomes, *J. Chem. Phys.*, $\underline{78}$, 3133 (1983).

(49)   J.A. Pople, *J. Chem. Phys.*, $\underline{24}$, 1111 (1956).

(50)   C.E. Johnson and F.A. Bovey, *J. Chem. Phys.*, $\underline{\underline{29}}$, 1012 (1958).

(51)   C.W. Haigh and R.B. Mallion, *Org. Magn. Reson.*, $\underline{4}$, 203 (1972).

(52)   S.J. Perkins and R.A. Dwek, *Biochem.*, $\underline{19}$, 245 (1980).

(53)   C. Giessner-Prettre and B. Pullman, *J. Theor. Biol.*, $\underline{\underline{27}}$, 87 (1970).

(54)   C. Giessner-Prettre and B. Pullman, *J. Theor. Biol.*, $\underline{\underline{27}}$, 341 (1970).

(55)   R.J. Abraham, S.C. Fell and K.M. Smith, *Org. Magn. Reson.*, $\underline{9}$, 367 (1977).

(56)   R.J. Abraham, K.M. Smith, D.A. Goff and J.J. Lai, *J. Amer. Chem. Soc.*, $\underline{\underline{104}}$, 4332 (1982).

AN INTRODUCTION TO NMR RELAXATION MECHANISMS

Edwin D. Becker and Cherie L. Fisk
National Institutes of Health
Bethesda, Maryland 20205, USA

ABSTRACT. The phenomena of spin-lattice and spin-spin relaxation
and their effect on NMR signals are described. Pulse methods for
measuring T_1 and T_2 are given. A simple picture of molecular motions
and of interactions between nuclei and randomly varying fields is
developed to provide a qualitative explanation of the observed phenomena. The various mechanisms for relaxation are discussed, with particular emphasis on those found most frequently in biological systems.

1. INTRODUCTION

An understanding of at least the rudiments of nuclear relaxation is
essential for an appreciation of both the advantages and the limitations of many NMR experiments. In this chapter we first discuss
relaxation from a simple, classical point of view that emphasizes
the relation between the behavior of the nuclear magnetization and
the observations made in the laboratory. We then describe the most
common methods by which pulse Fourier transform NMR is used to
measure relaxation times and the ways in which these experiments can
be used in NMR imaging. We next discuss the various mechanisms that
lead to nuclear relaxation and indicate the relaxation times to be
expected for different systems. Finally we comment on the effect of
exchange processes and the motions of biopolymers on observed relaxation times. Relaxation mechanisms are discussed in a number of standard texts, with various degrees of complexity. References 1-4 give
four sources in increasing order of sophistication.

2. RELAXATION PHENOMENA; MEASUREMENT OF T_1 AND T_2

In Chapter 1 we presented the classical picture of a nuclear magnetic
moment precessing at the Larmor frequency about an applied magnetic
field B_0. In a real sample there are, of course, a very large number
of nuclei. Such an ensemble of identical nuclei, all precessing at
the same frequency about an applied field B_0 is depicted in Figure 1.
Since the nuclei have no preferred orientation in the x or y direc-

39

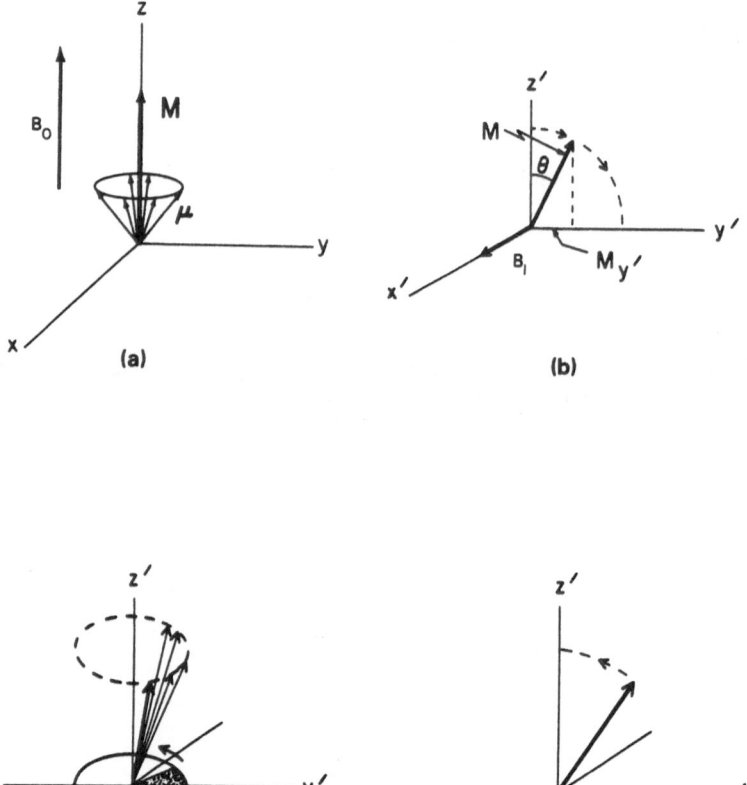

Figure 1.   (a) Ensemble of identical nuclei precessing about B_0, and the resultant macroscopic magnetization M. (b) M tipped in the rotating frame $y'z'$ plane by inter- action with the radio-frequency field B_1.   (c) Spin-spin relaxation: dephasing of the components of magnetiza- tion in the $x'y'$ plane.   (d) Spin-lattice relaxation: restoration of the z component of magnetization.

tions, their components of magnetization along these axes average to zero, and the net macroscopic magnetization M is, at equilibrium, directed along the z axis parallel to B_0. It is helpful to treat the motion of M not in the laboratory coordinate system, but in a coordinate system or frame of reference that rotates about B_0 at the Larmor frequency. In this rotating frame, with axes denoted by primes, a radio-frequency (RF) field, B_1, that is rotating at the Larmor frequency appears to be stationary along the x' axis. It can thus interact with M and cause a torque that leads to precession of M in the $y'z'$ plane of the rotating frame. This tipping of M away from the z' axis results in a decrease in $M_{z'}$, which is eventually restored to its equilibrium value by a first-order process in a time characterized by T_1, the longitudinal relaxation time. The components $M_{x'}$ and $M_{y'}$ relax to their equilibrium values of zero in a time characterized by T_2, the transverse relaxation time. It is clear that T_2 measures the time that it takes for the nuclei to get out of phase with each other and eventually reach the random phase characteristic of equilibrium. T_2 is also called the spin-spin relaxation time, since it is interactions between the spins that cause this relaxation process. The restoration of the z component with time constant T_1 requires a transfer of energy from the nuclear spin system to the surroundings, or lattice, so T_1 is also called the spin-lattice relaxation time.

The effect of relaxation on the observed NMR signals can be seen clearly from Figure 1. Decrease in $M_{y'}$ from dephasing of the components of magnetization results in decay of the free induction signal (see Chapter 1), so T_2 processes contribute to this decay. However, inhomogeneities in the applied magnetic field cause small differences in the precession frequencies of individual nuclei, so they dephase more rapidly. The observed decay time, T_2^*, thus has components from T_2 processes and from magnetic field inhomogeneity effects. Longitudinal relaxation has no effect on the free induction decay rate, but if another RF pulse is applied before M_z has been restored to its equilibrium value (a time of $5 \times T_1$ for 99.3% recovery), the next FID will be uniformly diminished in intensity.

NMR pulse techniques provide the easiest and most versatile methods for measuring relaxation times. To measure T_1 we must perturb the system to move the magnetization away from its equilibrium position, and then study the restoration of the z component of the magnetization. Figure 2 illustrates the most widely used and the most accurate method of measuring T_1, the inversion-recovery method. As part (a) of this Figure shows, a 180° pulse is applied to the spin system to invert the magnetization to the negative z' axis. The magnetization then spontaneously recovers by spin-lattice relaxation processes, passes through zero and ultimately reaches its initial equilibrium value along the positive z' axis. If we allow this process to go on only for some period of time, τ, and then apply a 90° pulse, we bring whatever portion of the magnetization exists at that time into the $x'y'$ plane, where it induces an NMR signal and gives a free induction decay. The free induction decay, after being Fourier transformed (as described in Chapter 1), then provides a spectrum which we could call a "partially relaxed spectrum," showing each of the nuclear signals with either

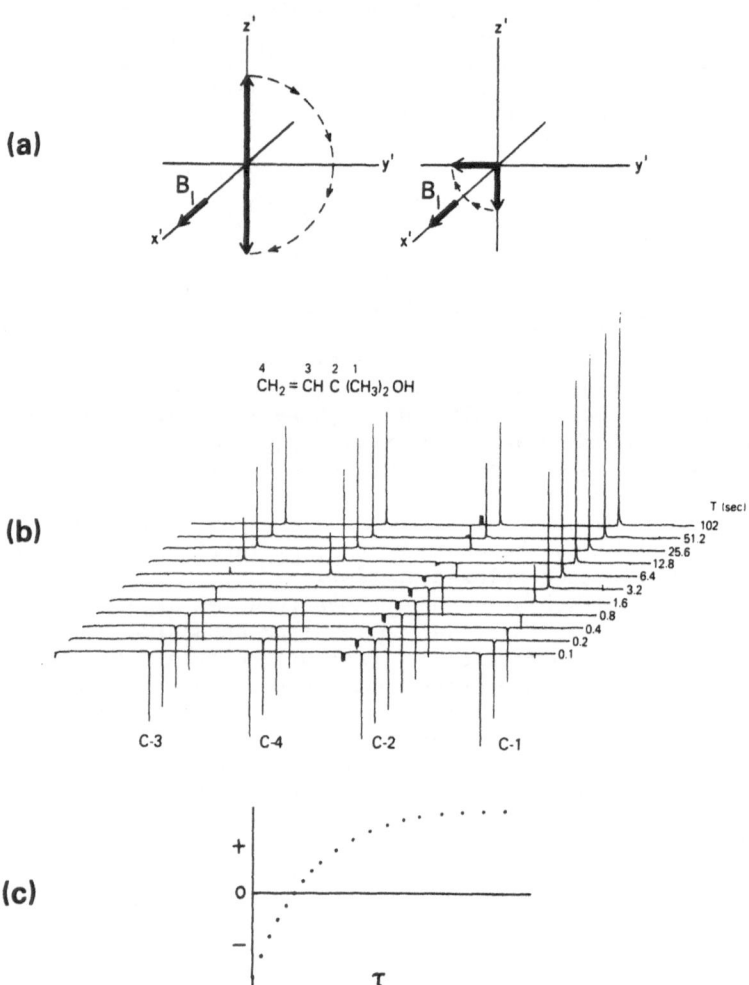

Figure 2. Inversion-recovery method for measuring T_1. (a) $180°$, τ, $90°$ sequence. (b) A set of partially relaxed spectra. (c) Time dependence of one of the lines in the partially relaxed spectra.

a positive or negative amplitude indicative of the orientation of the magnetization for that particular nucleus at time τ. After waiting for equilibrium to be reestablished, we can then go back and repeat the whole process with a different value of τ and thus obtain a set of spectra such as those shown in Figure 2b. Figure 2c illustrates that from these spectra, it is possible to trace out the recovery of any particular line in the spectrum and thus measure relaxation times for individual nuclei.

Note from Figure 2b that an FID at a particular value of τ may have a substantial contribution from one resonance frequency and very little from another if the longitudinal relaxation times are different. This fact is exploited in NMR imaging. Often water in adjacent tissues (e.g., normal and diseased) has different relaxation times, for reasons that we shall discuss later. With an appropriate value of τ, an inversion-recovery pulse sequence can thus be used to create an image in which the contrast between the tissues is enhanced. This method will be discussed extensively in later chapters.

We turn now to the measurement of T_2, the time constant for decay of the magnetization in the xy plane. If T_2 is very short, the rate of decay of the FID provides a good measure of T_2, but if magnetic field inhomogeneities contribute significantly then T_2 may be substantially longer than T_2^*. There are several methods for accurate measurement of T_2 itself; almost all depend on the formation of a spin-echo to overcome the effect of magnetic field inhomogeneity.

Figure 3 illustrates the formation of a spin-echo. Assume that the macroscopic magnetization oriented initially along the z axis is composed of a number of smaller macroscopic magnetizations (m_i), each arising from nuclei in different parts of the sample, which possibly have slightly different magnetic fields due to inhomogeneity in B_0. As indicated in Figure 3a, application of a 90° pulse (taken to be on resonance for simplicity) results in the entire magnetization of the sample being rotated to the y' axis. Nuclei that happen to be in fields slightly higher than the average will now precess more rapidly than the average. If the rotating frame is rotating at the average precession frequency of the nuclei, then those nuclei which precess faster than the average will always move clockwise in the rotating frame as viewed from the top, down the z axis. Initially, as in Figure 3b, these faster nuclei appear to be going toward the observer, while those moving more slowly than the average appear to be going away. The result is a dephasing, as indicated in Figure 3b, and the signal decreases with the time constant T_2^*. Suppose, after time τ, we apply a 180° pulse. Figure 3c shows that, as a result, each of these little macroscopic magnetizations is rotated 180° about the x' axis. Those that appeared to be closest to us in Figure 3b remain closest, but now are in the negative quadrant along the left-hand side. Since they are still rotating faster than the frame, they continue to move clockwise but now move back toward the negative y' axis, as indicated in Figure 3d. Meanwhile, the slower nuclei, still moving counterclockwise, also come toward the negative y' axis. After a

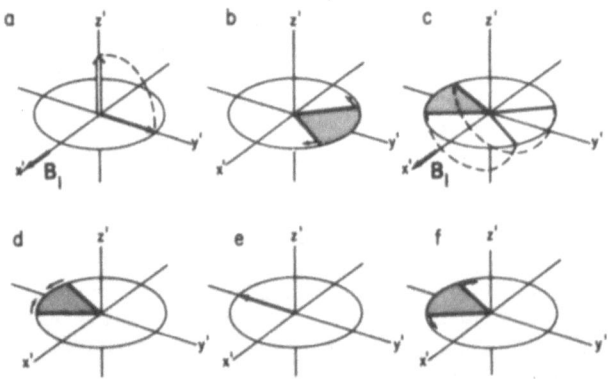

Figure 3.   Formation of spin-echoes.
(a) A 90° pulse applied along x' at time 0 causes
    M to tip to the positive y' axis.
(b) Macroscopic magnetizations, m_i, of nuclei in
    different parts of the sample dephase as a result
    of the inhomogeneity in B_0, with faster nuclei
    moving toward the observer.
(c) 180° pulse along x' at time τ causes all m_i
    to rotate 180° about the x' axis.
(d) The faster nuclei move away from the observer
    while the slower nuclei move toward the observer.
(e) At time 2τ the m_i rephase along the $-y'$ axis.
(f) At time >2τ the m_i again dephase.

time 2τ, the magnetizations all arrive at the negative y' axis,
as depicted in Figure 3e. We would observe this refocusing of the
magnetizations as a buildup of a signal and the formation of an
"echo." As the magnetization vectors go past the negative y' axis,
as illustrated in Figure 3f, the echo amplitude decays. If at a
time 3τ, we apply another 180° pulse, we can repeat the process,
now causing a refocusing along the <u>positive</u> y' axis and leading
to a second echo. We can thus get a whole series of echoes at time
2τ, 4τ, 6τ, etc. If spin-spin relaxation were not occurring, the
amplitudes of all these echos would be exactly the same. However,
relaxation processes <u>are</u> ocurring, and these are irreversible. It
is only the effects of magnetic field inhomogeneity that can be
reversed by the formation of spin echoes. For a single line
spectrum only amplitudes of the echoes are needed. In a
multi-line spectrum the echoes must be Fourier transformed
to provide partially relaxed spectra.

Like the inversion-recovery method, the spin echo pulse
sequence is used in NMR imaging. In this case the 90°, τ, 180°
sequence is used to create only the first echo, with the value of
τ chosen to accentuate the contrast between tissues on the basis of
differences in T_2, rather than T_1.

3. MECHANISMS OF RELAXATION

We turn now to consideration of the several mechanisms that
cause nuclei to relax. Our treatment is not rigorous but is
designed to identify the major factors involved in spin-lattice
relaxation processes. (These processes apply also to spin-spin
relaxation, but there are additional factors, mentioned below, in the
latter.) Figure 1 showed that application of an RF field B_1 causes M_z
to decrease from its equilibrium value, as energy is taken from B_1.
The process of spin-lattice relaxation requires that the nuclear spin
system give up energy to restore M_z to equilibrium. Just as a field
oscillating at the Larmor frequency was necessary to reduce M_z, so for
the most part some sort of moving magnetic field is needed to exchange
energy with the nuclear spin system to restore the magnetization to
its equilibrium value. The difference is that to study NMR we apply a
coherent radio frequency field at or near the Larmor frequency of the
nucleus, while the fields needed for relaxation are those that arise
from motions of molecules in a random fashion. For example, Brownian
motion of the molecules as they turn around carrying their nuclear
moments with them generate very small magnetic fields within the
sample. These fields are random in frequency and phase. A Fourier
analysis of the random motions shows what fraction are at or near the
Larmor frequency of the nuclei that are being relaxed; these motions
are most effective in bringing about spin-lattice relaxation.

The detailed mathematical treatment, which we shall not reproduce
here, is carried out in terms of a correlation time, τ_c, which is
roughly the time that it takes a molecule to rotate through about
one radian (or for an intermolecular process, the time for translation
through about one molecular diameter). The result, in general terms,
is that the component of the random motion at angular frequency ω is
proportional to

$$\frac{\tau_c}{1+\omega^2\tau_c^2}$$

For spin-lattice relaxation it is, as we have seen, the Larmor
frequency ω_0 that is of interest. (For some processes $2\omega_0$ also
turns out to be important, but we shall not discuss this point.)

We now ask what causes the fluctuating fields. There are
several distinct processes that lead to relaxation:

1. Magnetic dipole-dipole interaction

2. Electric quadrupole interaction

3. Chemical shift anisotropy

4. Spin-rotation interaction

5. Scalar coupling

Magnetic dipolar fields arise from the magnetic nuclei within a molecule. Thus as a molecule tumbles, the fluctuating magnetic field from one nucleus can relax another nucleus in the same molecule or in another molecule. With the formalism described previously to handle the average molecular motion, it is not difficult to derive an expression for the spin-lattice relaxation rate R_1 ($\equiv 1/T_1$) and the spin-spin relaxation rate R_2 ($\equiv 1/T_2$) for a nucleus relaxed by magnetic dipolar interaction with other nuclei of the same type within the molecule.

$$(R_1)_{rot.} = \frac{2\gamma^4\hbar^2 I(I+1)}{5r^6}\left[\frac{\tau_0}{1+\omega^2\tau_0^2}+\frac{4\tau_0}{1+4\omega^2\tau_0^2}\right],$$

$$(R_2)_{rot.} = \frac{\gamma^4\hbar^2 I(I+1)}{5r^6}\left[3\tau_0+\frac{5\tau_0}{1+\omega^2\tau_0^2}+\frac{2\tau_0}{1+4\omega^2\tau_0^2}\right].$$

Here r is the distance between the two nuclei and τ_c is the rotational correlation time. Note that the relaxation rate depends on the fourth power of γ. If the relaxing nucleus is a different species, a similar but more complex equation applies which depends on the squares of both magnetogyric ratios, so that nuclei with large magnetic moments play the dominant role. The inverse sixth power dependence on r means that nearby nuclei are by far the most significant. For example, a proton is normally relaxed by other nearby protons, but a ^{13}C nucleus (even in an enriched molecule with other nearby ^{13}C nuclei) is primarily relaxed by nearby protons, not other ^{13}C nuclei. A plot of T_1 and T_2 versus τ_c (Figure 4) shows the behavior predicted by our qualitative discussion of the frequency requirements for spin-lattice and spin-spin relaxation.

Spin-lattice relaxation is most efficient (T_1 shortest) when molecular tumbling occurs with a correlation time $\tau_c = 1/\omega_0$, while spin-spin relaxation becomes more efficient with increasing τ_c (eventually approaching a limit determined by a rigid crystal lattice). For sufficiently rapid molecular tumbling, such as that experienced by most small molecules in the liquid or gas phase, $T_1 = T_2$.

Intermolecular dipole-dipole relaxation can also occur. The expressions for T_1 and T_2 in this case are quite similar except that the correlation time is that for translational, rather than rotational, motion.

A phenomenon closely related to nuclear dipolar relaxation is the nuclear Overhauser effect (abbreviated NOE). The NOE is the change in intensity of a resonance line of nucleus A when some other

nucleus X is irradiated. The NOE arises from dipolar relaxation.
We shall not go into the details, but the rationale may become clear
from the diagrams of Figure 5, which show the energy levels of two
nuclei of spin 1/2, which relax each other by dipolar interactions.
Part (a) shows the spin orientation of nuclei A and X for the four
levels and the four RF transitions at frequencies ν_A and ν_X.
Part (b) shows that there are six paths for relaxation, four of
which involve the flip of only one nucleus and have probability
(or relative rates) of W_1 and W_1'. The others involve the simultaneous flip of both nuclei, leading to a change in total spin of
either two or zero. These double flips are not normally seen in
NMR spectral transitions, but they provide important paths for
relaxation. The relative rates W_2, W_0, W_1 and W_1' can be calculated. At equilibrium these competing processes result in a
Boltzmann distribution of nuclei among the four levels. If we
irradiate continuously at frequency ν_X with an RF field strong enough
to saturate, the populations of levels 1 and 3 become equal, and
those of 2 and 4 likewise become equal. The relaxation rates
remain unchanged, but with these additional constraints the populations readjust to a steady state in which those of levels 2 and 4
are higher. The result is an increase in intensity (η) of the ν_A
resonance line:

$$\eta = \frac{1}{2}\left[\gamma_X/\gamma_A\right] \cdot f\left(\tau_c, \omega_A, \omega_X\right)$$

$$I/I_o = 1 + \eta$$

where: η = nuclear Overhauser enhancement

I = intensity with double resonance

I_o = intensity without double resonance

The function of τ_c and the resonance frequencies is equal to unity
for molecules that tumble rapidly but can become smaller or negative
for large molecules. If A and X are the same (for example, both
protons) the intensity ratio is 1.50 (for small molecules), while
for X = H and A = C-13, the intensity ratio is nearly 3.0.
    If dipolar relaxation accounts for only a portion of the
relaxation pathways for a given nucleus, then the value of η is
only a proportional amount of the full NOE. This description of the
NOE experiment assumed a continuous irradiating field--the steady
state NOE. It is also possible to apply a selective pulse to one
nucleus and observe the NOE on other nuclei--the transient NOE.
Such experiments are particularly important in obtaining reliable
results for slowly tumbling molecules, such as polymers and solids,
where the rapid exchange of energy among nuclei (known as "spin
diffusion") can invalidate steady state NOE results.

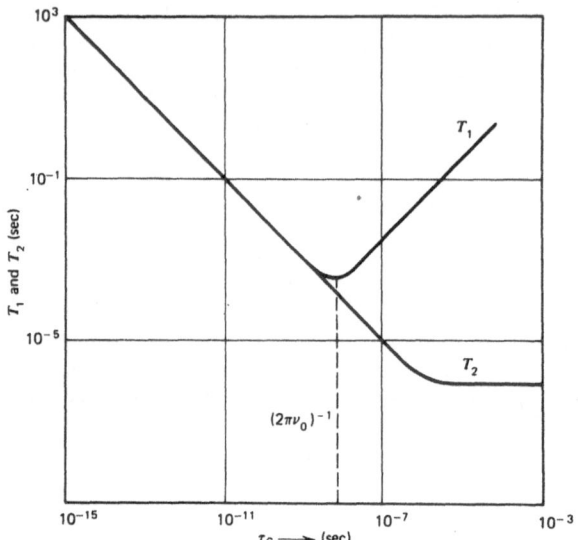

Figure 4. Dependence of T_1 and T_2 for magnetic
dipole-dipole relaxation on the correlation time
τ_c.

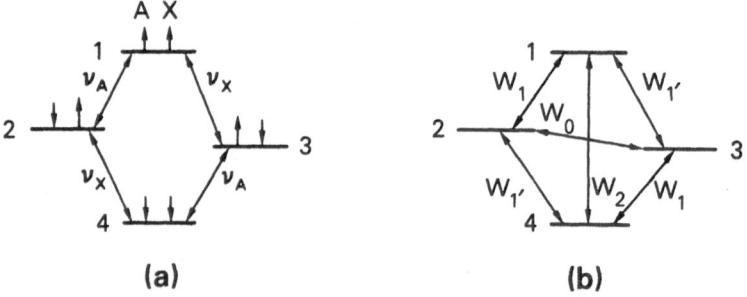

Figure 5. Energy levels for an AX spin system.
(a) Paths for transitions induced by absorption of
radiation at the resonance frequencies of A and X.
(b) Paths for spin-lattice relaxation, resulting in
a change in total spin (ΔF_z) of k for each pathway
indicated by W_k.

The dipolar fields required for magnetic dipole-dipole relaxation can also arise from unpaired electrons if they are present. Since the electron magnetic moment is about 658 times as great as the proton moment, and since the magnetic moment of the relaxing species enters the equation as the square, such relaxation can be very effective provided the distance r is small enough. Paramagnetic species present in low concentration, such as atmospheric oxygen, are rather effective in relaxing hydrogen nuclei in many compounds but much less effective in relaxing nuclei such as ^{13}C that lie in less exposed positions. Paramagnetic ions that can be complexed directly to a molecule are often very efficient; their use for increasing relaxation rates in NMR imaging is discussed in later chapters.

A nucleus with spin >1/2 possesses an electric quadrupole moment. If the electron environment around the nucleus is asymmetric, then the fluctuating electric field gradients at the nucleus induced by molecular tumbling permit nuclear relaxation. We shall not go into details of quadrupole relaxation, but qualitatively the situation is much like that for dipolar relaxation in terms of the dependence on correlation time. In particular, for the situation where molecular tumbling is rapid enough that $\tau_c \ll 1/\omega_0$,

$$R_1 = R_2 = \frac{3}{40} \frac{2I+3}{I^2(2I-1)} \left(1 + \frac{\eta^2}{3}\right) \left(\frac{e^2 Qq}{\hbar}\right)^2 \tau_c,$$

where η is an asymmetry parameter that measures the departure of the nuclear environment from cylindrical symmetry and $(e^2 Qq/\hbar)$ is the quadrupole coupling constant, which depends on the nuclear quadrupole moment Q and the electric field gradient q. Most quadrupolar nuclei relax predominantly by this means, and T_1's are often measured only in milliseconds, or even microseconds in some cases. The only exception is the situation where the electron distribution around the nucleus has tetrahedral or higher symmetry.

Of common quadrupolar nuclei, deuterium has a small quadrupole moment and, with only one electron, a small electric field gradient. Deuterium relaxation times for small molecules in liquids are rather long--of the order of 100 milliseconds. Other quadrupolar nuclei, such as sodium, potassium and chlorine, have much larger quadrupole moments, but in ionic form their aproximately spherical symmetry gives a very small electric field gradient. Nitrogen usually has a large quadrupole coupling constant, hence a T_1 of only a millisecond or less. In solids and in membranes, deuterium gives line widths of many kHz and can be studied readily, whereas most other quadrupolar nuclei have linewidths of several MHz and are extremely difficult to observe.

Chemical shift anisotropy can provide a mechanism for nuclear relaxation. In general the shielding factor σ is anisotropic, so that the local magnetic field at the nucleus varies as the molecule tumbles. The molecule tumbling rate in general is so rapid that only a single resonance line is seen, and the ordinary NMR spectrum measures the average value of the chemical shift. The fluctuating local field, however, may serve as a relaxation mechanism. For an axially symmetric situation,

$$R_1 = \tfrac{1}{15} \gamma^2 B_0{}^2 (\sigma_{\parallel} - \sigma_{\perp})^2 \frac{2\tau_c}{1 + \omega^2 \tau_c{}^2} \, ,$$

$$R_2 = \tfrac{1}{90} \gamma^2 B_0{}^2 (\sigma_{\parallel} - \sigma_{\perp})^2 \left\{ \frac{6\tau_c}{1 + \omega^2 \tau_c{}^2} + 8\tau_c \right\} \, ,$$

where $\sigma_{\parallel}$ and $\sigma_{\perp}$ are the values of σ along and perpendicular to the symmetry axis, respectively. Note that this relaxation mechanism is explicitly dependent on the value of B_0, since it is B_0 that induces the electron currents leading to the chemical shift. The quadratic dependence on B_0 suggests that this mechanism will be of importance principally at high fields, and that is indeed the case. For ^{31}P, chemical shift anisotropy relaxation often broadens lines above 150 MHz. On the other hand, ^{57}Fe, with a very long magnetic dipolar relaxation time, is best studied at high field so as to reduce T_1 to an optimum value. For many nuclei other mechanisms dominate relaxation, and chemical shift anisotropy relaxation is of little importance at presently attainable magnetic field strengths.

Spin-rotation relaxation arises from magnetic fields generated at the nucleus by the fluctuating motion of the molecular magnetic moment that is dependent on the overall electron distribution in the molecule. This effect is most significant for small, symmetric molecules that rotate rapidly or for similar portions of molecules, such as methyl groups. One important point to note regarding spin-rotation interaction is that it becomes more significant as the molecule increases its rotational rate; hence it is most effective for molecules in the gas phase or in liquids at high temperature. This mechanism is of little importance for most molecules of biological interest.

The ordinary spin-spin coupling (scalar coupling) that exists between two nuclei I and S can furnish a mechanism of relaxation for I if S relaxes at an appropriate rate, since relaxation by S alters the magnetic field experienced by I through the spin coupling. Scalar relaxation is most commonly found when S is a quadrupolar nucleus that relaxes rapidly. Even in this case, however, it is rare that scalar relaxation has much effect on T_1 unless the resonance frequencies ω_I and ω_S are nearly equal. T_2 is very commonly affected, however; line broadening (i.e., increase in $R_2{}^I$) in the ^1H spectrum of nuclei coupled to ^{14}N is commonly observed, for example.

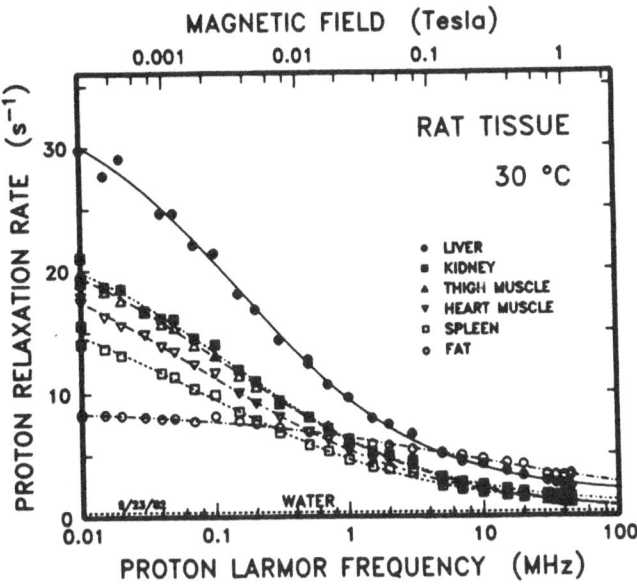

Figure 6. The magnetic field dependence of the proton relaxation rate (=1/T$_1$) in a variety of rat tissues, measured at 30°C. [Reprinted by permission from S.H. Koenig, R.D. Brown III, D. Adams, D. Emerson, and C.G. Harrison, Invest. Radiol. 19: 76 (1984). Copyright © 1984, J.B. Lippincott Co.]

4. OTHER FACTORS AFFECTING RELAXATION RATES

In many biological systems nuclei exchange among different
environments where their relaxation times may be very different.
For example, free chloride ion has approximately spherical symmetry
and a relatively long quadrupolar relaxation time, but when complexed
to a macromolecule the relaxation time may be shortened by several
orders of magnitude. When the nucleus exchanges rapidly between
different environments, the observed relaxation rate is the weighted
average of the rates in the individual sites (a situation quite
analogous to the averaging of chemical shifts by rapid exchange).
Thus

$$R_1(obs.) = p_A R_1(A) + p_B R_1(B) + \ldots,$$

where the p's give the fraction of time the nucleus spends in each
environment.

      In our initial discussion of the effect of molecular motion
on relaxation rates, we characterized the motion by means of a
correlation time τ_c. The use of a single correlation time is
clearly a gross approximation for most molecules, since the tumbling
of non-spherical molecules is anisotropic and must be represented
by two or three correlation times. Moreover, polymers often have
internal flexibility, so that the effective correlation time for one
portion of a molecule may be a composite of several correlation times.
The effects of multiple correlation times arising from complex molecular motions are best observed via a study of the dispersion of T_1
(i.e., its frequency dependence). Relaxation times of water in
biological tissues are found to be highly frequency dependent because
the water, in exchanging rapidly with many macromolecular species,
acquires in its own relaxation behavior the characteristics of the
molecules with which it interacts. Figure 6 shows the dispersion of
T_1 for several types of excised tissues. The frequency dependence of
T_1 in tissues has important consequences in NMR imaging for optimizing
the contrast between different tissues and minimizing the time required
to obtain an image. Later chapters will cover this aspect in more
detail.

REFERENCES

(1) E.D. Becker, High Resolution NMR (2nd ed.), (Academic Press,
     New York, 1980), Chapter 8.
(2) T.C. Farrar and E.D. Becker, Pulse and Fourier Transform NMR,
     (Academic Press, New York, 1971), Chapter 4.
(3) C.P. Slichter, Principles of Magnetic Resonance, (2nd ed.),
     (Springer-Verlag, Berlin 1978).
(4) A. Abragam, The Principles of Nuclear Magnetism, (Clarendon
     Press, Oxford, 1961).

SOME CALCULATIONS OF NUCLEAR SPIN-SPIN COUPLINGS

G. A. Webb
Department of Chemistry
University of Surrey·
Guildford
Surrey U.K.

"I pass with relief from the tossing sea of Cause and Theory to the firm ground of Result and Fact".
W.S. Churchill, "The Story of the Malakand Field Force", Hamlyn, London, 1898.

ABSTRACT. The theoretical background to the spin-spin coupling inter-actions of light nuclei was presented by Ramsey. Contributions from contact, orbital and dipolar interactions can be important for couplings not involving protons. At the semi-empirical MO level, proton couplings are due to contact interactions only. Couplings for heavier nuclei require a relativistic theory for their interpretation. The importance of both non-specific and specific medium effects on spin-spin couplings is discussed. Examples are presented which illus-trate the more chemically interesting aspects of the various coupling phenomena considered.

INTRODUCTION

Spin-spin coupling interactions between neighbouring nuclei occur in-directly through the intervening electrons. Thus the values of spin-spin couplings are very sensitive to variations in molecular electronic structure.

It is generally considered that spin-spin coupling depends upon the first nucleus perturbing the electrons in the bonds joining the spin coupled nuclei; due to a resulting partial imbalance of electron spin a magnetic field is produced at the second nucleus by the bonding electrons. Thus calculations of nuclear spin-spin coupling inter-actions are based upon models of molecular electronic structure.

The energy of the spin-spin interaction between nuclei A and B, E_{AB}, is given by equation (1).

$$E_{AB} = hJ_{AB}\bar{I}_A{}'\bar{I}_B \tag{1}$$

T. Axenrod and G. Ceccarelli (eds.), NMR in Living Systems, 53–65.
© 1986 by D. Reidel Publishing Company.

Where I_A and I_B refer to the spins of nuclei A and B respectively and J_{AB} is the spin-spin coupling between them.   The value of J_{AB} is inde-pendent of the magnitude of the magnetic field used in the NMR experi-ment.   Consequently the gauge problem, experienced in calculations of nuclear shielding, does not arise in discussions of spin-spin couplings. In contrast to the nuclear shielding parameter, values of J are directly obtainable from the analysis of a given NMR spectrum.

Since nuclear spin-spin couplings are dependent upon electronic structure a satisfactory coupling theory will have a number of struc-tural applications in chemistry.   The difficulties encountered in formulating acceptable spin-spin coupling models and in evaluating them are similar to those noted for nuclear shielding (1).   Normally, either the SOS or FPT approach is adopted to evaluate the spin-spin coupling interaction.   For small molecules ab initio calculations, based on the coupled Hartree Fock (CHF) procedure, appear to be very promising (2).   However, calculations on larger molecules are per-formed at the semi empirical level.   Normally such calculations involve the use of INDO parameters (1).

In order to be able to concentrate on the electronic factors involved in nuclear spin-spin couplings, the reduced coupling, K_{AB}, is used;

$$K_{AB} = \frac{2\pi J_{AB}}{h\gamma_A\gamma_B}$$ (2)

Where γ_A and γ_B are the magnetogyric ratios of the coupled nuclei.

Basic Spin-Spin Coupling Interactions

The model normally used in calculations of nuclear spin-spin couplings is that due to Ramsey (3).   This assumes that there may be three types of electron coupled interactions between the nuclei and electrons of the molecule concerned.   These comprise orbital, dipolar and contact interactions.

The total nuclear spin-spin coupling energy, E_{AB}, is obtained in Ramsey's approach from second order perturbation theory (3).   Such that

$$E_{AB} = \sum_B \frac{<o|\mathcal{H}|n><n|\mathcal{H}|o>}{E_o - E_n}$$ (3)

Where $<o|$ and $<n|$ refer to the ground and excited molecular electronic states with energies of E_o and E_n respectively, E_{AB} is related to J_{AB} and K_{AB} via equations (1) and (2).

The Hamiltonian operator, $\mathcal{H}$, in equation (3) is defined by,

$$\mathcal{H} = \overset{(a)}{\mathcal{H}_1} + \overset{(b)}{\mathcal{H}_1} + \mathcal{H}_2 + \mathcal{H}_3$$ (4)

(a)   (b)

Where H_1 and H_1 represent the orbital interaction between the nuclear magnetic moments and the field produced by the orbital motion of the electrons; H_2 accounts for the dipole-dipole interaction between the nuclear and electron spins and H_3 refers to the electron-nucleus contact interaction. The forms of these various operators are as follows:-

$$H_1^{(a)} = \frac{\mu_o^2 \mu_B^2 e \hbar}{16\pi^2} \sum_k \sum_A \sum_B \gamma_A \gamma_B \left(\frac{\bar{I}_A \cdot \bar{r}_{kA}}{r_{kA}^3} \right)$$

$$\times \left(\frac{\bar{I}_B \cdot \bar{r}_{kB}}{r_{kB}^3} \right) \tag{5}$$

$$H_1^{(b)} = \frac{\mu_o \mu_B \hbar}{2\pi i} \sum_k \sum_A \gamma_A \left(\frac{\bar{I}_A \cdot \bar{r}_{kA}}{r_{kA}^3} \right) \times \nabla_k \tag{6}$$

$$H_2 = \frac{\mu_o \mu_B \hbar}{2\pi} \sum_k \sum_A \gamma_A \left[\frac{3(\bar{S}_k \cdot \bar{r}_{kA})(\bar{I}_A \cdot \bar{r}_{kA})}{r_{kA}^5} - \frac{\bar{S}_k \cdot \bar{I}_A}{r_{kA}^3} \right] \tag{7}$$

$$\text{and} \quad H_3 = \frac{4\mu_o \mu_B \hbar}{3} \sum_k \sum_A \gamma_A \, \delta(\bar{r}_{kA})(\bar{S}_k \cdot \bar{I}_A) \tag{8}$$

Where μ_B is the Bohr magneton, $\bar{I}$ is the nuclear spin operator, $\bar{S}$ is the electron spin operator, r_{kA} refers to the separation between electron k and nucleus A, ∇_k is del, the vector operator for electrons and $\delta(\bar{r}_{kA})$ is the Dirac delta function which picks out the value of the electronic eigenfunction at the nucleus in an integration over the coordinates of electron K.

From the shapes of equations (5), (6) and (7) it is apparent that their evaluation over electronic eigenfunctions will involve a knowledge of $<r^{-3}>$. At the semi empirical molecular orbital level the requirement is that $<r^{-3}>$ relates to orbitals with some angular momentum, thus it refers to p, d, f etc electrons. In contrast equation (8) depends upon the nucleus and electrons in question being in direct contact. In the semi empirical formulation this implies S electrons only and the contact interaction depends upon the S electron densities at the coupled nuclei.

Ab initio CHF coupling calculations reveal that, the neat division between S electrons contributing to the contact interaction only, while the non-contact terms depend only on electrons with non-zero orbital angular momenta is not strictly valid (2) However, the assumption that such a division is applicable is probably no worse than many of the other approximations which are normally included in semi empirical MO perturbation calculations.

In the previous chapter we have noted that $<r^{-3}>$p varies periodically, the S electron density varies in a similar manner for comparable reasons. Consequently heavy nuclei are expected to have large spin-spin couplings with significant contributions from orbital, dipolar and contact interactions. In contrast to this couplings involving hydrogen nuclei, and those of other Groups I and II elements, are predicted to have contact contributions only and hence to be much smaller. Thus the ubiquitous hydrogen nuclei are the exception, rather than the rule, when it comes to a consideration of the factors controlling both their spin-spin couplings and their shieldings.

As in the case of calculations of nuclear shielding, one difficulty experienced in the use of equation (3) is the requirement of infinite summations over excited electronic states including those of the continuum. In SOS calculations this problem may be dealt with by using a truncated set of excited states or by means of an average excitation energy approach as noted for calculations of nuclear shielding (4)(5). The alternative procedure of FPT calculations avoids this problem by not requiring the explicit calculation of excited state functions (6)(7). Self consistent perturbation theory (SCPT) calculations are analogous in this regard (8), and are often less demanding than FPT calculations on computer time.

Relationships between Spin-Spin Couplings and Molecular Structure

The dependence of the non contact spin-spin coupling contributions on $<r^{-3}>$p, as implied by equations (5), (6) and (7), suggests that the orbital and dipolar interactions will assume a greater importance for multiply bonded nuclei. This is demonstrated to be the case for some N-C and N-N couplings in Table I. The data presented here are obtained as a result of some SCPT-INDO coupling calculations.

A significant contribution to the contact term is made by lone pair electrons (9)-(12). This may be demonstrated from a comparison of the $^1J(^{15}N-^{13}C)$ results for pyridine and the pyridinium ion. In the former case the contact contribution is predicted, by SOS-INDO calculations to be 0.04 Hz whereas -14.49 Hz is calculated for the latter (9). The corresponding experimental values are 0.45 Hz and -11.9 Hz respectively. The difference between the two contact contributions arises from a low energy n→π* transition in pyridine which corresponds to a large positive contribution to the contact term and thus almost cancels the effects of other negative contributions. The absence of the lone pair in the pyridinium ion removes the n→π* transition and the large negative coupling contributions remain.

Table I

Some calculated contributions to $^{15}N-^{13}C$ and $^{15}N-^{15}N$ Couplings in Hz (9)(10)

Molecule	Coupling	Contact	Orbital	Dipolar	Total	Experimental
CH_3CN	$^1J(N\equiv C)$	2.33	-9.29	-14.95	-21.91	-17.5
	$^2J(N-C)$	3.21	0.25	0.09	3.55	+ 3.0
CH_3NC	$^1J(N\equiv C)$	14.85	-7.89	-12.44	- 5.48	- 8.8
	$^1J(N-C)$	-13.20	0.29	- 0.15	-13.05	-10.6
Ph-NC	$^1J(N\equiv C)$	13.97	-6.55	-12.22	- 4.80	(7.3)
	$^1J(N-C)$	-14.71	0.33	- 0.14	-14.52	(18.5)
O-di(Me)-Phenyl-CNO	$^1J(N\equiv C)$	-29.81	-22.84	-19.53	-72.18	(77.5)
$Ph-N=N-N(CH_3)_2$	$^1J(N=N)$	- 8.45	-7.62	0.24	-15.83	(12.8)
	$^1J(N-N)$	-13.69	-0.34	0.52	-13.52	(14.0)
O_2N-NO	$^1J(N-N)$	-23.01	1.17	6.35	-15.49	(11.7)
$[O_2N=NO]^{2-}$	$^1J(N=N)$	-10.40	-7.01	1.16	-16.25	(16.9)
$Ph-NH-NHCOCH_3$ Z isomer	$^1J(N-N)$	2.31	0.90	0.64	3.85	(3.6)

   In general, singly bonded $^{15}N-^{13}C$ couplings are predicted to be negative in sign, in agreement with experiment.   The coupling contribution of a lone pair with S character, on one of the coupled nuclei, is in opposition to that of the bonding electrons.   Thus, the presence of a lone pair with S character on nitrogen tends to lead to a small and positive contact term.   This point is also demonstrated by the results given in Table I.
   In the case of $^1J(N-N)$ positive values are anticipated when there are no valence shell lone pairs present in S orbitals (13).   The data in Table I illustrate this point and show that a negative contribution is produced by a lone pair with S character.
   Due to the often significant contributions from non contact interactions and the variability of the contact contribution on account of non bonding electrons, a simple empirical relationship, such as equation (9), between coupling and S character of the intervening bond is not expected to be generally applicable to couplings involving nitrogen and other atoms bearing lone pairs.

$$80\left|^1J(^{15}N-^{13}C)\right| = \%S_N \, \%S_C \tag{9}$$

Some SCPT-INDO calculations of $^1J(P-N)$, $^1J(P-C)$, $^1J(P-F)$, $^1J(Si-C)$ and $^1J(Si-F)$ support this conclusion as shown in Table II (14)-(16).

Table II

Some calculated contributions to spin-spin couplings involving Phosphorus and Silicon in Hz

Molecule	Coupling	Contact	Orbital	Dipolar	Total	Experimental
F_2PNPF_3	$^1J(P-N)$	67.87	10.39	-0.67	77.58	+93.8
F_2PNH_2	$^1J(P-N)$	66.04	7.01	-0.41	72.63	(73.0)
$Cl_2PN(CH_3)_2$	$^1J(P-N)$	76.20	7.34	-0.54	83.01	(89.4)
$F_2PN=\overset{*}{P}F_3$	$^1J(P≡N)$	-35.92	4.06	-0.64	-32.50	-53.2
$[(CH_3)_2N]_3PO$	$^1J(P-N)$	-19.23	2.46	-1.66	-18.43	-26.9
CH_3PCl_2	$^1J(P-C)$	-47.99	-7.53	2.31	-53.22	-45.0
$(C_2H_5)_2PCl$	$^1J(P-C)$	-34.47	-4.53	1.85	-37.15	(28.8)
$(CH_3)_4P^+$	$^1J(P-C)$	65.09	-5.01	0.97	61.05	+55.5
$(CH_3)_3PS$	$^1J(P-C)$	66.15	-4.81	0.91	62.16	+56.1
PF_3	$^1J(P-F)$	-809.32	-557.84	24.81	-1342.34	(1400-1440)
F_3PO	$^1J(P-F)$	152.76	-1289.43	73.20	-1063.47	(1055-1080)
F_3PS	$^1J(P-F)$	102.48	-1274.58	15.29	-1156.81	(1170-1184)
$Si(CH_3)_3H$	$^1J(Si-C)$	-49.53	2.56	-0.49	-47.56	(50.8)
$Si(C_2H_5)_4$	$^1J(Si-C)$	-52.17	2.42	-0.48	-50.23	(50.2)
$Si(CHCH_2)Cl_3$	$^1J(Si-C)$	-112.26	2.41	-0.86	-110.72	-113 ±1
$SiFH_3$	$^1J(Si-F)$	-98.97	366.24	-14.91	252.36	(281.0)
$SiF_3(NCO)$	$^1J(Si-F)$	-220.22	414.77	-16.83	177.72	(181.0)

These calculations also reveal the importance of including d orbitals on phosphorus and silicon in a description of these couplings. The role of the d orbitals is particularly important for $^1J(P-F)$ and $^1J(Si-F)$ on account of $p_\pi-d_\pi$ back bonding interactions.

Another simple empirical relationship between spin-spin coupling and molecular structure is that of the Karplus-type equation (17).

For saturated X-C-C-Y fragments the value of ^3J(X-Y) may be related to the dihedral angle, ϕ, by an expression similar to equation (10). In

$$^3J(X-Y) \ = \ A \cos 2\phi + B \cos \phi + C \tag{10}$$

this equation A, B and C are empirical constants, usually B is negative, and $|A| > |B|$. Consequently values of ^3J(X-Y) are at a maximum when $\phi = 180°$ and a minimum when ϕ is close to $90°$. In general relationships comparable to equation (10) are fairly satisfactory for ^3J(H-H) data. However, some SOS-INDO calculations on fluoroethanes (18) show that the dependence of ^3J(F-F) upon the F-C-C-F dihedral angle is much more complicated than accounted for by equation (10). These calculations show significant, and non-sinusoidal, coupling contributions from the non contact expressions (18).

Other theoretical studies, by means of FPT-INDO calculations, on $^3J(^{13}C-^1H)$ and $^3J(^{13}C-^{13}C)$ have considered the contact interaction only (19)-(21). These investigations reveal that nonbonded interactions can have a substantial effect on the contact contribution to couplings involving ^{13}C; thus important deviations from angular dependencies of the Karplus type are expected (20). The presence of substituents on the γ carbon atom can cause a perturbation of the nonbonded interactions and a further non-Karplus type variation of the contact contribution to $^3J(^{13}C-^1H)$ and $^3J(^{13}C-^{13}C)$ data (21).

SCPT-INDO calculations on $^3J(^{13}C-^{13}C)$ data show three distinct patterns for the dihedral angle dependence of the contact contribution to the coupling (22). The patterns depend upon the degree of double bonding present in the coupling path and on $\sigma-\pi$ exchange. The contact term is usually dominant except for conjugated systems where the magnitude of the dipolar term is highly dependent upon the dihedral angle (22).

Calculations of proton couplings in sugar fragments have been reported (23)(24). It is clearly shown that any attempt to establish the conformation about an isolated bond, on the basis of observed ^3J(H-H) data and a Karplus type relationship, can lead to erroneous conclusions unless the influence of the remainder of the molecule is properly taken into account.

Consequently, couplings not involving protons are often unlikely to follow a Karplus type relationship due to the presence of non-contact coupling contributions and subtle molecular electronic effects. ^3J(H-H) interactions are more likely to follow a Karplus type relationship but great care is required in the estimation of conformational data.

Relativistic Effects on Spin-Spin Couplings

As noted for calculations on nuclear shieldings, relativistic effects are expected to be significant when considerations of the NMR parameters of heavier nuclei are being made. Ramsey's spin-spin coupling theory is a non-relativistic one in that it assumes that Russell-Saunders coupling applies to the electronic spin and orbital angular momenta and that the vector potential of a nucleus may be represented by a point dipole. Pyykkö has presented a relativistic analogue of Ramsey's theory (25). In this approach the terms $\mathcal{H}_1^{(b)}$, $\mathcal{H}_2$ and $\mathcal{H}_3$ in equation (4) are replaced by a single hyperfine Hamiltonian. The term $\mathcal{H}_1^{(a)}$ is obtained by means of a second-order contribution from positron-like intermediate states.

Relativistically parameterised extended Hückel (REX) MO calculations of reduced one bond couplings have been reported for some hydrides and other simple compounds of elements from Groups IV to VII of the periodic table (26). Comparison of the results obtained from the non-relativistic extended Hückel theory (EHT) provides an estimate of the importance of relativistic influences on the couplings for the heavier nuclei considered, as shown in Table III.

Table III (26)

Some values of reduced one bond couplings, in $10^{19} J^{-1} T^2$, obtained from semi-empirical MO calculations, REX and EHT, and experiment

Molecule	Coupling	EHT Value	REX Value	Experimental Value
SiH_4	$^1K(Si-H)$	53.1	53.1	84.8
SnH_4	$^1K(Sn-H)$	219.0	289.0	430.0
PbH_4	$^1K(Pb-H)$	373.0	844.0	938.0
$Sn(CH_3)_4$	$^1K(Sn-C)$	103.0	143.0	300.0
$Pb(CH_3)_4$	$^1K(Pb-C)$	164.0	465.0	396.0
$Tl(CH_3)_3$	$^1K(Tl-c)$	151.0	519.0	1096.0
$Tl(CH_3)_2^+$	$^1K(Tl-C)$	262.0	831.0	1420.0 to 1648.0
$(CH_3)_3P=Te$	$^1K(Te-P)$	-274.0	-444.0	-1113.0

Analysis of the various contributions to the spin coupling interactions reveals that, the term corresponding to the non-relativistic contact interaction, usually dominates the spin-spin couplings at the relativistic level (26). Thus, as in the case of nuclear shieldings, we conclude that an account of relativistic effects must be incorporated into discussions involving spin-spin couplings of heavy nuclei.

Solvent Effects on Spin-Spin Couplings

Analogous to the case of nuclear shielding solvent effects on spin-spin couplings can be divided into non-specific and specific categories.

The solvaton model (1)(27) has been applied to calculations of spin-spin couplings with some success.   The reaction field, and other similar models, have also been employed in conjunction with a study of variations in the contact contribution to couplings as the medium changes (28).

In general, spin-spin couplings are less sensitive to a change of solvent than are nuclear shieldings.   This is exemplified in Table IV

Table IV (29)(30)

Results of some FPT-INDO calculations incorporating the solvaton model of the effect of the Dielectric (ε) of the medium on some values of $^1J(N\equiv C)$ and $^1J(N-C)$ in Hz

Molecule	Coupling	ε	Contact	Orbital	Dipolar	Total
CH_3NH_2	$^1J(N-C)$	1	-13.05	0.87	-0.29	-12.47
		4	-12.94	0.88	-0.29	-12.35
		8	-12.92	0.88	-0.29	-12.33
		20	-12.91	0.88	-0.29	-12.32
		40	-12.90	0.88	-0.29	-12.31
		80	-12.90	0.88	-0.29	-12.31
$(NH_3)_2CO$	$^1J(N-C)$	1	-17.43	1.62	0.08	-15.73
		4	-17.97	1.68	0.06	-16.23
		8	-18.06	1.70	0.05	-16.31
		20	-18.11	1.71	0.05	-16.37
		40	-18.14	1.71	0.05	-16.38
		80	-18.15	1.71	0.05	-16.39
CH_3NC	$^1J(N\equiv C)$	1	14.82	-8.43	-12.58	-6.19
		4	14.07	-8.37	-12.63	-6.93
		8	13.94	-8.36	-12.64	-7.07
		20	13.85	-8.36	-12.65	-7.16
		40	13.82	-8.36	-12.65	-7.19
		80	13.81	-8.36	-12.65	-7.20
CH_3CN	$^1J(N\equiv C)$	1	2.32	-9.33	-15.02	-22.04
		4	1.77	-9.11	-14.78	-22.12
		8	1.68	-9.06	-14.74	-22.13
		20	1.62	-9.04	-14.71	-22.13
		40	1.60	-9.03	-14.70	-22.13
		80	1.59	-9.02	-14.70	-22.14
PhNC		1	13.72	-5.63	-11.33	-3.24
		4	12.94	-5.63	-11.38	-4.08
		8	12.79	-5.63	-11.39	-4.24
		20	12.70	-5.64	-11.40	-4.34
		40	12.70	-5.64	-11.41	-4.37
		80	12.65	-5.64	-11.41	-4.39

by the results of some FPT-INDO calculations of $^1J(N\equiv C)$ and $^1J(N-C)$ incorporating the solvaton model (29)(30). As ε, the dielectric of the medium, varies from 1 to 80 the value of $^1J(N\equiv C)$ may change by up to 2 Hz.

The variation predicted for $^1J(N-C)$ values over the same range of changes in ε, is much smaller than for $^1J(N\equiv C)$. The major variation in the total coupling, as a function of ε, is usually due to the contact interaction even when it is not the dominant spin coupling mechanism. The isocyanide couplings are predicted to be more sensitive to a change in ε, than are those of the cyanides. This is consistent with the normally held view of a greater polar character for the isocyanides.

Due to the importance of solute-solvent interactions for protein structure and stability, specific medium effects on spin-spin couplings have been studied as demonstrated by same $^5J(H-H)$ data for cis-N-Methylacetamide (31). FPT-INDO calculations of the isolated amide predict that the $^5J(H-H)$ cis and trans values are -0.37 and -0.41 Hz respectively. Using a model containing five waters of hydration, based on an optimised structure for trans-N-Methylacetamide (32), both the cis and trans $^5J(H-H)$ values are predicted to be +0.12 Hz. The positive increase in the couplings with hydration of the amide bond is consistent with experimental data for cyclo-(Gly-Phgly) taken on solutions containing increasing amounts of water (31).

Similar calculations on the planar form of cyclo-(Gly-Gly)·10H$_2$O show that the presence of the ten water molecules results in an increase of the cis and trans $^5J(H-H)$ values by 1.7 and 1.3 Hz respectively (31).

Protonation not only has a very strong influence on couplings involving the protonated atom, but also on couplings between pairs of neighbouring atoms. This is demonstrated by means of some FPT-INDO calculations on pyridine and the pyridinium ion (33) as shown in Table V.

Table V   (33)

Some calculated and observed $^1J(^{13}C-^1H)$ data, in Hz, for pyridine and the pyridinium ion

		Pyridine		Pyridinium Ion
C_2-H_2	calculated	163.94		182.93
C_2-H_2	observed	177.37		190.7
Protonation Effect (ΔJ)		+19.0	calculated	
		+13.3	observed	
C_3-H_3	calculated	145.98		162.11
C_3-H_3	observed	162.11		173.95
Protonation Effect (ΔJ)		+16.2	calculated	
		+11.8	observed	
C_4-H_4	calculated	145.31		158.15
C_4-H_4	observed	158.15		169.43
Protonation Effect (ΔJ)		+12.8	calculated	
		+11.3	observed	

Analysis of the data reveals that the main structural change upon protonation is a reduction of the internal CCN angle by 3.8°. This results in an increase in the 2S-1S bond order of the C-H bonds and thus an increase in the contact contribution to ^1J(C-H) upon protonation.

The satisfactory agreement between the calculated and observed effects on ^1J(C-H) due to protonation of pyridine (Table V) raises the possibility of determining tautomeric ratios from calculated spin-spin couplings.

In the case of purine the mole fraction of the N-7H tautomer is predicted to be 0.47 and 0.32 for the neutral system in D_2O and DMSO respectively while for the monocation in 20% D_2SO_4 the fraction is predicted to be 0.50 from a consideration of the coupling data. This compares with empirical values of 0.51, 0.32 and 0.47 for analogous solutions of methylpurines. A similar study on adenine gives the mole fraction of the N-9H tautomer as 0.19 in DMSO from the spin-spin coupling results whereas independent data suggest 0.15 (34) and 0.22 (35). Thus calculated spin-spin coupling results can be satisfactorily employed for estimating protonation tautomer equilibria.

CONCLUSIONS

It is to be hoped that to some extent, at least, the sentiments expressed by Churchill in his account of the Malakand Field Force have not been too accurately reflected in the discourse presented here. On the contrary it would be comforting to think that an attempt has been made to bridge the apparent gap between the, more theoretical and the more experimental, extremes of the field of NMR parameters.

In the case of spin-spin couplings Ramsey's model appears to be satisfactory for couplings involving only light nuclei. The relativistic modifications proposed by Pyykkö seem to be necessary for a discussion of couplings involving heavier nuclei.

In general simple empirical relationships between spin-spin couplings and molecular parameters must be treated with caution. Lone pair effects, non-contract contributions and non-bonded interactions render such relationships open to doubt. Solvent effects can also be important and are readily available to study by theoretical methods.

The question of whether to choose ab initio or semi empirical MO methods for calculations of spin-spin couplings is largely answered by the nature of the problem in hand. Perhaps the situation is best summed up by Occam's Razar (36), Entia non sunt multiplicanda praeter necessitatem.

However, as is often the case, perhaps the final word rests with Hippocrates, "Declare the past, diagnose the present, foretell the future" (37).

References

1.   I. Ando and G.A. Webb, 'Theory of NMR Parameters', Academic Press,
     London (1983)
2.   J. Kowalewski in 'Annual Reports on NMR Spectroscopy', G.A. Webb,
     ed., Academic Press, London, Vol. 12, p.81 (1982).
3.   N.F. Ramsey, Phys. Rev., 91, 303 (1953).
4.   J.A. Pople and D.P. Santry, Mol. Phys., 8, 1 (1964).
5.   A.D.C. Towl and K. Schaumberg, Mol. Phys., 22, 49 (1971).
6.   J.A. Pople, J.W. McIver and N.S. Ostlund, J. Chem. Phys., 49, 2960
     (1968).
7.   J.A. Pople, J.W. McIver and N.S. Ostlund, J. Chem. Phys., 49, 2965
     (1968).
8.   A.C. Blizzard and D.P. Santry, J. Chem. Phys., 55, 950 (1971).
9.   Tun Khin and G.A. Webb, Org. Magn. Reson., 10, 175 (1977).
10. Tun Khin and G.A. Webb, J. Magn. Reson., 33, 159 (1979).
11. Tun Khin and G.A. Webb, Org. Magn. Reson., 11, 487 (1978).
12. J.M. Schulman and T. Venanzi, J. Amer. Chem. Soc., 98, 4701 (1976).
13. J.M. Schulman, J. Ruggio and T. Venanzi, J. Amer. Chem. Soc., 99,
     2045 (1977).
14. S. Duangthai and G.A. Webb, Org. Magn. Reson., 20, 33 (1982).
15. S. Duangthai and G.A. Webb, Org. Magn. Reson., 20, 225 (1982).
16. S. Duangthai and G.A. Webb, Org. Magn. Reson., 21, 125 (1983).
17. M. Barfield and M. Karplus, J. Amer. Chem. Soc., 91, 1 (1969).
18. K. Hirao, H. Nakatsuji and H. Kato, J. Amer. Chem. Soc., 95, 31
     (1973).
19. M. Barfield, J.L. Marshall, E.D. Canada and M.R. Willcott, J. Amer.
     Chem. Soc., 100, 7075 (1978).
20. M. Barfield, J. Amer. Chem. Soc., 102, 1 (1980).
21. M. Barfield, J.L. Marshall and E.D. Canada, J. Amer. Chem. Soc.,
     102, 7 (1980).
22. M.L. Sevenson and G.E. Maciel, J. Magn. Reson., 57, 248 (1984).
23. A. Jaworski, I. Ekiel and D. Shugor, J. Amer. Chem. Soc., 100,
     4357 (1978).
24. A. Jaworski and I. Ekiel, Int. J. Quant. Chem., 16, 615 (1979).
25. P. Pyykkö, Chem. Phys., 22, 289 (1977).
26. P. Pyykkö and L. Wiesenfeld, Mol. Phys., 43, 557 (1981).
27. I. Ando and G.A. Webb, Org. Magn. Reson., 15, 111 (1981).
28. M. Barfield and M.D. Johnston, Chem. Rev., 73, 53 (1973).
29. S.N. Shargi and G.A. Webb, Org. Magn. Reson., 19, 126 (1982).
30. S.N. Shargi, G.A. Webb, I. Ando and S. Watanabe, J. Mol. Struct.,
     91, 325 (1983).
31. M. Barfield, F.A. Al-Obeidi, V.J. Hruby and S.R. Walter, J. Amer.
     Chem. Soc., 104, 3302 (1982).
32. S. Scheiner and C.W. Kern, J. Amer. Chem. Soc., 99, 7042 (1977).
33. M. Schumacher and H. Günther, J. Amer. Chem. Soc., 104 4167 (1982).
34. M.T. Chenon, R.J. Pugmire, D.M. Grant, R.P. Panzica and L.B.
     Townsend, J. Amer. Chem. Soc., 97, 4636 (1975).
35. M. Dreyfus, G. Dodin, O. Bensaude and J.E. Dubois, J. Amer. Chem.
     Soc., 97, 2369 (1975).

36. Attributed to William of Occam 1300–1349, (present day Ockham in the County of Surrey, U.K.), "It is vain to do with more what can be done with less".

37. Hippocrates of Kos <u>ca</u> 460 to 357 B.C., <u>Epidemics</u>, Book 1, section 11.

TWO-DIMENSIONAL NMR SPECTROSCOPY

Ad Bax
Laboratory of Chemical Physics
National Institute of Arthritis, Diabetes
and Digestive and Kidney Diseases
National Institutes of Health
Bethesda, Maryland 20205, USA.

ABSTRACT. Two-dimensional (2D) NMR spectroscopy has been developed during the past decade to become an extremely powerful tool, greatly expanding the applicability of NMR to chemical and biochemical structural problems. The fundamental aspects of 2D NMR will be discussed and some of the basic pulse schemes will be treated in more detail. The application of 2D spectroscopy to the imaging of macroscopic objects will not be treated here, but is, at least in principle, very similar to some of the pulse schemes that will be discussed.

1. INTRODUCTION

The concept of two-dimensional Fourier transformation in NMR was first introduced by Jeener (1) in 1971. Since that time, several hundred different 2D pulse schemes have been proposed in the literature. The selection of experiments that will be described is based on the insight they provide into the basis and generality of 2D NMR, and also on the importance for solving the most common types of problems.

The experiments that will be described here are (a) 2D homonuclear shift correlation through scalar coupling (COSY), (b) 2D cross relaxation spectroscopy based on the nuclear Overhauser effect (NOESY) and (c) heteronuclear chemical shift correlation of ^{1}H and ^{15}N chemical shifts through multiple quantum coherence.

Before addressing those experiments, an introduction into the principles and general aspects of two-dimensional NMR will be presented. The original 2D experiment, proposed by Jeener (1), will be discussed for the simple case of non-coupled nuclear spins, for example, the protons in chloroform. This will illustrate how a 2D Fourier transformation is accomplished and also which type of data

T. Axenrod and G. Ceccarelli (eds.), NMR in Living Systems, 67–94.
© *1986 by D. Reidel Publishing Company.*

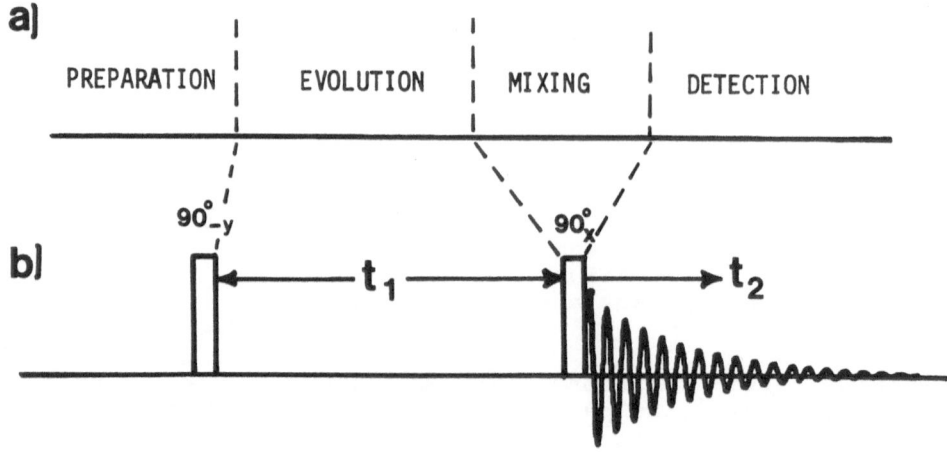

Figure 1.   (a) General subdivision of the time axis of a
two-dimensional NMR experiment. (b) Pulse scheme of the
Jeener experiment.

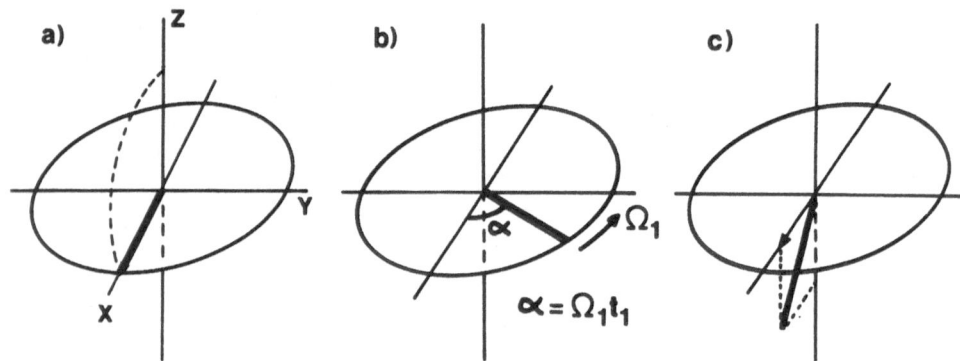

Figure 2.   Evolution of the magnetization of a set of
isolated spins during the pulse scheme of Fig. 1b. (a) The
$90°_{-y}$ pulse rotates the z magnetization to the x axis. (b)
During the evolution period, t_1, the magnetization rotates
through an angle $\alpha = \Omega_1 t_1$. (c) The second 90° pulse rotates
the transverse magnetization into the xz plane, leaving a
transverse component proportional to $\sin(\alpha)$ parallel to the
x axis.

presentation (absorptive / dispersive / absolute value) is
generally preferrable. Jeener's original sequence is
depicted in Figure 1. At the end of the preparation period,
which is sufficiently long to establish a (close to) thermal
equilibrium situation, a 90° pulse applied along the -y axis
of the rotating frame ($90°_{-y}$ pulse) rotates the
magnetization to a position parallel to the x axis (Fig. 2a).
The system then evolves (usually in an unperturbed fashion)
for a time t_1, which is generally referred to as the
evolution period. During this period the magnetization
rotates through an angle $\Omega_1 t_1$, where Ω_1 is the angular
resonance frequency of the magnetization considered
(Fig. 2b). At the end of the evolution period, a $90°_x$ pulse
rotates the magnetization into the xz plane (Fig. 2c). At
this point in time a transverse component proportional to
$\cos(\Omega_1 t_1)$ is left parallel to the x axis of the rotating
frame. During the detection period, t_2, a signal $s(t_1, t_2)$
will be detected that is in amplitude proportional to
$\cos(\Omega_1 t_1)$. If quadrature detection is employed during the
detection period, the signal is described by:

$$s(t_1, t_2) = M_0 \cos(\Omega_1 t_1) \exp(i \Omega_2 t_2) \exp(-t_1/T_2^{(1)}) \exp(-t_2/T_2^{(2)})$$
$$[1]$$

where Ω_1 and Ω_2 denote the angular frequencies of the
magnetization during the times t_1 and t_2, respectively.
$T_2^{(1)}$ and $T_2^{(2)}$ are the decay constants of the
magnetization during the times t_1 and t_2. Of course, in this
simple experiment, $\Omega_1 = \Omega_2$ and $T_2^{(1)} = T_2^{(2)}$. However in
many other experiments this is not necessarily the case, and
therefore different labels are used.

Fourier transformation with respect to t_2 of the FID's
acquired for the various t_1 values gives a set of spectra
with amplitude proportional to $\cos(\Omega_1 t_1)$:

$$s(t_1, \omega_2) = M_0 \cos(\Omega_1 t_1)[A_2(\omega_2) + i D_2(\omega_2)] \exp(-t_1/T_2^{(1)}) \quad [2]$$

where $A_2(\omega_2)$ and $D_2(\omega_2)$ are the absorptive and dispersive
parts of the resonance, given by

$$A_2(\omega_2) = T_2^{(2)} / \{1 + [T_2^{(2)}(\omega_2 - \Omega_2)]^2\} \quad [3a]$$

$$D_2(\omega_2) = T_2^{(2)}(\omega_2 - \Omega_2) A_2(\omega_2) \quad [3b]$$

The absorptive parts of a set of those spectra, obtained for
different values of t_1, are sketched in Figure 3a. Cross
sections parallel to the t_1 axis through the data matrix of
Figure 3a show a cosine modulation with angular frequency
Ω_1, if taken near $\omega_2 = \Omega_2$, and consist of near zero intensity
for other ω_2 values. Usually the data matrix of Figure 3a is
transposed in the computer memory, in order to facilitate a

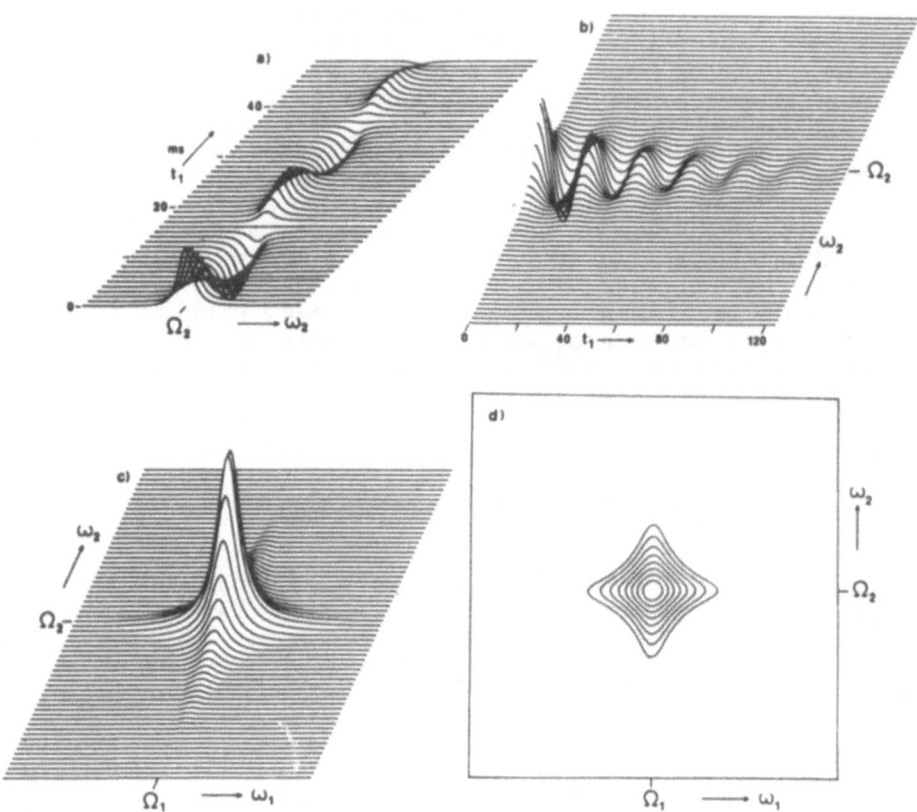

Figure 3.   (a) A set of spectra obtained with the sequence
of Fig. 1a for increasing durations of the evolution period,
t_1. (b) Transposed data matrix of Fig. 3a. (c) Fourier
transform of the interferograms of Fig. 3b, resulting in a
two-dimensional stacked line spectrum. (d) The spectrum of
Fig. 3c, represented as a contour plot.

Fourier transformation with respect to t_1 (Fig. 3b). Fourier transformation of those t_1 sections, generally referred to as <u>interferograms</u> (2), gives the final 2D spectrum, shown in Figure 3c. Usually such a spectrum is presented as a contour plot (Fig. 3d), rather than a stacked line representation, since this simplifies measuring coordinates of the resonance and avoids the possibility of low intensity resonances to be hidden behind intense resonances.

1.1 Sampling frequency and sensitivity

In conventional one-dimensional Fourier transform NMR experiments, the spectral width after Fourier transformation equals $1/(2\Delta t)$, or $\pm 1(2\Delta t)$ in the case of complex Fourier transformation, where Δt is the time between sampling points. Analogously, if consecutive t_1 values are separated by an amount Δt_1, this will give a spectral width equal to $1/(2\Delta t_1)$ after Fourier transformation with respect to t_1.

In a regular one-dimensional Fourier transform experiment, the signal-to-noise ratio for a single time-domain data point can be very poor; however, the Fourier transformation takes the signal energy of all data points and puts it all into one (or several) narrow resonance line(s). Similarly, if for each t_1 value in a 2D experiment a spectrum with poor signal-to-noise ratio is obtained, the second Fourier transformation with respect to t_1 combines the signal energy of a particular resonance from all spectra obtained for different t_1 values, and concentrates it into one narrow line in the 2D spectrum. Therefore, the sensitivity of 2D NMR is not necessarily lower than for the one-dimensional experiment.

In certain types of spectroscopy one tries to transfer magnetization from one resonance to another by means of a coherent process or by means of cross relaxation or chemical exchange (to be discussed later). In this case the sensitivity of 2D NMR can become rather poor if the transfer process is not very efficient (as is the case in coherent transfer through non-resolved couplings or in the case of slow cross relaxation or chemical exchange). However, the analogous one-dimensional experiment also suffers in sensitivity in this case.

If sensitivity is a crucial problem, the two rules that should always be obeyed are :
1. The acquisition time in the t_2 dimension, $t_{2\,max}$, should be at least equal to 1.5 T_2.
2. The acquisition time in the t_1 dimension, $t_{1\,max}$, should be chosen as short as possible, i.e. not longer than absolutely necessary to obtain enough resolution in the ω_1 dimension after Fourier transformation. Since the signal decays as a function of the time t_1, spectra taken for short t_1 values contribute more to the 2D resonance intensity (and

sensitivity) than spectra obtained for t_1 values on the
order of $T_2^{(1)}$ or longer.

More discussions on sensitivity of 2D NMR can be found in
the literature (3-6).

1.2 Lineshapes and transform techniques

The spectrum in Figure 3c represents the cosine Fourier
transform with respect to t_1 of the real part of Eq. [2]. If
interferograms through the real and imaginary halves of the
$S(t_1, \omega_2)$ are Fourier transformed separately, this gives:

$$S(\omega_1, \omega_2) = A_1(\omega_1)A_2(\omega_2) + iA(\omega_1)D_2(\omega_2) +$$
$$+ jD_1(\omega_1)A_2(\omega_2) + j iD_1(\omega_1)D_2(\omega_2) \qquad [4]$$

where "j" has the same meaning as "i", but refers to the
imaginary data in the F_1 dimension. $A_1(\omega_1)$ and $D_1(\omega_1)$ are
defined analogous to Eq. [3]. The four terms at the right
hand side of Eq. [4] are also known as S^{CC}, S^{CS}, S^{SC}
and S^{SS} in the older literature (2,7). Clearly, only one
of the four parts (S^{CC}) shows the desirable 2D absorption
mode lineshape.

The signal of Eq. [2] is modulated in amplitude by a
cosine function. It is impossible to tell from the second
Fourier transformation whether the modulation frequency, Ω_1,
is positive or negative. Of course, for this simple case one
knows that $\Omega_1 = \Omega_2$, and if quadrature detection during t_2 is
employed, the sign of the modulation frequency is
determined. However, in many experiments this is not the
case and in order to avoid confusion, one has to make sure
that all modulation frequencies have the same sign by
positioning the transmitter frequency at either the low or
high field side of the spectrum. Because of sensitivity
considerations, quadrature detection in the t_2 dimension is
always necessary, and data storage space is wasted if the
transmitter frequency is not set at the center of the
spectrum.

A simple way around this problem is the introduction of
artificial phase modulation, to be described below. If a
second experiment, "$90°_{-y} - t_1 - 90°_y -$ acquire (t_2)" is
performed, the signal detected in this second experiment
will start out along the y axis (at $t_2 = 0$) and is modulated
in amplitude by $\sin(\Omega_1 t_1)$:

$$s'(t_1, t_2) = M_0 \sin(\Omega_1 t_1)\exp[i(\Omega_2 t_2 + \pi/2)] \times$$
$$\times \exp(-t_1/T_2^{(1)})\exp(-t_2/T_2^{(2)})$$
$$= iM_0 \sin(\Omega_1 t_1)\exp(i\Omega_2 t_2) \times$$
$$\times \exp(-t_1/T_2^{(1)})\exp(-t_2/T_2^{(2)}) \qquad [5]$$

Adding the results of the two experiments, Eqs. [5] and [1],
directly together and omitting the relaxation terms gives :

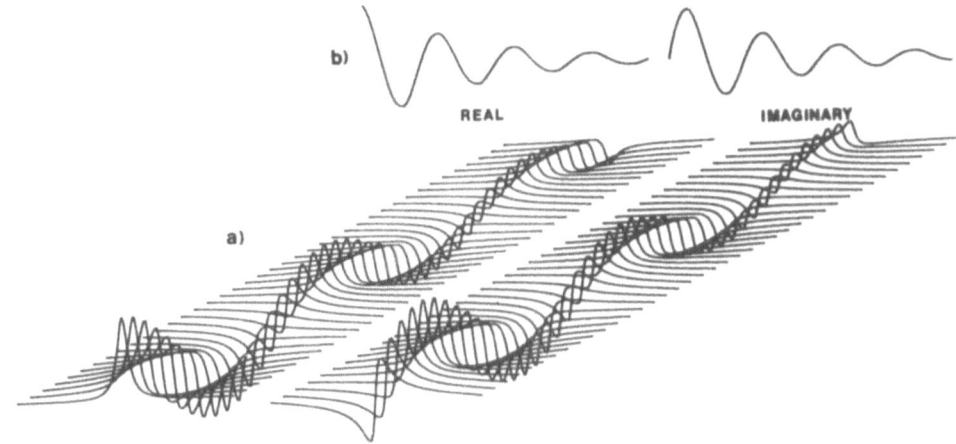

Figure 4.   (a) A set of phase-modulated spectra. The phase
of the resonance is a linear function of the duration of the
evolution period, t_1. Both the real and imaginary halves of
the spectra are shown. (b) Complex interferogram taken at
$\omega_2 = \Omega_2$. The first half of the interferogram represents a t_1
section through the real halves of the spectra in Fig. 4a,
and the second half is the interferogram through the
imaginary halves. A quadrature Fourier transform of this
complex interferogram determines the sign and the magnitude
of the modulation frequency.

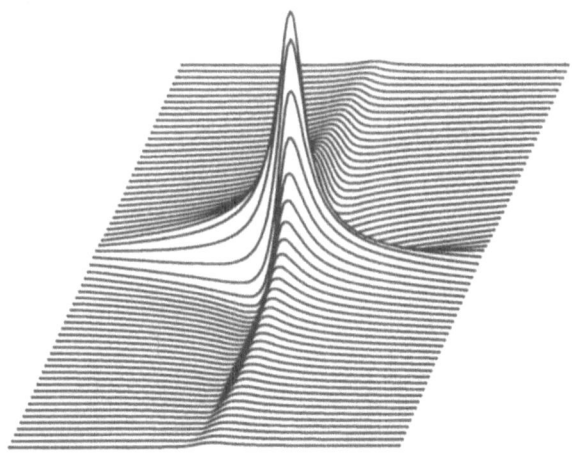

Figure 5.   Phase-twisted line shape obtained by Fourier
transformation of the matrix of Fig. 4a.

$$s^+(t_1, t_2) = M_0 \exp(i\Omega_1 t_1) \exp(i\Omega_2 t_2) \qquad [6]$$

Eq. [6] represents a signal of which the phase at time $t_2 = 0$ is a linear function of the duration of evolution period, t_1. Fourier transformation with respect to t_2 will yield a resonance at $\omega_2 = \Omega_2$, and with phase $\Omega_1 t_1$:

$$S^+(t_1, \omega_2) = M_0[\cos(\Omega_1 t_1) A_2(\omega_2) - \sin(\Omega_1 t_1) D_2(\omega_2)] +$$
$$+ iM_0[\cos(\Omega_1 t_1) D_2(\omega_2) + \sin(\Omega_1 t_1) A_2(\Omega_2)] \qquad [7]$$

A set of spectra obtained this way for a series of t_1 values, is sketched in Figure 4. Both the real and imaginary halves of those spectra are shown. An interferogram taken at $\omega_2 = \Omega_2$ does not contain any of the dispersive components since $D_2(\Omega_2) = 0$, and this interferogram is described by:

$$S^+(t_1, \Omega_2) = M_0[\cos(\Omega_1 t_1) + i\sin(\Omega_1 t_1)] T_2^{(2)} \qquad [8]$$

where the real part represents the interferogram taken through the real part of Eq. [6], and the imaginary part of Eq. [8] is the interferogram taken through the imaginary parts of the $s^+(t_1, \Omega_2)$ spectra. This complex interferogram is sketched in Figure 4b. A complex Fourier transformation of Eq. [8] can be made, and the sign of the modulation frequency, Ω_1, is automatically determined. Any interferogram taken at an ω_2 value different from Ω_2, will have non-zero contributions from $D_2(\omega_2)$, and Fourier transformation will yield a resonance in the F_1 dimension that is 90° out of phase relative to the interferogram taken at $\omega_2 = \Omega_2$. The full 2D Fourier transform of Eq. [8] is given by:

$$S^+(\omega_1, \omega_2) = M_0[A_1(\omega_1) A_2(\omega_2) - D_1(\omega_1) D_2(\omega_2)] +$$
$$+ iM_0[A_1(\omega_1) D_2(\omega_2) + D_1(\omega_1) A_2(\omega_2)] \qquad [9]$$

Clearly, both the real and imaginary part of this function are mixtures of absorption and dispersion. The real part of Eq. [9] is sketched in Figure 5. The resonance shows a so-called "phase twist" lineshape (2), and cannot be phased to the pure absorption mode. In practice, an absolute value mode calculation is usually made before display:

$$\text{Absolute value} = [\text{Re}^2 + \text{Im}^2]^{1/2} \qquad [10]$$

Since the tails of an absolute value mode resonance decrease proportional to $1/|\omega - \Omega)|$, this resonance shows undesirable tails, decreasing resolution.

Nevertheless, this artificially induced phase modulation is currently the most common way of operation for most 2D experiments. The software of most commercial spectrometers assume data in a 2D experiment to be phase-modulated, and

the data matrix transposition routine automatically places
the imaginary half of the interferogram behind the real half
(as depicted in Figure 4b), ready for a second complex
Fourier transformation, this time with respect to t_1.

The strong tailing of the absolute value mode lineshape
can be suppressed by the use of appropriate digital
filtering. All those filters have in common that they
reshape the envelope amplitude of the time domain data to
become decaying in a near symmetrical fashion from the
midpoint of the FID (8). Filters commonly used for this
purpose are the sine bell function (9), the "pseudo-echo
window" (10) and the convolution difference filter (11).
Figure 6 compares the contour plots for a regular absolute
value mode line-shape, and one that has been obtained after
the time domain data were multiplied by a sine bell in both
dimensions. Unfortunately, the sensitivity generally suffers
severely from the use of such resolution enhancement
filtering functions (the COSY experiment, to be discussed
later, is an exception to this rule).

Although phase modulated experiments are experimentally
very convenient, sensitivity and resolution suffer. Another
disadvantage of artificial phase modulation, not discussed
above nor mentioned explicitly in the literature, is that
only half of the available signal is used: If the difference
of the two experiments (Eq. [1] and Eq. [5]) were taken, this
gives a signal of the shape:

$$s^-(t_1, t_2) = M_0 \exp(-i\Omega_1 t_1)\exp(i\Omega_2 t_2) \qquad [11]$$

The noise in Eqs. [6] and [11] is in principle independent.
If only the sum, or the difference, is taken, half of the
available signal is wasted !

1.3 Two-dimensional quadrature and absorption mode

As explained above, absorption mode 2D spectra can only be
recorded if the transmitter is placed at either the low or
high field side of the spectrum. Since data acquisition
during t_2 has to be done in quadrature (for sensitivity
reasons), this type of experiment is very inefficient as far
as data storage is concerned. Also, pulse imperfections due
to resonance offset can become severe. A more efficient way
to obtain a 2D absorption mode spectrum in 2D quadrature,
was first introduced by Freeman et al. (12) and States et
al. (13) and will be described below.

Consider again the pulse sequence of Figure 1 and the
signal of Eq. [1]. A second experiment, $90°_{-x} - t_1 - 90°_x$
- acquire (t_2), is performed. The signal in the second
experiment is initially ($t_2 = 0$) also along the x axis, but is
modulated in amplitude by $\sin(\Omega_1 t_1)$. The FID's obtained in

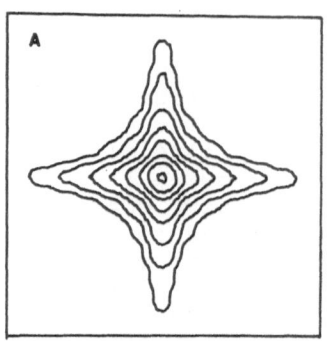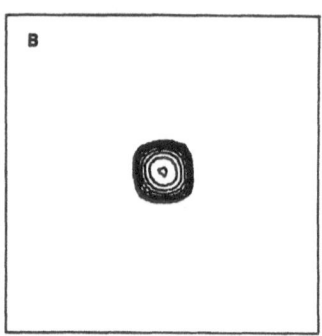

Figure 6.   Comparison of the contour plots of absolute value
mode line shapes. (a) Line shape obtained after an absolute
value mode calculation of a signal that has been multiplied
by a negative exponential with a time constant T_2 = AT/3,
where AT is the duration of the acquisition time. (b) Line
shape obtained if the time domain signal is multiplied by a
sine bell function. The lowest contour level is taken at
1/24 of the peak height.

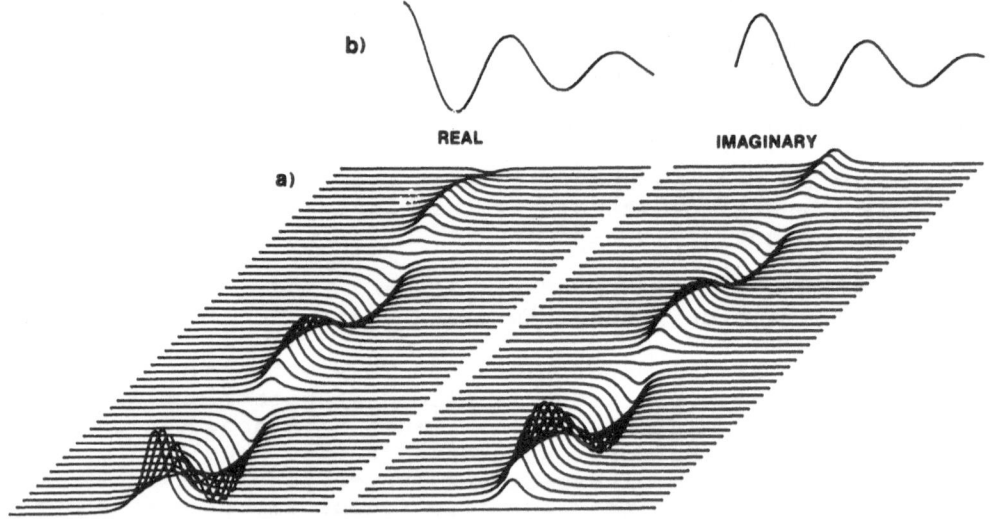

Figure 7.   (a) The left halves of the spectra are the
absorption parts of the spectra obtained with an experiment
where the resonance is modulated in amplitude by a cosine
function. The dispersive parts of those spectra have been
replaced by the absorptive part of the spectra obtained with
a second experiment, where the resonances are modulated in
amplitude by a sinusoidal function. (b) Complex
interferogram taken at $\omega_2 = \Omega_2$.

the two experiments, $s(t_1,t_2)$ and $s'(t_1,t_2)$, are <u>not</u>
co-added this time, but stored in separate locations in
memory. Hence, for every t_1 value, two spectra are recorded,
one modulated by a cosine and the other one by a sine
function. Fourier transformation of the two sets of spectra
gives:

$$S(t_1,\omega_2) = M_0\cos(\Omega_1 t_1)[A_2(\omega_2)+iD_2(\omega_2)] \qquad [12a]$$

$$S'(t_1,\omega_2) = M_0\sin(\Omega_1 t_1)[A_2(\omega_2)+iD_2(\omega_2)] \qquad [12b]$$

The simple but crucial trick is to replace the imaginary
part of $S(t_1,\omega_2)$ by the real part of $S'(t_1,\omega_2)$, yielding:

$$S^t(t_1,\omega_2)= M_0\exp(i\Omega_1 t_1)A_2(\omega_2) \qquad [13]$$

A set of those spectra is shown in Figure 7. Complex Fourier
transformation with respect to t_1 of Eq.[13] gives for the
real part:

$$S^t(\omega_1,\omega_2) = M_0 A_1(\omega_1)A_2(\omega_2) \qquad [14]$$

which represents a 2D absorption mode resonance. Undoubtedly
this will become the accepted way of data processing for
most 2D NMR experiments in the near future.

1.4 Coherence transfer by means of radiofrequency pulses

Classical vector pictures have been used for over three
decades to explain the mechanisms on which many NMR
experiments rely (14). However, for a description of many of
the newer type pulse sequences, applied to coupled spin
systems, straightforward application of those vector
pictures leads to erroneous results. Ernst and co-workers
(15) have introduced a formalism that does allow the use of
vector pictures to analyze the behavior of a coupled spin
system. This operator formalism based vector picture is more
complicated than is the use of the classical picture based
on the Bloch equations, but is much less tedious than use of
the density matrix formalism. The new approach will be
briefly discussed for a homonuclear weakly coupled two-spin
system. For a more detailed treatment the reader is referred
to the literature (15). Two weakly coupled spins, A and B,
will be considered.

The total net magnetization of spin A equals the vector
sum of the magnetizations of the two doublet components. As
in the classical vector picture, this total magnetization is
represented by a vector I_A that can be decomposed in the
standard fashion into its components along the principal
axes of the rotating frame (Fig.8):

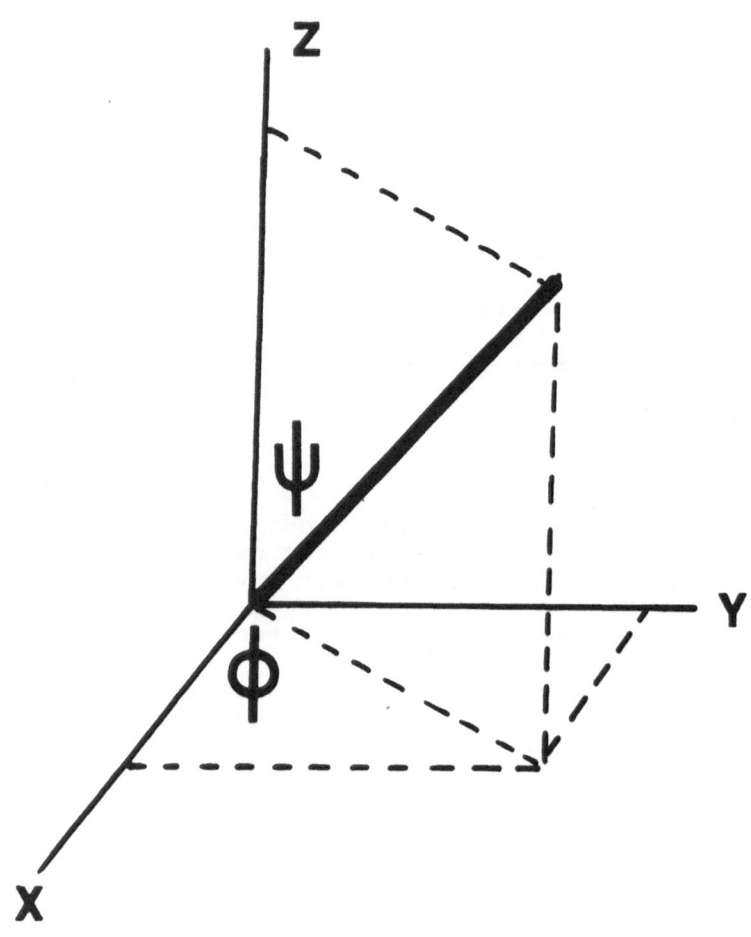

Figure 8. Decomposition of a magnetization vector in its three components along the axes of the rotating frame.

$$I_A = \cos(\psi)I_{zA} + \sin(\psi)\cos(\phi)I_{xA} + \sin(\psi)\sin(\phi)I_{yA} \qquad [15]$$

The antiphase components of the two doublet magnetization vectors do not contribute to I_A in this picture. Since those components are opposite to each other, they do not contribute to macroscopic observable magnetization. Of the antiphase components, one component corresponds to spin B in the $m=1/2$ spin state, and the other to the $m=-1/2$ state. This antiphase magnetization can then formally be written as $2I_AI_{zB}$. The factor "2" in this product is needed for normalization. The new formalism treats the individual terms in such a product as normal magnetization, in the classical way.

In order to make the description more explicit: consider the effect of a $90°_x$ pulse applied to the two-spin system that is initially in thermal equilibrium. The magnetization $(I_{zA} + I_{zB})$ gets rotated to a position parallel to the y axis, and thus creates $(I_{yA}+I_{yB})$. The magnetization of the two nuclei can be considered separately, and we will concentrate on the fate of the A spin magnetization. This will rotate with angular frequency, Ω_A, about the z axis and the two doublet components will periodically (with period $1/J$) get in antiphase. These two processes can be considered separately:

$$I_{yA} \xrightarrow{\Omega_A I_{zA}t} I_{yA}\cos(\Omega_A t) - I_{xA}\sin(\Omega_A t) \qquad [16a]$$

$$I_{yA} \xrightarrow{2\pi J I_{zA} I_{zB}t} I_{ya}\cos(\pi Jt) - 2I_{xA}I_{zB}\sin(\pi Jt) \qquad [16b]$$

$$I_{xA} \xrightarrow{2\pi J I_{zA} I_{zB}t} I_{xa}\cos(\pi Jt) + 2I_{yA}I_{zB}\sin(\pi Jt) \qquad [16c]$$

Substitution of Eqs.[16b] and [16c] in [16a] then gives the complete evolution of the magnetization. The interesting terms in Eq.[16] are the products $I_{xA}I_{zB}$, and $I_{yA}I_{zB}$. Consider a 90° pulse applied to such a term:

$$I_{xA}I_{zB} \xrightarrow{\quad 90°_y \quad} -I_{za}I_{xB} \qquad [17a]$$

$$I_{xA}I_{zB} \xrightarrow{\quad 90°_x \quad} I_{xA}I_{yB} \qquad [17b]$$

Eq.[17a] shows how antiphase A spin magnetization gets converted into antiphase B spin magnetization by a 90° pulse applied perpendicular to the doublet magnetization vectors. This important result is the basis of Jeener's original experiment when applied to a homonuclear coupled spin system. Eq. [17b] contains the product $I_{xA}I_{yB}$ and is harder to visualize; this term represents so-called two-spin coherence, a combination of zero- and double quantum coherence. The time evolution of the product equals the product of the time evolution of the individual terms; i.e. the time evolution of $I_{xA}I_{yB}$ is given by

$$I_{xA}I_{yB} \xrightarrow{\Omega_A t I_{zA} + \Omega_B t I_{zB}} [\cos(\Omega_A t)I_{xA} + \sin(\Omega_A t)I_{yA}] \times$$
$$\times [\cos(\Omega_B t)I_{yB} - \sin(\Omega_B t)I_{xB}] \qquad [18]$$

The operator formalism is easily extended to more spins by
considering product terms of all spins involved.

2. HOMONUCLEAR SHIFT CORRELATION THROUGH SCALAR COUPLING

Jeener's original 2D pulse scheme can be considered as a
convenient alternative for the conventional one-dimensionanl
double resonance experiments, and is often referred to as
the COSY (COrrelated SpectroscopY) experiment. A complete
quantum mechanical description of the experiment was
presented by Aue et al.(16) but did not contribute much to
the popularity of the experiment. Only in the early 1980's
the wide-spread applicability of this technique was realized
(17-21). The basic pulse scheme has already been discussed
in the previous sections. Here a $90°_x$ - t_1 - $90°_\phi$ -
acquire (t_2) pulse scheme is used, where the phase ϕ of the
final pulse and the mode of data acquisition are selected as
indicated in Table 1. This means that a minimum of four
experiments is performed for each t_1 value with the phase of
the final 90° pulse incremented by 90° each time and data
alternately added to and subtracted from memory. This way of
phase cycling results in detection of the $s^-(t_1, t_2)$ signal
of Eq.[11], often referred to as the coherence transfer echo
(22). The occurrence of the echo is easily understood by
considering that in Eq.[11], Ω_1 and Ω_2 have approximately
the same value (in the laboratory frame). Therefore, at time
$t_1 = t_2$, the phase of the magnetization, $\exp[i(\Omega_2 t_2 - \Omega_1 t_1)]$, is
to first order independent of the magnetic field strength,
i.e. independent of magnetic field inhomogeneity, and
consequently an echo will occur. The entire four-step
experiment is often repeated four times with the phases of
all radiofrequency pulses and receiver incremented by 90°
each time. This additional so-called CYCLOPS cycling (23)
eliminates imperfections in the quadrature detection system
of the spectrometer which otherwise may cause small mirror
image signals about the $\omega_2 = 0$ and $\omega_1 = 0$ axes.
    The COSY experiment relies on transfer of magnetization
from spin A to spin X by the second 90° pulse in Jeener's
experiment, and can only occur if spin A and X are mutually
coupled. The mechanism for this magnetization transfer has
been discussed in the previous section : Eq.[17a] shows how
spin A doublet components that are in antiphase with respect
to spin X are transferred into X spin doublet components
that are in antiphase with respect to spin A. The amount of
antiphase A-spin magnetization present before the second 90°
transfer pulse depends on $\sin(\pi J_{AX} t_1)$. The magnetization

Table 1. Cycling of the phase of the observe pulse, ϕ, and
of the receiver in the various steps of the COSY experiment
in order to obtain phase modulation and to detect the
coherence transfer echo.

Step	ϕ	Receiver
1	x	+
2	y	−
3	−x	+
4	−y	−

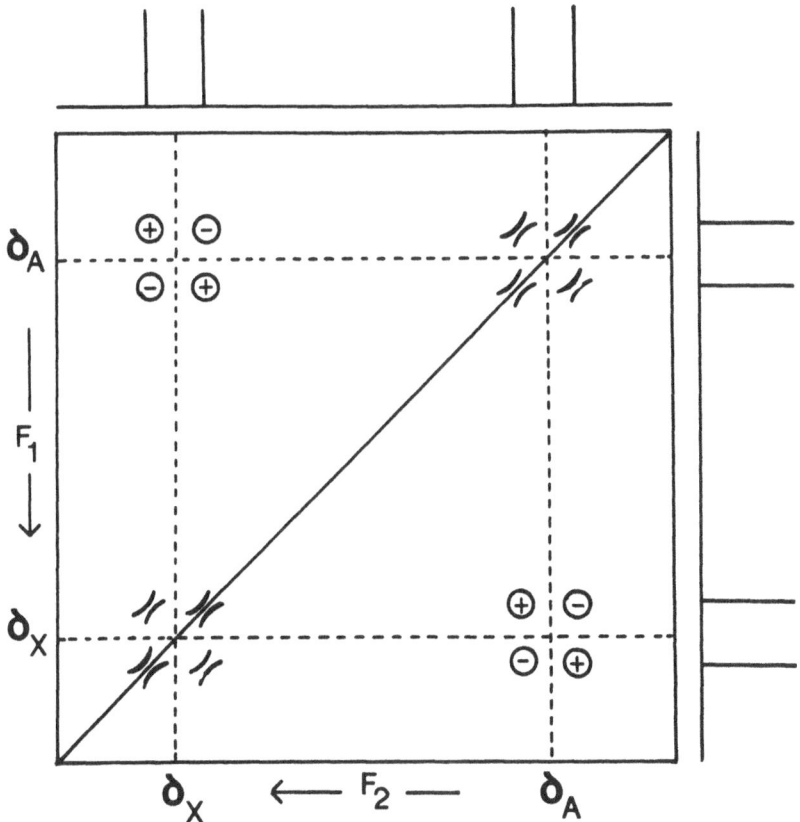

Figure 9.   Schematic diagram of the 2D COSY spectra of AX
spin system. The four components of the AX cross multiplet
are pairwise in antiphase, whereas the four diagonal
multiplet components are 90° out of phase in both dimensions
relative to the cross peaks.

observed during t_2 starts out in antiphase and is
proportional to $\sin(\pi J_{AX} t_2)$. The time domain signal for
the magnetization transferred from A to X is given by

$$s^-_{AX}(t_1, t_2) = M_0 \sin(\pi J_{AX} t_1)\sin(\pi J_{AX} t_2)\exp(-i\Omega_A t_1)\exp(i\Omega_X t_2)$$
[19]

Note that for very short t_1 values only very little
magnetization is transferred from A to X. Rewriting:

$$\sin(\pi Jt) = i[\exp(i\pi Jt) - \exp(-i\pi Jt)]/2$$
[20]

and substitution in Eq. [19] shows that the Fourier
transformed signal $S^-(\omega_1, \omega_2)$ will show four peaks at
$(\omega_1, \omega_2) = (\Omega_A \pm \pi J_{AX}, \Omega_X \pm \pi J_{AX})$, and that those resonances
show antiphase relationships, as schematically indicated in
Figure 9. Also indicated in Figure 9 are the "diagonal
resonances", due to magnetization that is not transferred
from A to X or from X to A, and which are 90° out of phase
relative to the cross peaks. It is therefore impossible to
phase this spectrum to the 2D absorption mode (unless the
pulse scheme is altered (24)), and an absolute value mode
calculation before display is therefore commonly used. The
artificial phase modulation scheme (discussed before)
therefore does not degrade performance of the experiment
very much. Also, since the cross peak time domain signal has
an envelope amplitude proportional to $\sin(\pi J_{AX} t_1)$ x
$\sin(\pi J_{AX} t_2)$, and acquisition times in the t_1 and t_2
dimension are typically 100-300 ms, use of a sine bell
digital filter is close to a matched filter for those
signals and favors the sensitivity of the cross multiplets,
meanwhile cutting down the intensity of redundant diagonal
peaks which have a $\cos(\pi J_{AX} t_1)\cos(\pi J_{AX} t_2)$ dependence.

Figure 10 shows the COSY spectrum for the compound
sketched at the top of that figure, recorded on a Nicolet
500 MHz spectrometer. 512 t_1 increments of 300 μsec each
were used, and 512 complex data points were acquired for
each t_1 value. The artificial phase modulation scheme (Table
1) was employed and the total measuring time was 4 h. Note
that in the regular one-dimensional spectrum many of the
couplings are not or poorly resolved. However, a wealth of
cross peaks can be observed in the 2D spectrum. For example,
it is seen that proton 1 is coupled to methyl group 38
(broken line in Fig. 10).

Many users of the COSY experiment are often puzzled by
the absence or low intensity of certain cross peaks. For
example, the cross peaks between protons 1 and 2 in Fig. 10
have too low an intensity to be observed in the contour
plot. In general, it is hard to calculate exactly how
intense a cross multiplet will be, but two factors that are
of major importance will be mentioned below.

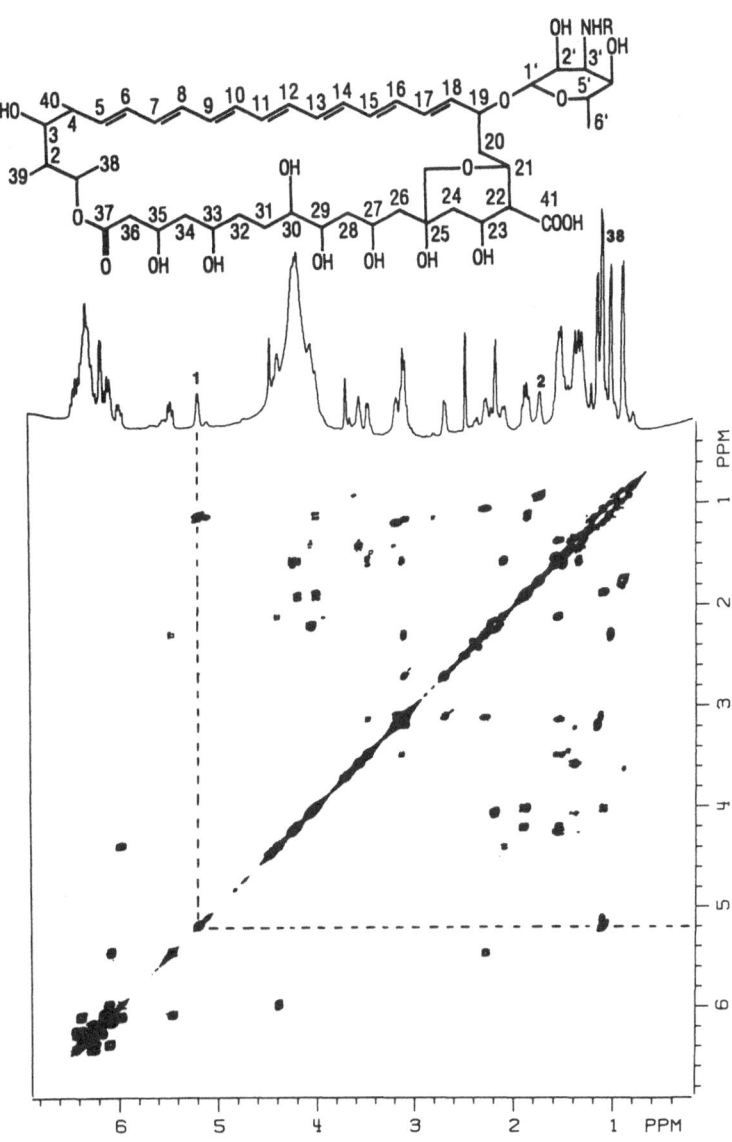

Figure 10.   500 MHz absolute value mode COSY spectrum of a
sample of amphotericin B in DMSO-d6. 16 experiments were
performed for each t_1 value, and the total duration of the
experiment was 4 h. A sine bell has been used in both
dimensions prior to Fourier transformation.

1. A proton that is coupled to a large number of other protons will show rather low intensity for its individual 1D multiplet components. In the COSY experiment, this low intensity will now be redistributed among all protons to which it is coupled by the 90° mixing pulse, giving very low intensity for the cross multiplets. The effect is particularly severe for cross peaks between two multiplets that both have a complicated multiplet structure.
2. If transverse relaxation times, T_2, are short compared with J_{AX}^{-1}, the transferred magnetization in Eq. [19] will never assume a large value and therefore only (vanishingly) low intensity cross peaks can be observed.

From point 1, it is clear that a large coupling does not necessarily give rise to an intense cross peak. However, if acquisition times $t_{1\,max}$ and $t_{2\,max}$ are chosen short (<100 ms) this will relatively emphasize cross peaks due to large scalar couplings.

3. HOMONUCLEAR CHEMICAL SHIFT CORRELATION THROUGH CROSS RELAXATION

In the COSY experiment, magnetization is transferred from one proton to another through the scalar coupling mechanism. This experiment relies on the existence of (partially) resolved scalar couplings. Another way to transfer magnetization between nuclei is the cross relaxation mechanism, which relies on the internuclear dipolar interaction. This mechanism is generally referred to as the nuclear Overhauser effect (NOE). The 2D pulse scheme that is based on the NOE effect is generally known as the NOESY experiment. This experiment was first proposed by Ernst, Jeener et al. (25, 26). It is mentioned here that the same experiment can also be used for the investigation of chemical exchange processes. Obviously, no resolved couplings are needed for this experiment; the experiment tends to work very well for macromolecules which have a slow tumbling rate and therefore less ideal averaging of the dipolar coupling mechanism. This is the reason for strong cross relaxation and causes line broadening in the conventional 1D spectrum and also in the 2D spectrum.
The pulse scheme is sketched in Fig. 11 and the mechanism on which this 2D experiment relies will be briefly discussed below. Assume for reasons of simplicity that all pulses in the scheme are applied along the x axis of the rotating frame, and consider a molecule with two spins A and B that have no mutual scalar coupling. The longitudinal magnetization of spin A, just after the second 90° pulse, is given by:

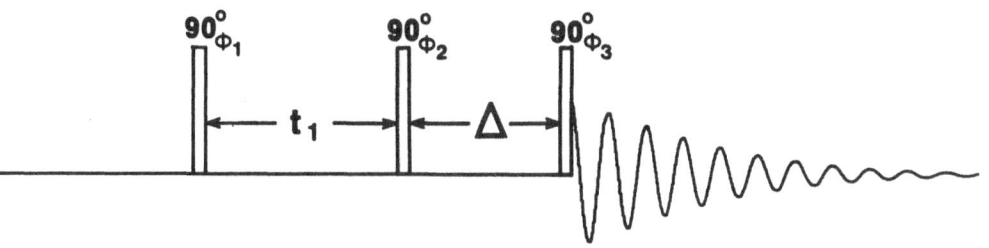

Figure 11.   Pulse scheme of the 2D experiment to detect homonuclear cross relaxation and chemical exchange. The phases of the r.f. pulses, ϕ_1 and ϕ_2, and of the receiver are cycled according to Table 2, and the results of the odd and even steps are stored in separate locations in memory and processed as described in the text in order to obtain an absorption mode spectrum.

Table 2.   Phases ϕ_1 and ϕ_2 of the pulses in Fig. 11 in the various steps of the experiment. Data of odd and even steps are stored separately in the computer memory.

Step	ϕ_1	ϕ_2	Receiver
1	x	x	x
2	y	x	x
3	-x	x	-x
4	-y	x	-x
5	x	y	y
6	y	y	y
7	-x	y	-y
8	-y	y	-y
9	x	-x	-x
10	y	-x	-x
11	-x	-x	x
12	-y	-x	x
13	x	-y	-y
14	y	-y	-y
15	-x	-y	y
16	-y	-y	y

$$M_{ZA}(t_1) = -M_{OA}\cos(\Omega_A t_1) \tag{21}$$

During the mixing period of duration, Δ, cross relaxation
with spin B takes place, changing the longitudinal B spin
magnetization by an amount $C[M_{ZA}(t_1)-M_{ZB}(t_1)]$ and the A
spin magnetization by the opposite amount, where C is a
constant depending on the cross relaxation rate, the
longitudinal relaxation rates, and the duration, Δ. Just
before the final pulse, the longitudinal B spin
magnetization is thus given by

$$M_{ZB}(t_1) = f[M_{ZB}(t_1)] + C \, M_{ZA}(t_1) \tag{22}$$

where $f[M_{ZB}(t_1)]$ is a function depending on the relaxation
of proton B during the delay, Δ, and on the modulation of
the B spin magnetization by the first two pulses in the
sequence. It is the second term at the right hand side of
Eq. [22] that is the term of interest, since this term is due
to cross relaxation from nucleus A to B. The final 90° pulse
converts this term into transverse B magnetization which
follows from Eqs. [21] and [22]:

$$s_{AB}(t_1,t_2) = C \, M_{OA} \cos(\Omega_A t_1)\exp(i\Omega_X t_2) \tag{23}$$

This signal is of the same shape as Eq. [1], and 2D Fourier
transformation will therefore give a resonance at
$(\omega_1,\omega_2)=(\Omega_A,\Omega_B)$. In contrast with the COSY experiment,
all peaks in the 2D spectrum will have the same phase, and
it is therefore strongly desirable to record the spectrum in
the absorption mode, using the procedure outlined in section
1.4. In order to eliminate transfer through scalar coupling
(the COSY mechanism) further phase cycling is necessary. In
practice a 16-step sequence (Table 2) is used and
additionally, this 16-step sequence is repeated four times
in the CYCLOPS mode (23) in order to eliminate quadrature
artefacts. Remaining coherent transfer through zero and
triple quantum coherence, that is not cycled out this way
can be eliminated by random fluctuation of Δ by a small
amount (5%).

   If the cross relaxation is slow compared to the
longitudinal relaxation, maximum transfer from spin A to B,
and vice versa, occurs for a mixing time on the order of the
shortest T_1 of the two spins involved. Hence, from a
sensitivity point of view, a mixing time on the order of T_1
is optimum for the detection of cross peaks. However, if one
wants to obtain quantitative information about the
relaxation rates, one has to consider that the cross peak
buildup rate (as a function of Δ) is non-linear (25-29). The
simplest way around this problem is to consider only short
mixing times, for which the NOE buildup is still in the
linear region (28,29), but this approach necessarily leads

to smaller cross peaks, i.e. lower sensitivity.

As an example, Fig.12 shows part of the 2D NOE spectrum
of the octamer [d-(5'GGAATTCC3')]$_2$, showing a number of
cross peaks, obtained for a mixing time of 200 ms. A full
analysis of the 2D NOE spectrum of this molecule is given by
Broido et al.(30). Analysis of the cross peak network does
not only provide assignment for all ^{1}H resonances in this
compound, but also gives information regarding the
three-dimensional structure in solution.

4. INDIRECT DETECTION OF ^{15}N THROUGH MULTIPLE QUANTUM COHERENCE

Detection of ^{15}N shifts is limited by its low NMR
sensitivity, which is due to the small and negative value of
the magnetogyric ratio and to the low natural abundance
(0.37%). The fact that the magnetogyric ratio, γ, is
negative can cause signal cancellation in the case of
incomplete nuclear Overhauser enhancement. NMR sensitivity
is approximately proportional to $\gamma^{5/2}$ (31) and is
therefore about a factor of 300 lower for ^{15}N than for
protons, which implies a factor of 100000 difference in
measuring time. It has been demonstrated that the INEPT
experiment can alleviate this problem to a certain extent,
but nevertheless detection remains difficult. Bodenhausen
and Ruben (32) demonstrated that the ^{15}N frequency could
be measured indirectly _via_ the protons directly coupled to
the ^{15}N nucleus. Their rather complicated sequence
transfers proton magnetization to the ^{15}N, which then
evolves during the evolution period of the 2D experiment,
before being transferred back to the protons which are
detected during the acquisition time in this experiment. A
much simpler alternative, that relies on the same principle
as the "Bodenhausen experiment" has been proposed rather
recently (33,34). Experimental results indicate that with
this new experiment the theoretical enhancement factor of
300 really can be obtained. The experiment works only for
protonated ^{15}N nuclei. Consider the energy level diagram
of an isolated ^{1}H-^{15}N pair (Fig.13). The broken lines
represent the two (weak) ^{15}N transitions. The solid lines
represent the (intense) proton transitions. The basic
concept of the new experiment is to generate the dotted
transitions (zero and double quantum), that resonate with
frequencies $\Omega_H \pm \Omega_N$. If those frequencies are measured
indirectly, with a 2D experiment, the ^{15}N frequency can be
calculated since the proton frequency, Ω_H, is known.

The pulse scheme of the experiment is shown in Fig.14.
The ^{1}H 180° pulse at the center of the evolution period
and the ^{15}N decoupling during data acquisition are
optional and will, at first, not be taken into account. The

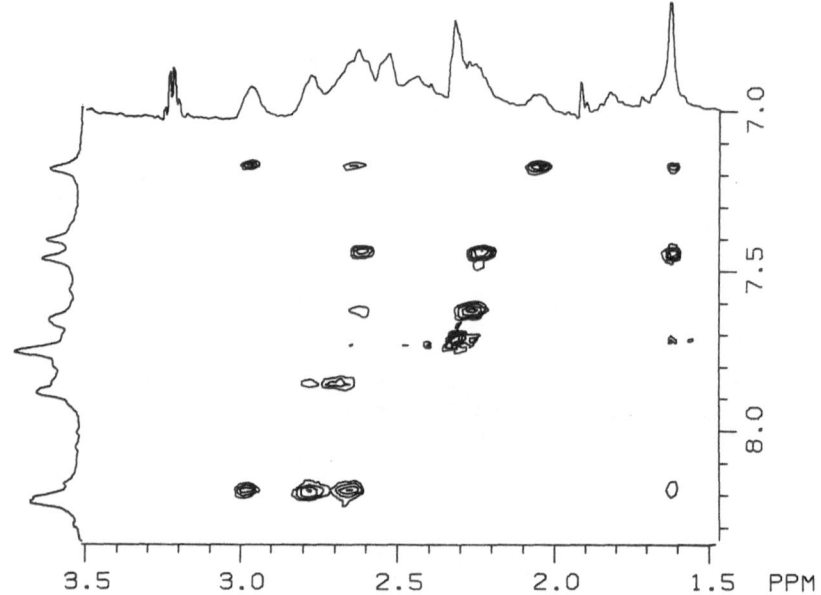

Figure 12.   Part of the 500 MHz 2D NOE spectrum of the
octamer [d-(5'GGAATTCC3')]₂, obtained for a mixing time of
200 ms. 5 mg of the compound were dissolved in 0.5 ml D_2O,
0.16 M NaCl, at 20° C.

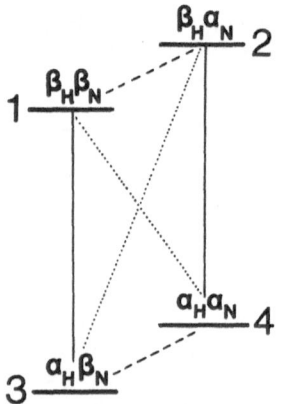

Figure 13.   Energy level diagram and wave functions for a
[15]H-^{1}H spin pair. The insensitive ^{15}N resonances
(broken lines) are measured indirectly by measuring the zero
and double quantum resonance frequencies (dotted lines) via
the proton resonances (solid lines).

theory of the experiment is most easily described with the operator formalism, treated in section 1.4. The proton 90° pulse creates magnetization along the y axis of the rotating frame, which then evolves, for a time Δ:

$$I_{yH} \xrightarrow{(\Omega_H + 2\pi J_{NH}I_{zH}I_{zN})\Delta}$$

$$\{I_{yH}\cos(\Omega_H\Delta) - I_{xH}\sin(\Omega_H\Delta)\}\cos(\pi J_{NH}\Delta) +$$
$$+ \{-I_{xH}\cos(\Omega_H\Delta) - I_{yH}\sin(\Omega_H\Delta)\}\sin(\pi J_{NH})I_{zN} \qquad [24]$$

If the delay, Δ, is set to $1/(2J_{NH})$, only the second term at the right hand side of expression [24] survives, and a $90°_x$ ^{15}N pulse applied at this time will generate product terms $I_{xH}I_{yN}$ and $I_{yH}I_{yN}$. The sine and cosine coefficients will be omitted to simplify the expressions. During the evolution period, those product terms evolve according to:

$$I_{xH}I_{yN} \xrightarrow{\Omega_H t_1 + \Omega_N t_1} [\cos(\Omega_H t_1)I_{xH} + \sin(\Omega_H t_1)I_{yH}] \times$$
$$\times [\cos(\Omega_N t_1)I_{yN} - \sin(\Omega_N t_1)I_{xN}] \qquad [25]$$

The final 90° ^{15}N pulse converts those two-spin coherences back into observable ^1H magnetization. If all terms are taken into account, a $90°_x$ ^{15}N pulse generates as observable signal:

$$s(t_1, t_2) = M_{OH}\exp[i(\Omega_H \pm \pi J_{NH})(t_1 + t_2)]\cos(\Omega_N t_1) \qquad [26a]$$

and a $90°_y$ ^{15}N pulse generates

$$s(t_1, t_2) = M_{OH}\exp[i(\Omega_H \pm \pi J_{NH})(t_1 + t_2)]\sin(\Omega_N t_1) \qquad [26b]$$

If either of those two signals is used separately to calculate a 2D spectrum, two resonances in the ω_1 dimension, at $\Omega_H \pm \Omega_N$, will appear, denoting the zero and double quantum frequencies, respectively. The results of Eqs. [26a] and [26b] can be combined in the usual fashion (Eqs. [6] and [11]) to give either the double or the zero quantum frequency in the 2D spectrum. Because the zero quantum resonance in the 2D spectrum is centered at $(\omega_1, \omega_2) = (\Omega_N + \Omega_H, \Omega_H)$, the computer can subtract a frequency ω_2 from all ω_1 coordinates, to yield a pure chemical shift correlation map, with resonances centered at (Ω_N, Ω_H). Broad-band ^{15}N decoupling during the detection period can be used to eliminate the effect of heteronuclear coupling in this experiment.

If the final ^{15}N 90° pulse is applied along the -x axis, the signal of Eq. [26a] will be detected with opposite sign. Since signals from protons not coupled to ^{15}N will not know about this phase shift and their shape will be unchanged in the two experiments, subtraction of the two

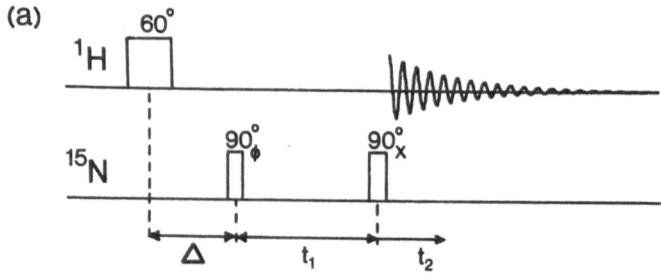

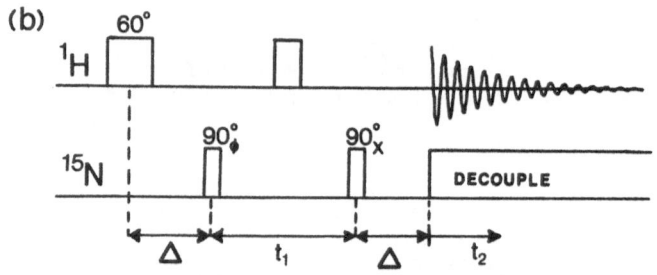

Figure 14.   Pulse scheme of the experiment for indirect
detection of ^{15}N through multiple quantum coherence. The
first pulse applied to the protons can be of the Redfield
type or of the 1-3-3-1 type and does not require additional
phase cycling. (b) The 180° ^{1}H pulse applied at the center
of the evolution period interchanges zero and double quantum
coherence and causes elimination of the ^{1}H frequency
contribution in the F_1 dimension, leading to a regular
heteronuclear shift correlation spectrum.   The ^{15}N
decoupling during acquisition removes heteronuclear coupling
from the F_2 dimension and, in principle, doubles the
sensitivity of the experiment. In both (a) and (b), the
phase of the first 90° ^{15}N pulse is cycled according to
Table 3.

Table 3.   Phase of the first ^{15}H pulse in the pulse scheme
of Fig. 14 and the mode of data collection for detection of
the double (DQ) and of the zero quantum (ZQ) component.

Step	ϕ	DQ	ZQ
1	x	x	x
2	y	y	y
3	-x	-x	-x
4	-y	y	-y

experiments will thus give cancellation of the signals of protons that are not coupled to ^{15}N. Hence, the ^{15}N satellites in the ^{1}H spectrum can therefore be detected, not hampered by the 600 times stronger signal from protons coupled to ^{14}N. In total four experiments will be performed for every t_1 value, with the phase of the final ^{15}N pulse cycled along all four axes.

As an example, Figure 15 shows the heteronuclear chemical shift correlation spectrum of a 0.3 M solution of a uridine derivative, in $CDCl_3$, in a 5 mm sample tube. Spectra were recorded on a modified Nicolet 360 MHz instrument, and the total measuring time was approximately 1 hr. The signals of Eqs. [26a] and [26b] were stored in separate locations and spectrum (a) was computated from the double quantum signals and (b) was computated from the zero quantum signals, using the same two sets of acquired data.

As pointed out in section 1, it is desirable to record spectra in the absorption mode, both from a viewpoint of sensitivity as well as resolution. However, in this experiment the data are really phase modulated (not artificially induced). Conversion to amplitude modulation is possible by insertion of a 180° pulse at the center of the evolution period. However, in the case where the proton also has homonuclear coupling, phase modulation cannot be avoided and pure absorption mode spectra cannot be recorded. A nice feature of the simplest form of the experiment is that it utilizes only one pulse for the observed protons. This pulse can be of arbitrary flip angle; a small flip angle will allow a faster repetition rate and consequently somewhat higher sensitivity. More important is the fact that any type of pulse can be used for this proton excitation. For example, a Redfield water suppression or a 1-3-3-1 water suppression pulse can be used, making it feasible to use this experiment in H_2O solution.

5. Discussion

Although only a small number out of the large collection of two-dimensional NMR experiments has been treated here, it will be clear that the 2D approach extends the capabilities of NMR experiments enormously. Many applications of 2D NMR in organic and biochemistry have appeared in the recent literature. On modern NMR spectrometers, utilization of the various two-dimensional experiments has become rather simple by the introduction of suitable support software and spectrometer documentation. The main problem the inexperienced spectroscopist has to face is which experiment to choose and which results to expect. A comprehensive guide on this subject has not yet appeared, but in general it is usually a good idea to apply the standard experiments before

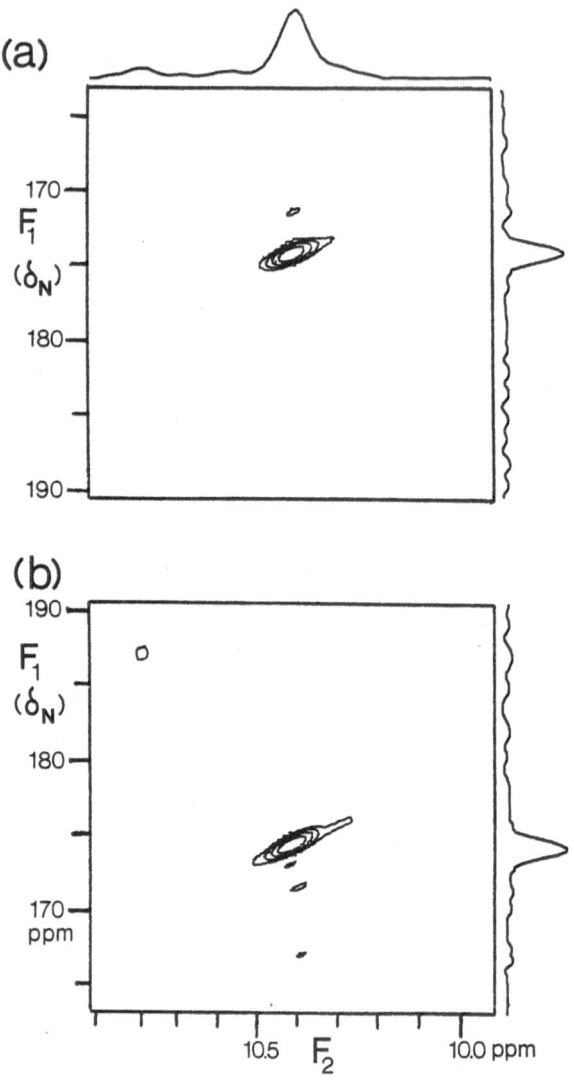

Figure 15.   Chemical shift correlation spectra of
2',3',5'tri-o-benzoyl-4-thiouridine (a) obtained from the
double quantum spectrum and (b) from the zero quantum
spectrum. The projections on the F_1 axes, representing ^{15}N
chemical shift spectra, are shown along the vertical axes.
The projections on the F_2 axes, representing the proton
chemical shift spectra, are similar for the two 2D spectra,
and such a projection is shown. ^{15}N shifts are given with
respect to ammonia at 25°C.

attempting to use a more sophisticated version of those experiments.

Acknowledgment
I wish to thank Ingrid Pufahl for typing and editing most of the manuscript.

References

(1) J. Jeener, Ampere International Summer School, Basko Polje, Yugoslavia (1971).
(2) G. Bodenhausen, R. Freeman, R. Niedermeyer and D.L. Turner, J. Magn. Reson. 26, 133 (1977).
(3) W.P. Aue, P. Bachmann, A. Wokaun and R.R. Ernst, J. Magn. Reson. 29, 523 (1978).
(4) A. Bax and T.H. Mareci, J. Magn. Reson. 53, 360 (1983).
(5) G. Wider, S. Macura, A. Kumar, R.R. Ernst and K. Wuethrich, J. Magn. Reson. 56, 207 (1984).
(6) D.L. Turner, J. Magn. Reson. 58, 500 (1984).
(7) P. Bachmann, W.P. Aue, L. Mueller and R.R. Ernst, J. Magn. Reson. 28, 29 (1977).
(8) A. Bax, A.F. Mehlkopf and J. Smidt, J. Magn. Reson. 40, 213 (1980).
(9) A. de Marco and K. Wuethrich, J. Magn. Reson. 24, 201 (1976).
(10) A. Bax, G.A. Morris and R. Freeman, J. Magn. Reson. 43, 333 (1981).
(11) I.D. Campbell, C.M. Dobson, R.J.P. Williams and A.V. Xavier, J. Magn. Reson. 11, 172 (1973).
(12) R. Freeman, S.P. Kempsell and M.H. Levitt, J. Magn. Reson. 34, 663 (1979).
(13) D.J. States, R.A. Haberkorn and D.J. Ruben, J. Magn. Reson. 48, 286 (1982).
(14) See, for example, T.C. Farrar and E.D. Becker, Pulse and Fourier Transform NMR, Academic Press, New York (1971).
(15) O.W. Sorensen, G.W. Eich, M.H. Levitt, G. Bodenhausen and R.R. Ernst, Progr. in NMR Spectroscopy 16, 163 (1983).
(16) W.P. Aue, E. Bartholdi and R.R. Ernst, J. Chem. Phys. 64, 2229 (1976).
(17) A. Bax and R. Freeman, J. Magn. Reson. 44, 542 (1981).
(18) K. Nagayama, A. Kumar, K. Wuethrich and R.R. Ernst, J. Magn. Reson. 40, 321 (1980).
(19) A. Bax, R. Freeman and G.A. Morris, J. Magn. Reson. 42, 164 (1982).
(20) G. Wider, S. Macura, A. Kumar, R.R. Ernst and K. Wuethrich, J. Magn. Reson. 56, 207 (1984).
(21) D. Marion and K. Wuethrich, Biochem. Biophys. Res. Commun. 113, 967 (1983).

(22) A. Bax, Two-Dimensional NMR in Liquids, Reidel, Boston (1982), Chapter 2.

(23) D.I. Hoult and R.E. Richards, Proc. Roy. Soc. London A.344, 311 (1975).

(24) U. Piantini, O.W. Sorensen and R.R. Ernst, J. Am. Chem. Soc. 104, 6800 (1982).

(25) J. Jeener, B.H. Meier, P. Bachmann and R.R. Ernst, J. Chem. Phys. 71, 4546 (1979).

(26) S. Macura and R.R. Ernst, Mol. Phys. 41, 95 (1980).

(27) W. Braun, G. Wider, K.H. Lee and K. Wuethrich, J. Mol. Biol. 169, 921 (1983).

(28) W. Braun, C. Boesch, L.R. Brown, N.Go and K. Wuethrich, Biochem. Biophys. Acta 667, 377 (1981).

(29) S. Macura, K. Wuethrich and R.R. Ernst, J. Magn. Reson. 46, 269 (1982).

(30) M.S. Broido, G. Zon and T.L. James, Biochem. Biophys. Res. Commun. 119, 663 (1984).

(31) A. Minoretti, W.P. Aue, M. Reinhold and R.R. Ernst, J. Magn. Reson. 40, 175 (1980).

(32) G. Bodenhausen and D.J. Ruben, Chem. Phys. Lett. 69, 185 (1980).

(33) A. Bax, R.H. Griffey and B.L. Hawkins, J. Am. Chem. Soc. 105, 7188 (1983).

(34) A. Bax, R.H. Griffey and B.L. Hawkins, J. Magn. Reson. 55, 301 (1983).

NMR DATA PROCESSING IN COMPUTERS

Dieter Ziessow
I.N. Stranski-Institut, Technical University of Berlin
Str. des 17. Juni 112 (ERH)
1000 Berlin 12, Germany-West

ABSTRACT. NMR signals are invariably processed with the aid of digital computers. Main steps are the collection, storage, transformation, and communication of data. The involved basic principles are discussed with particular emphasis on spectral analysis of time-limited signals. Current trends in computer construction are reviewed.

1. Introduction

The majority of NMR experiments are conducted in such a way that the detector delivers an output voltage which is a superposition of free induction decay signals. Each FID k is a harmonic wave with frequency F_k and phase P_k which decays according to the function l(t). The FID intensity $I_k = l(0)$ is determined by the spin concentration as well as experimental time delays with respect to the T_1 relaxation time. Frequently, l(t) is given by $\exp(-t/T2 (k))$ where T_2 comprises spin-spin relaxation and B_o inhomogeneity.

The purpose of NMR data processing is to extract the parameters F_k, P_k, and I_k from the recorded signal and to deduce from this parameter set information about the molecular composition and physical state of the molecular assembly (viscosity, heterogeneity, etc) in a specified volume and its spatial dependence (topical NMR, imaging). Fairly large amounts of data are subjected to simple but extensive calculations which invariably are performed in computers. It is the purpose of this chapter to discuss the basic underlying principles for the collection, storage, spectral analysis, and communication of NMR data. The usage of data banks will not be treated here. A considerable body of knowledge has been accumulated for the given subjects in the last decade and recently surveyed in an excellent review article (1). New trends and subjects not covered in Ref.(1) are therefore treated in this chapter.

T. Axenrod and G. Ceccarelli (eds.), NMR in Living Systems, 95–107.

2. Instrumention for Digital Signal Processing (DSP)

The basic units of DSP are shown in Fig. 1. Analogue-to-digital con-

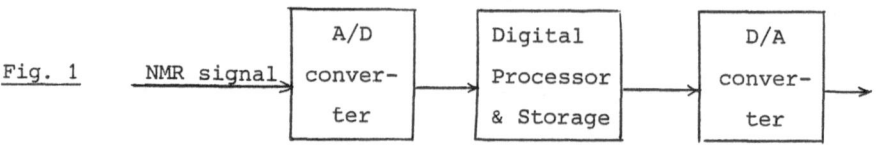

| Fig. 1 | NMR signal | A/D conver-ter | Digital Processor & Storage | D/A conver-ter |

version is achieved by comparing the NMR voltage U_s with suitable reference voltages U_r. The result is an n-bit digital word with sign bit spanning the integer range from $-(2^n-1)$ to $+(2^n-1)$. The conversion may be done by applying U_s to the plus-input of (2^n-1) comparators. Their minusinput is sequentially adjusted from 0 to U_r in steps of $U_r/(2^n-1)$ with the aid of a ladder of (2^n-1) laser-trimmed resistors. This so-called flash conversion is performed in one comparison step and is therefore extremely rapid (20 to 50 MHz sampling rate at 8 bits). It requires however high accuracy of the resistor ladder.

A less demanding but slower method is to utilize only one comparator and to repeat the comparison n times with reference voltages $U_r(i)$ which are adjusted according to the result of step (i-1). Typical conversion times are 1 to 50 μs with 12 to 15 bit accuracy. This method of succes-sive approximation is commonly employed in NMR spectroscopy although the first method might be used to digitize the intermediate frequency NMR signal of the heterodyn detector.

The amplification of the FID has to be adjusted in such a way that the rms value of the superposed detector noise is close to the smallest possible voltage increment $U_r/(2^{n-1})$ of the A/D converter. This might not be feasible for strong signals in which case weak signals may be obscured by digitization noise. Solvent supression methods are frequent-ly used in such a situation although other excitation schemes such as rapid scan or stochastic rf modulation also provide remedy (c.f. Ref.(2)).

In the extreme case where the FID is completely buried in the de-tector noise, a 1-bit A/D conversion is sufficient. This is demonstra-ted in Fig. 2 for a S/N ratio of 1/20. Shown is one signal scan (a), the

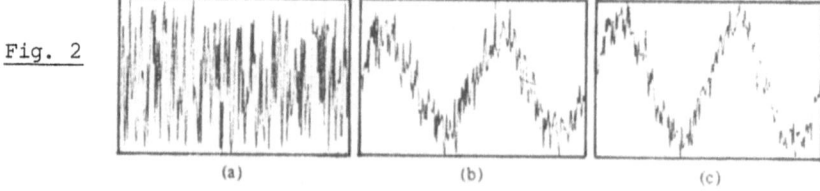

Fig. 2

(a)   (b)   (c)

average of 10^4 transients after 1-bit conversion (b), and a test signal
obtained by averaging 10^4 noise traces and addition of the signal multiplied by 10^4. It is clear from this example that the effective A/D accuracy can be improved by averaging noisy signals. Flash conversion of
intermediate frequency signals might therefore be used to reduce dynamic
range problems.

In the last step of DSP, data are either stored in a suitable memory (floppy disk, winchester disk, cassettes, or tapes), read out
(tables or text), or plotted. In the last case, an n-bit word is converted to an analogue voltage (D/A) which is done by adding n currents
in an operational amplifier. The current values reflect the weight of
the bit positions of the digital word, where a "1" or "0" switches the
current on or off, respectively.

The basic units for the treatment of digital data are shown in Fig. 3.
The main processor unit (and also special processors for Fourier transformation and display) is in general built by the NMR manufacturers. In
future constructions, however, general purpose microprocessor chips such
as 68020, 16032, or 32032 will be used since they provide extremely high
computing power at moderate expense due to their large production number.

Fig. 3

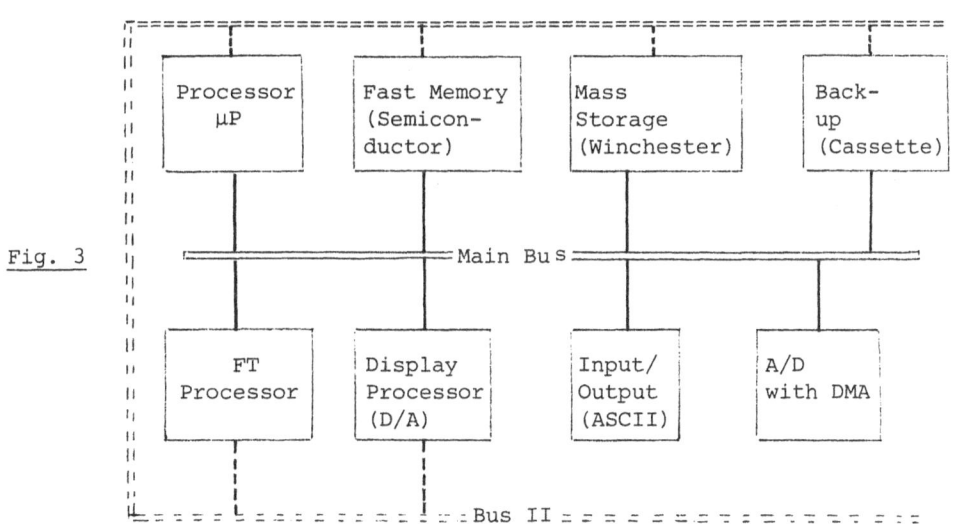

These µP's work on digital words up to 32 bits and may directly address
up to 16 Mbyte (4 Gigabyte, respectively). This allows highly efficient
programming for data transformations and retrieval. Personal computers
based on the 16032 chip (supported by the arithmetic extension chip
16031) already achieve a computation speed which is only by a factor
100 slower than in the mainframe computer CRAY-1. Even faster processings
units are to be expected in NMR instruments when the chips 32032 or
68020 will be used.

Digital words are transferred between the various devices in Fig. 3 with the aid of a "bus". This stands for a bunch of wires for data (16, 24, or 32 bits), memory addresses (16, 22, 24, or 32 bits) and control signals. The actual voltage on each line at a given time ("bus state") is governed by the bus protocol which is a set of rules how to choose these voltages in order to achieve the required transfer from one device to another. At the moment, many protocols exist but it is to be expected that only two or three will find world-wide acceptance. One good candidate is the VME bus which derives from the Motorola Versabus. This opens the possibility to tailor (and later up-grade) NMR instruments with standardized VME circuit boards from a vast number of hardware and software manufacturers (distributed processors; semiconductor memory; floating-point processors; array processors; controllers for in/output; etc). The benefit will be a considerable increase in DSP speed at acceptable expense.

Standardization of hardware will also contribute to take advantage of general operating systems such as for example the UNIX system (or derivatives of it) which provides many software tools for editing, programming, file handling, and communication to other computers in the department, university, city, or country. At present, UNIX is not able to handle real-time tasks such as the control of experiments (pulse sequences in 2D NMR, imaging) and data acquisition. It may, however, serve co-processors with appropriate firmware for these operations which will be supplied by the NMR manufacturers.

The bus structure has originally been introduced to ease tailoring and up-grading of computer systems. Its primary disadvantage is that at a given time only two devices can exchange digital words for control and data. For example, the µP cannot access a device without being interrupted when data are collected, i.e. when digital words are transferred from the A/D converter to memory under the mode of direct memory access (DMA) every other sampling period (ca. 50 µs). Delays thus occur which decrease the overall processing speed.

The bottleneck of a single bus structure may be opened by adding more busses to the computer system. Typical examples are special I/0 busses (Fig. 3, dotted line) or the direct connection of a µP or another device to the fast memory via a second input (dual-ported memory). Yet another solution would be to implement a double-bus structure (Fig. 3, double-dashed line). Then parallel processes are fully supported at the price of additional control hardware.

3. Digital Processing of NMR Data

Once the data have been acquired and stored in memory or on disk,
NMR DSP takes place. It may be classified as follows:

(a) <u>Data combination</u> according to specific pulse sequences
    (averaging, phase cycles, etc)

(b) <u>Data refinement</u>
    (filtering for S/N improvement or resolution enhancement; base-
    line corrections; line shapes, e.g. pseudo echo; zero-filling;
    etc)

(c) <u>Spectral or spatial analysis</u>
    (transformation of time into frequency data; phase correction;
    back-projection reconstruction)

(d) <u>Spectral evaluation</u>
    (derivation of the molecular structure and/or composition of the
    sample; use of data banks; etc)

(e) <u>Documentation</u>

Step (a) requires simple operations for restoring, adding, or subtracting of data. It depends on the specific experiment and is not discussed here.

There are many methods for the refinement of NMR data (b) which have
recently been reviewed (1). Apart from zero-filling, which will be discussed in chapter 4, their commonly involve the multiplication of the
FID with a suitable window function which weights the data with respect
to the desired improvement. To increase the S/N ratio in the spectrum,
the weighting coefficients for instance may be chosen to be proportional
to the decay function l(t). Data thus contribute to spectral analysis
according to their instantaneous S/N ration in the time domain. Likewise, resolution may be enhanced at the expense of S/N when the window
suppresses FID contributions which broaden the spectral line, i.e. when
data at the beginning of the observation are de-emphasized with respect
to later data. An equivalent method is to subtract from a spectrum
appropriate amounts of higher derivatives of the spectrum (3).

After spectral or spatial analysis (c.f. chs. 4 and 5), NMR data
need to be evaluated on the basis of prior knowledge (chemical shift
tables, data or spectra banks) and documented. This process is supported
by DSP but strongly depends upon the nature of the problem and the availability of data banks. Therefore, only the more general aspect of data
communication will be discussed here any further (ch. 6).

A general comment with regard to the digital representation of
numbers is in order at this point. Word lengths of 32 bits will allow
the user to choose either one of two common number formats. In both
cases, the most significant bit (MSB, left-justified) is the sign bit.

For fixed-point (FXP) numbers, the remaining 31 bits are used to code
the magnitude in binary fractions 1/2, 1/4, 1/8,... as noted by
0.111...01 with 31 positions after the binary point. The total number
range is equivalent to decimal rational numbers from 0 to $\pm$0.99....9
with a count of decimal fractions between 9 and 10. For a floating-
point (FLP) number, the magnitude is coded as $0.110...11 \times 10^P$. The 8-bit
exponent p is adjusted in such a way that the first binary fraction
(1/2) is <u>always a one</u>. For that reason a FLP number is stored without
the first binary fraction, i.e. the mantissa of the number 0.10011...
10×10^P is stored as 0.0011...10. For actual calculations, however, this
bit is restored either by software or hardware. FLP numbers cover a
range over many orders of magnitude at the expense of the reduced
accuracy of the mantissa with respect to FXP numbers, the count of decimal positions being between 6 and 7. As a consequence, the numbers
10^{-8} and 1 cannot be added in FLP format contrary to the FXP format. It
seems that this feature makes FXP numbers more attractive to NMR DSP
since the nature of the experiments does not necessitate the huge number
range of the FLP format. On the other hand, FLP numbers ease programming
and have a wider application range than FXP numbers, which accounts for
the availability of FLP array processors at relatively low costs.

4. Spectral Analysis of NMR Data

The purpose of spectral analysis is to determine the parameter set
F_k, P_k, and I_k, k=1,2,... from the observed FID signal (c.f. ch. 1).

<u>Fig. 4</u>   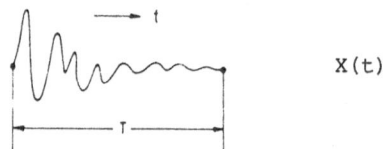   X(t)

The common approach is the discrete complex Fourier analysis (CFT)

$$A(m) = \sum_{n=0}^{N-1} X(n) \exp(-2\pi mn/N) \qquad m = 0...N-1$$

where X(m) is the digital record of the FID sampled at times m Δt with
m = 0,...N-1 for an observation period from t=0 to T=(N-1)Δt. From the
complex spectrum A(m) one obtains the required parameter from those values which are well above the noise level, say m=k then F_k=k/T for instance. The FID is correctly digitized when all resonance frequencies
in the rotating frame obey the relation $-1/2\Delta t \leq F_k \leq +1/2\Delta t$ (sampling
theorem).

The spectrum A(m) may be used to re-calculate the complex time series
according to

$$X'(n) = \sum_{m=0}^{N-1} A(m) \cdot \exp(2\pi \cdot m \cdot n/N) \tag{2}$$

(inverse or plus-CFT). The resulting X'(n) is exactly equal to the
original X(n) except for rounding errors. When the calculation is extended to times less than zero or greater than T (by using in equ. (2)
m 0 and m N-1), a periodic signal is obtained. This is shown in Fig.5
for a non-decaying sine wave for the cases $F_k = k/T$ and $F_k = (k+0.5)/T$. In
the first case, observation beyond T and calculated signal X' matches
exactly. In the second case, X and X' are not alike. This is generally
the case when the natural frequencies F_k are in between the values of
the discrete frequency axis.

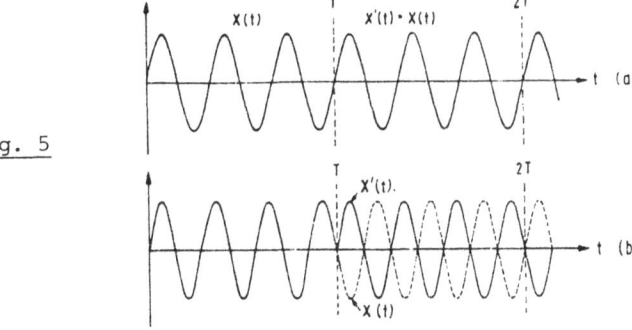

Fig. 5

Under these conditions, severe intensity and phase anomalies may result.
This is shown in Fig.6 for the cases $F_k = (k+b)/T$, b=0;0.125;0.25;0.375;
0.5. For decaying signals such as in NMR this problem is less pronounced
as shown in Fig.7a,b for exponential decrease to 50 % and 1 %, respectively. It is important to note that even for a decay down to 1 %. line
heights differ notably for FID components with the same intensity
(Fig. 7b). Another consequence of time-limited records is the difficulty
to distinguish two resonance lines when $F_k - F_{k'}$ is of the order of 1/T.

The inherent feature of periodicity of the CFT is of particular concern when the FID has been generated after some preparation period such
that the signal is zero for times less than zero. Here some remedy is
achieved by appending N zero's to the digitized signal. This procedure
adds information not considered in the first place and re-establishes to
a good deal the relationship between the imaginary and real part of A(m)
due to the causality of the experiment, namely that the signal is zero
prior to the irradiation of the rf pulse. Zero-filling also increases
somewhat the apparent resolution in plots of A(m).

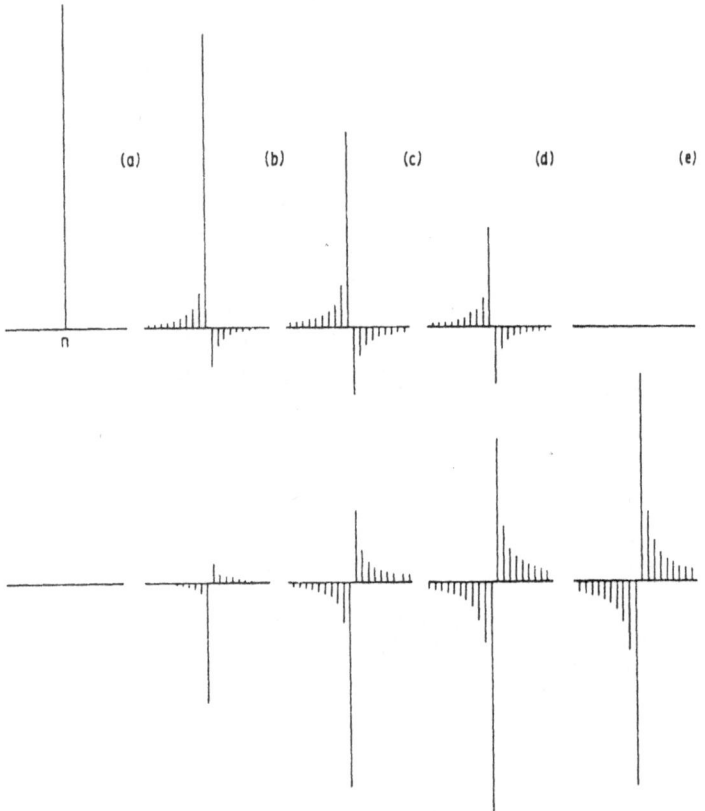

Fig. 6 Real and imaginary spectra for resonance lines with interdigital
        resonance frequencies $F_k=(k+b)/T$ with respect to the discrete
        frequency axis m/T. k is an arbitrary integer value and b is
        given by 0, 0.125, 0.25, 0.375, 0.5 for (a), (b), (c), (d), and
        (e) respectively. The time domain signal is a non-decaying sine
        wave FID.

Whether zero-filling is applied or not, the Fourier transformation of a
time-limited, not fully decayed FID (as considered in Figs. 6 and 7) is
not the optimum choice for spectral analysis since for times greater
than T it is a tacit assumption that the signal is periodic (or zero
when zero-filling has been used). The question therefore arises whether
there are alternatives routes from the time to the frequency domain
which make no assumptions with regard to times beyond the observation
time period. Such methods in fact exist and have been successfully
applied in areas other than NMR. They are commonly referred to as non-
linear spectral analysis since the recorded date enter the algorithm

not linearly as in Fourier transform methods eqn. (1). With respect
to 1D NMR, there has in fact been little interest in applying these
methods since sufficiently long observation times T are readily
accomplished in these experiments. In 2D NMR or imaging, however,
suitable algorithms might be developped which result a considerable decrease in the total measurement time without sacrifying pertinent spectral information. It remains to be seen how they actually cope with NMR
practise.

It is beyond the scope of this chapter to give a detailed account of
the present status of nonlinear spectral analysis. As an introductory
example, however, the following filter is discussed. Assume a linear
combination of the digitized FID as given by

$$(a_2 x_{n-2} + a_1 x_{n-1} + a_0 x_n) - x_{n+1} = e_n . \tag{3}$$

This equation gives the error value e_n when the fourth data point is
tried to be calculated on the basis of the three previous data points.
Many values of e_n are obtained when the calculation is repeated by shifting n as far as possible through the recorded data. The process is
stopped for n+1=N, i.e. when x_{n+1} is just one sampling time interval
out of the observation period. An optimum choice for the unknown coefficients a_j may be determined by minimizing the sum of squares $(e_n)^2$.
On the basis of these coefficients, data can be calculated with eqn.(3)
for a certain time length beyond T. This process of linear prediction
is demonstrated in Fig.8 for the FID signal of an AB spin system. The
coefficient a_j have been calculated according to the Burg algorithm
(c.f. FORTRAN program given in Ref.(4)). Considerable time savings may
be realized when this approach is extended to 2D NMR. This is demonstrated in Fig.9 for an homonuclear COSY experiment. Further improvement of nonlinear algorithm seems feasible particularly in view of the
fact that information from 1D NMR measurements might be incorporated in
the least square evaluation schemes.

5. Spatial Analysis of NMR Data

NMR images are calculated from digitized FID signals with the aid of
the Fourier transformation and back-projection reconstruction. The purpose of this chapter is to give an elementary introduction to the latter
method. We start with a spin density distribution in a 2x2 points planar
sample. Upon application of a magnetic field linear gradient in the direction of the x and y axis one obtains the following integral intensities (projections):

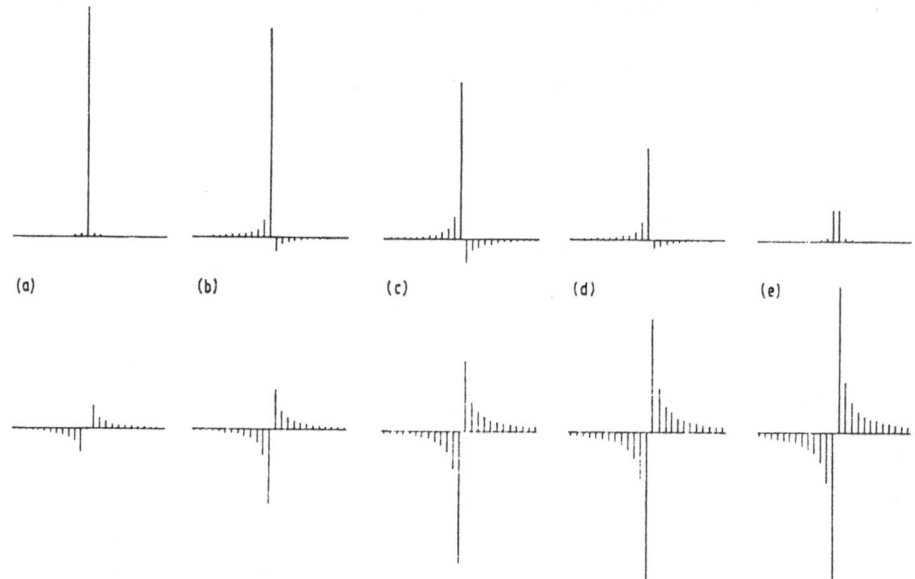

Fig. 7a   Exponential decay down to 50 %

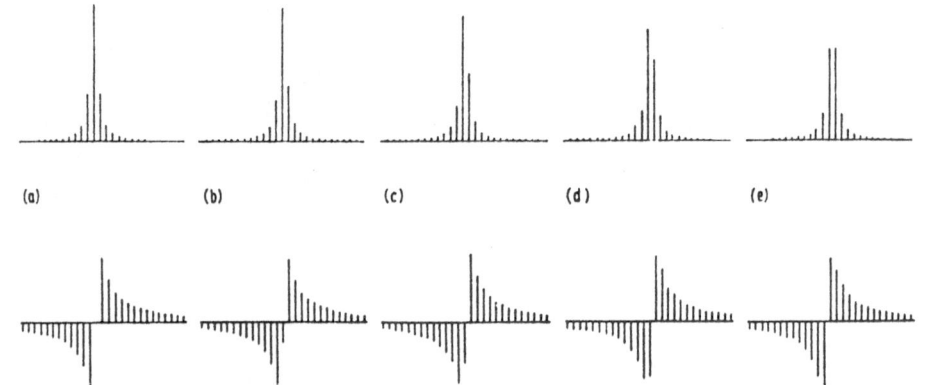

Fig. 7b Exponential decay down to 1 %

Fig. 7   Real and imaginary spectra for resonance lines with interdigital
         frequencies F_k with respect to the discrete frequency axis m/T,
         $m=0,1,\ldots N-1$. Decay of the FID signal as indicated in a,b.
         (c.f. legende of Fig. 6)

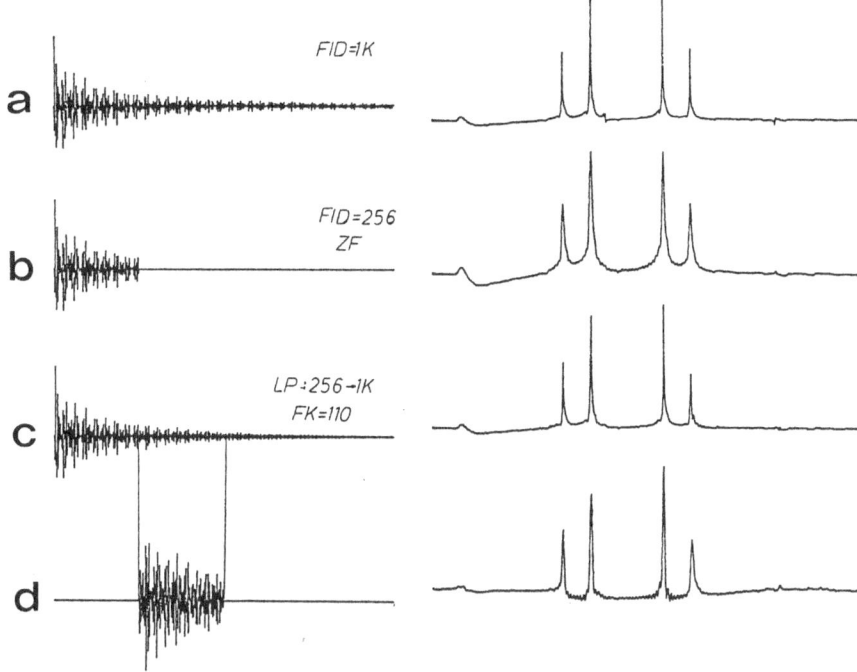

Fig. 8   FID signals and their Fourier transforms of an AB spin system.
         (a) Original data, 1K points. (b) Truncated FID with zero filling
         (c) Truncated FID extended to 1K data points by linear prediction
         (d) First 256 predicted data points and their Fourier transform

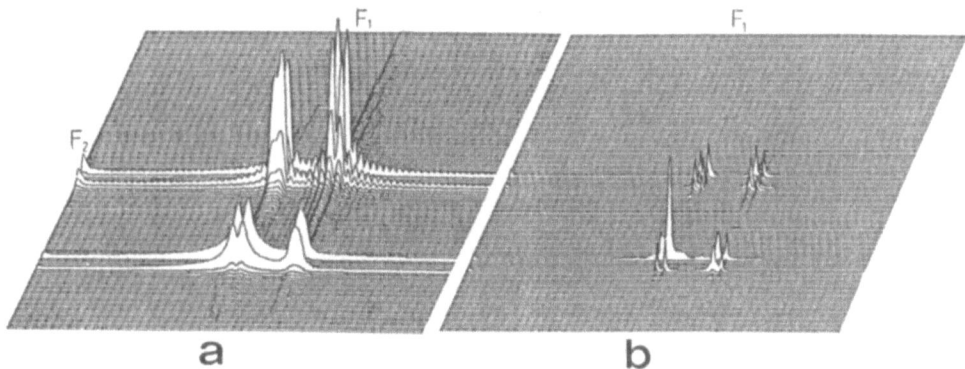

Fig. 9   2D COSY experiment for an AB spin system, 128 and 512 data points
         in the t_1 and t_2 domain, respectively. (a) 2D Fourier transform
         after zero filling to 512 points in the t_1 domain. (b) 2D Fourier
         transform after extension to 512 data points in the t_1 domain
         with linear prediction

One might think that from these four projection values the four densities can be reconstructed by solving a linear algebraic system with
four unknowns. It is immediately obvious that this analysis fails since
the following density distribution yields the same projection values:

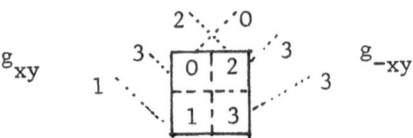

It is easy to prove that the linear set of equations has no unique solution since the respective determinant is zero. Further projections
are therefore required in order to reconstruct the density distribution:

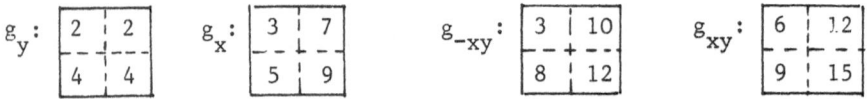

An image may now be constructed simply by adding the integral intensities from the four projections to the respective pixel elements which
at the beginning are all set to zero:

g_y: | 2 | 2 |
        |---|---|
        | 4 | 4 |

g_x: | 3 | 7 |
        |---|---|
        | 5 | 9 |

g_{-xy}: | 3 | 10 |
           |----|----|
           | 8 | 12 |

g_{xy}: | 6 | 12 |
          |---|----|
          | 9 | 15 |

The resulting density distribution is transformed into the original one
by subtracting 6 from each pixel followed by multiplication with 1/3.
For larger number of pixels, more projections need to be taken. For
instance, for a 3x3 image four projections along the gradients given
above yield 12 integral densities from which the image cannot yet be
reconstructed. The number of projections which are actually needed has
been subject to mathematical studies as early as 1917 (6). Practical
techniques were first reported in 1956 (7). In view of the acquired
data and the large number of additions it is quite clear that the fixed-
point number format is well suited for back-projection methods.

6. Distributed Digital Signal Processing

Computation needs have increased in NMR spectroscopy with the introduction of complex rf pulse sequences (2D NMR) and imaging techniques. They
may further increase when more sophisticated algorithms than the Fourier
transformation find use for spectral analysis with the ultimate goal to
reduce the measurement time (in the sense of time required for a sample
to be in the NMR magnet). Apart from up-grading the computer in the spectrometer, adequate computation equipment may be accessed via local area
networks for computer and analytical instruments. Digital data from one
instrument can be passed on to idling computers in other areas or to
computer centers. Pertinent results then are retransmitted to the source.
At the moment, many implementations for such networks exist which differ
with respect to number of stations, speed of transmission, and data link
protocols. As a rule of thumb, expenses are directly related to the

speed of data transfer. When financial constraints impose the dominant
design feature, particularly when computers from various manufacturers
(including personal computers in scientific laboratories) need to be
connected, then a star configuration has been shown to be of practical
advantage (8). It is based on the RS 232 interface which is part of or
can easily added to virtually any computer, peripheral device, or analytical instrument. The idea is to open the communication line between
a computer an a terminal

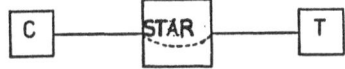

and insert a central or star (communication) computer. Devices with the
RS 232 interface are directly connected to the star computer.

The resulting star network can be connected to other networks or computer centers with the aid of a package-assembler-disassembler (PAD).

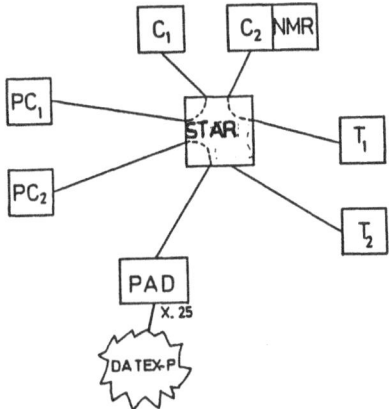

The star computer uses the UNIX operating system which is a time-sharing
multi-user system with hierarchical file system. These features have
been utilized to establish software links between the various stations
of the star net. Several connections may be maintained in parallel.

References

(1) J.C. Lindon and A.G. Ferrige, Progr.NMR Spectr. 14, 27 (1980)
(2) B. Bluemich and D. Ziessow, J. Magn. Res.
(3) D. Ziessow, "On-line Rechner in der Chemie", de Gryuter, Berlin 1973
(4) J.F. Claerbout, "Fundamentals of Geophysical Data Processing",
    McGraw-Hill, N.Y., 1976
(5) J.P. Burg, NATO ASI on Signal Processing, Enschede, 1968
(6) J. Radon, Ber.Saechs.Akad.Wiss. Leipzig, Math.Phys. 69, 262 (1917)
(7) R.N. Bracewell, Australian J. Phys. 9, 198 (1956)
(8) Research Report, IFP-6/2, Technical University Berlin, 1984

THE PHYSICAL BASIS OF NMR TOMOGRAPHY

F. De Luca, B.C. De Simone, B. Maraviglia
Dipt. di Fisica, Università di Roma "La Sapienza",
00185 Roma, Italy
and National Research Council
R. Campanella and C. Casieri
Dipt. di Fisica, Università di Roma "La Sapienza",
00185 Roma, Italy

ABSTRACT. Most of the naturally existing matter is heterogeneous, whereas spectroscopic techniques can in general be applied only to homogeneous systems. In this paper the main physical aspects, which have
made NMR spectroscopy applicable to heterogeneous systems study, will
be described. Particular attention will be devoted to the approaches
which have been successful in producing NMR parameters maps of biomedical interest.

1. INTRODUCTION

The use of NMR spectroscopy has produced results of great relevance in most areas of condensed matter research. In particular its role
has been crucial in the investigation of biochemical structures and
processes, due to its peculiarity of been able to select the wanted
fraction (resonant) of the whole nuclear magnetization. Besides the
use of a coherent radiation and the great number of photons associated with a R.F. pulse make NMR spectroscopy extremely versatile and
in continuous progress. In this paper, following others which introduced the general aspects of NMR spectroscopy, we will analyze the
basis that in the last decade have allowed the study of heterogeneous
systems. Of course the enormous relevance of the knowledge of the
structure and functioning of human beings has pushed most of the research towards the production of NMR parameter distributions, which
will in general be called either maps or images. These images are already applied for medical diagnosis in several medical areas and will
surely evolve towards a sophisticated research tool in biomedical research.

As NMR parameters are several, we will limit ourselves to the
study of the most relevant ones in NMR Imaging (tomography). Moreover
we will consider only cases of spin $\frac{1}{2}$, which include protons, phospo-
rus-31, etc. Infact protons are almost the only nuclei used to form
images. Spin greater than $\frac{1}{2}$ have a more complicated spectroscopy, but
most of the aspects discussed below for spin $\frac{1}{2}$ can be extended to
other nuclei.

T. Axenrod and G. Ceccarelli (eds.), NMR in Living Systems, 109–116.

In heterogeneous systems the spin density, ρ , spin-lattice relaxation T_1 time and spin-spin relaxation time T_2 are functions of space coordinates and thus they will be written respectively as:

$$\rho(\vec{r}); \quad T_1(\vec{r}); \quad T_2(\vec{r})$$

The original idea of P. Lauterbur[1], which has brought to the birth of NMR tomography, consisted in adding a weak magnetic field gradient $\vec{G}$ to the intense static magnetic field Ho. The addition of this gradient, as it will be seen later, introduces a spread of the resonant frequencies arising from different positions in space. Let us now consider in general the behaviour of a spin system under the action of magnetic field gradients, after having been excited by R.F. pulses.

The Bloch equation[2], in a heterogeneous system, is thus given in the laboratory frame by:

$$\frac{\partial}{\partial t}\, \vec{m}(\vec{r},t)=\gamma\vec{m}(\vec{r},t)\cdot\vec{H}(\vec{r},t)-\{m_x(\vec{r},t)\vec{i}+m_y(\vec{r},t)\vec{j}\}/T_2(\vec{r})-\{(m_z(\vec{r},t)-m_0(\vec{r}))\vec{k}\}/$$

$$/T_1(\vec{r}) \tag{1}$$

Where γ is the gyromagnetic ratio for the chosen nucleus, $m_0(\vec{r})$ is the local equilibrium nuclear magnetization and in general

$$H(\vec{r},t)=H_{1x}(t)\vec{i}+H_{1y}(t)\vec{j}+(H_0+\vec{r}\cdot\vec{G}(t))\vec{k} \tag{2}$$

H_{1x} and H_{1y} being the components of the magnetic field produced by the R.F.pulse, H_0 the homogeneous static magnetic field and $\vec{G}(t)$ the magnetic field gradient, which in general can be time dependent. After the R.F. pulse (2) becomes:

$$\vec{H}(\vec{r},t)=\left[H_0+\vec{r}\cdot\vec{G}(t)\right]\vec{k} \tag{3}$$

It is an excellent approximation the assumption that

$$\vec{G}(t)\simeq \frac{\partial H_z(t)}{\partial x}\,\vec{i}+ \frac{\partial H_z(t)}{\partial y}\,\vec{j}+ \frac{\partial\, H_z(t)}{\partial z}\vec{k} \tag{4}$$

By integrating the Bloch equation (1), the transverse magnetization, defined as

$$m_\perp(\vec{r},t)=m_x+i\ m_y$$

is given by:

$$m_\perp(r_G,t)=m_0(r_G)\exp\{-i\omega_0 t-i\gamma\int_{t_1}^{t_1+t}\vec{r}\cdot\vec{G}(t')dt'- \frac{t}{T_2(r_G)}\} \tag{5}$$

where $\omega_0 = \gamma H_0$ is the Larmor frequency, the time is set $t=o$ at the end
of the exciting $\pi/2$ R.F. pulse and the gradient $\vec{G}$ is switched on at t_1.
Equation (5) holds for monochromatic spins, which produce the equilibrium magnetization

$$m_0(r_G) = \int_{r_G} \rho(x,y,z) \, dx\,dy\,dz \tag{6}$$

of the plane $\vec{r} \cdot \vec{G} =$ const. perpendicular to $\vec{G}$ and intersecting $\vec{G}$ at the
position r_G. Of course $\rho(x,y,z)$ is the resonating spin density. The
total equilibrium magnetization M_0 is then

$$M_0 = \int_{L_G} m_0(r_G)\,dr_G \tag{7}$$

where L_G is the maximum dimension of the sample along $\vec{G}$.
    At the same way the FID generated by the whole sample is given by

$$S(t) = \int_{L_G} m_\perp(r_G,t)\,dr_G \tag{8}$$

    Where $m_+(r_G,t)$ is expressed by (5). What has been discussed so far
is quite general and the experimental determination of (8) should in
principle contain all informations required by NMR spectroscopy for a
heterogeneous sample. In practice the way the magnetic field gradients
are excited and the whole R.F. pulse sequence can vary appreciably
among the several proposed imaging methods. Here we will limit ourselves to the description of the most relevant methods.

2. NMR IMAGING METHODS

    The first approach[1] to NMR imaging was also the first to be successful
for whole body imaging[3]. This method, called projection-reconstruction
(PR), is infact still used and, although largely replaced by other procedures, it deserves consideration because of its high efficiency.

2.1. Projection Reconstruction

The typical feature of PR method is the use of time independent magnetic
field gradients. Then if

$$\vec{G} = \frac{\partial H_z}{\partial x}\vec{i} + \frac{\partial H_z}{\partial y}\vec{j} + \frac{\partial H_z}{\partial z}\vec{k} = \text{const}$$

that means

$$\frac{\partial H_z}{\partial x} = \text{const}; \quad \frac{\partial H_z}{\partial y} = \text{const}; \quad \frac{\partial H_z}{\partial z} = \text{const}$$

the integral at the exponent in equation (5) will easily be solved as follows:

$$\int_{t_1}^{t_1+t} \vec{r} \cdot \vec{G}(t') dt' = \int_0^t \vec{r} \cdot \vec{G} \ dt' = (\vec{r} \cdot \vec{G}) t \tag{9}$$

From (9) and (5) it derives that all spins with

$$xG_x + yG_y + zG_z = const \tag{10}$$

generate a single frequency in the spectrum. The relation (10) represents a plane orthogonal to $\vec{G}$ which contains the monochromatic spins.

The Fourier Transform (FT) of equation (5), through the value of $m_0(r_G)$, gives the amplitude of the spectral component associated to the plane given by (10). The real part of the FT of (5) becomes then

$$m_\perp^c (r_G, \omega) \propto 2m_0(r_G) T_2(r_G) \{1 + T_2^2(r_G) \left[\omega - (\omega_0 + \gamma \vec{r} \cdot \vec{G})\right]^2\}^{-1} \tag{11}$$

To obtain the whole spectrum of frequencies it is necessary to sum up all the planes orthogonal to $\vec{G}$ and resonating at different frequencies. In other words we must integrate along $\vec{G}$ over the whole sample. The total spectrum is thus

$$S(\omega) = \int_{L_G} m_\perp(r_G, \omega) dr_G \tag{12}$$

where L_G is the maximum dimension of the sample along $\vec{G}$. Equation (11) represents, within the whole spectrum, a lorentzian line produced by the plane (10) and centered at the frequency

$$\omega = \omega_0 + \gamma \vec{r} \cdot \vec{G} \tag{13}$$

with half width $(\pi T_2)^{-1}$ and amplitude $2m_0(r_G) T_2(r_G)$. Equation (12) instead says that the total spectrum (when $\vec{G}$=const) is a continuum of superimposed lorentzian lines, the spectrum itself representing the spin density profile along $\vec{G}$. This last statement is true only if the following condition is satisfied:

$$\frac{\gamma |\vec{G}| L_G}{N} > \frac{1}{\pi T_{2m}} \tag{14}$$

where T_{2m} is the minimum T_2 contained in our sample and $\gamma |\vec{G}| L_G$ is the frequency broadening produced by $\vec{G}$ over the total lenght of the sample. The ratio L_G/N is the space resolution, where N is an integer number.

The PR method makes use of a whole set o projections, as expressed by (13), each one obtained at a different direction of $\vec{G}$, namely by changing Gx, Gy, Gz while leaving $|\vec{G}|$ constant.

From the set of projections, by using reconstruction techniques similar to the ones used in X-ray tomography, the image can be easily obtained. The image represents a 3D or 2D space distribution of $m_0 T_2$. These maps are usually called spin density images, although we have demonstrated that they produce an $m_0 T_2$ map. The reduction from 3D to 2D images is normally obtained by means of a selective R.F. irradiation, which excites only a slice of wanted thickness, let us say in the x, y plane. Then the projections are produced by rotating $\vec{G}$ within the x, y plane, over a whole set of equally spaced angles.

Images with T_1 or T_2 contrast can be generated by using different pulse sequences. For the spin density image in principle just a $\pi/2$ pulse sequence would be enough but for technical reasons the spin-echo (SE) sequence is used, with a delay between the $\pi/2$ and π pulses short with respect to T_2. If this delay time is made longer a higher contrast in T_2 is obtained. The T_1 contrast is generally produced by appling a π pulse before the spin-echo sequence. The delay before the spin-echo should be comparable with T_1. This T_1 contrasting sequence is called inversion-recovery (IR).

2.2. Fourier zeugmatography

Fourier zeugmatography,proposed by R. Ernst[4], is the base of the methods which nowadays are prevailing. It is infact a special case of multi dimensional FT spectroscopy. This technique uses pulsed field gradients after the RF pulse. Immediately after the $\pi/2$ pulse a magnetic field gradient G_x is applied along x for a certain time interval $o < t < t_x$, then a field gradient G_y is applied along y for the time interval $t_x < t < t_x + t_y$ and finally a field gradient G_z is applied along the z axis for time $t > t_x + t_y$. All these times must be contained within the same FID produced by the $\pi/2$ pulse. The recorded data $S(t)$ are only those of the fraction of FID during the third time interval. To summarize the procedure the z-component of the total magnetic field is given by:

$$H_o + G_x \cdot x \qquad\qquad o < t < t_x$$

$$H_o + G_y \cdot y \qquad\qquad t_x < t < t_x + t_y$$

$$H_o + G_z \cdot z \qquad\qquad t > t_x + t_y$$

For a 3D image N^2 FID's recorded at $t > t_x + t_y$ will be needed for a complete set of values of t_x and t_y.

It is necessary to demonstrate at this stage that the 3D FT of the observed signal represents the space distribution of the spin density.

The recorded FID is a function of t_x, t_y and t_z, where $t_z = t - (t_x + t_y)$, thus,

$$S(t) = S(t_x, t_y, t_z) \tag{15}$$

The experiment is repeated for a full set of regularly incremented t_x and t_y values. Of course the function $S(t)$ can be expressed as a sum of the contributions arising from each volume element $dV = dx\,dy\,dz$, thus:

$$S(t) = \int \rho(\vec{r})s(\vec{r},t)dV \tag{16}$$

where $s(\vec{r},t)dV$ is the contribution to the FID generated by the volume element dV at position $\vec{r}$; $\rho(\vec{r})$ is the spin density at position $\vec{r}$. The 3D FT of $S(t)$ is denoted by $S(\omega)$ then:

$$S(\omega) = \iiint S(t)\exp(-i\omega t)dt_x dt_y dt_z \tag{17}$$

The function $S(\omega)$, like its FT conjugate can be expressed as an integral over volume elements as follows:

$$S(\omega) = \int \rho(\vec{r})s(\vec{r},\omega)dV \tag{18}$$

where $s(\vec{r},\omega)$ is the FT of $s(\vec{r},t)$. Now the change of variables

$$s(\vec{r},\omega) = s(o,\omega+\gamma\vec{G}\cdot\vec{r}) \tag{19}$$

allows us to rewrite (18) in the following way:

$$S(\omega) = \int \rho(\vec{r})s(o,\omega+\gamma\vec{G}\cdot\vec{r})dV \tag{20}$$

and by writing ω as a function of coordinates $\vec{r}'$ we can finally write (20) as follows:

$$S(\omega) = \bar{\rho}(\vec{r}')=\int \rho(\vec{r})s(o,\gamma\vec{G}\cdot(\vec{r}'-\vec{r}))dV \tag{21}$$

Equation (21) demonstrates that the 3D FT of the measured signal $S(t)$ yields a spin density space distribution $\bar{\rho}(\vec{r}')$, which is a convolution of the real spin density distribution $\rho(\vec{r})$ with the lineshape function. This result is very similar, as it is to be expected, to that obtained with the PR method. Of course here too if the broadening caused by the magnetic field gradient is much greater than the natural linewidth (the lineshape function) it will be reasonable to assume $\bar{\rho}(\vec{r}')\approx\rho(\vec{r})$. This corresponds to having the condition (14) satisfied. Of course this is always the chosen experimental situation. The reduction to a 2D image is done here too by means of selective irradiation.

The technique used commonly today is a modification[5] of the Fourier Zeugmatography, which is currently called "spin warp". Infact the spin phase accumulation caused by the gradient G_x is given by:

$$\int_{o}^{t_x} G_x(t)dt \tag{22}$$

as it is clear form equation (5). But the value of the integral (22) can be changed either by varing the time interval t_x while leaving G_x constant or viceversa. In the two cases we have then

Fourier Zeugmatography $\quad\begin{cases} G_x = \text{const.} \\[6pt] t_x \text{ varied by steps} \end{cases}$

Spin warp $\quad\begin{cases} G_x \text{ varied by steps} \\[6pt] t_x = \text{const.} \end{cases}$

The reasons which have made the spin warp method preferable are essentially technical. Infact it is much easier to keep all the time delays fixed and change the gradient amplitude rather than varying the times. The complete spin warp sequence is shown in Fig. 1.

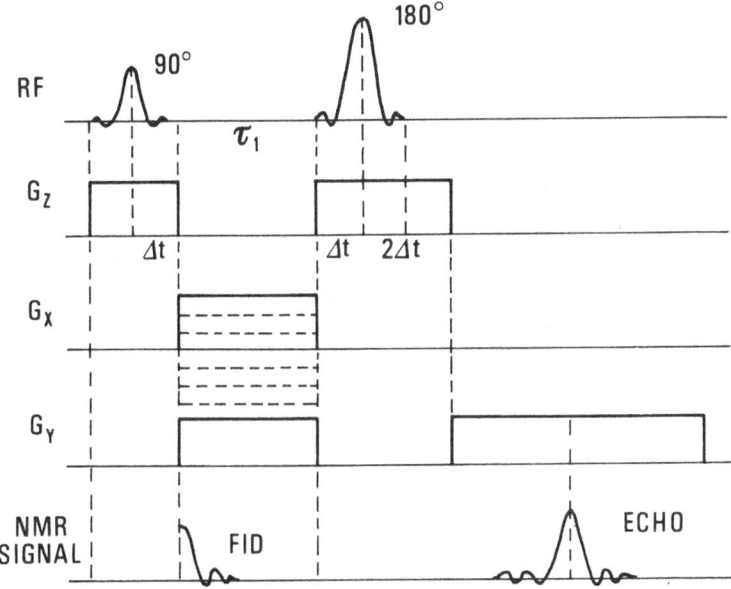

Figure 1. Typical spin warp sequence. It is a spin echo with both se-lective pulses. The gradient G_z is switched on to select a x, y slice during R.F. irradiation. The G_y gradient is the reading gradient, which is on while the echo is recorded. G_y introduces the frequency spread along y. The phase enconding gradient G_x is applied with a whole set of amplitudes (e.g. 128) and for each one the echo is recorded. The 2D FT of the recorded signal gives the spin density map of course here too T_1 contrast can be generated by appling an extra selective π pulse before the spin echo sequence (IR).

Other techniques which are of relevant interest are the echo pla-nar method[6] and the rotating frame zeugmatography[7]. The echo planar method is the only real time imaging technique but its signal to noise ratio is quite worse. Fot this reason it has been so far rather negle-

cted. The rotating frame zeugmatography has instead relevant features
in principle but it implies very serious technical problems.

3. REFERENCES

1) Lauterbur, P.C. 'Image formation by induced local interaction: Examples employing nuclear magnetic resonance' Nature, 242, 190 (1973).
2) Abragam, A. The principles of nuclear magnetism. Oxford Press, 1961.
3) Holland, G.N.; Hawkes, R.C.; Moore, W.S. 'Nuclear Magnetic Resonance
   (NMR) Tomography of the brain: coronal and sagittal sections' J. of
   Comp. Ass. Tomography, 4, 429 (1980).
4) Kumar, A.; Welti, D.; Ernst, R.R. 'NMR Fourier zeugmatography' J. of
   Magn. Res. 18, 69 (1975).
5) Hutchinson, J.M.S.; Edelstein, W.W.; Johnson, G. 'A whole body NMR
   imaging machine' J. Phys. E. Sci. Instrum 13, 947 (1980).
6) Mansfield, P.; Morris, P.G. NMR Imaging in biomedicine Supplement 2
   Advances in Magnetic Resonance, Academic Press, 1982.
7) Hoult, D.I. 'Rotating frame zeugmatography' J. of Magn. Res. 33, 183
   (1978).

THE SENSITIVITY OF THE NMR IMAGING EXPERIMENT

D. I. Hoult
Biomedical Engineering and Instrumentation Branch,
Division of Research Services. Building 13, Room 3W13
National Institutes of Health,
Bethesda, Maryland   20205, USA

ABSTRACT. Commencing with the signal-to-noise ratio of the free induction decay from the hydrogen in a human being, the various factors which influence the signal-to-noise ratio of a medical NMR image are examined. It is shown that the chemical shift range inherent in human tissue and the considerable variation of longitudinal relaxation times with frequency ω_0 profoundly affect any analysis, causing, for a fixed resolution and given imaging time, the image signal-to-noise ratio to vary only as approximately $\omega_0^{1/4}$. The power deposited in the human body by the r.f. pulses is also considered, and it is shown that, above about 60 MHz, the heating produced in the torso (under the conditions pertaining to multi-slice examination) exceeds recommended values. Techniques for reducing the power absorption are briefly considered, and the use of multiple echoes at medium field strengths ($\sim$0.7T) is advocated as a possible method of improving image quality.

INTRODUCTION

Considerable controversy has recently developed in the medical NMR community over the choice of an optimal field for diagnostic imaging. The controversy has been fueled by the opposing claims of various commercial companies, the lack of hard evidence and the complexity of the topic. Optimization involves not merely signal-to-noise ratio in an image, but also patient throughput, contrast, versatility and resolution, and it is not trivial to discern how these various factors interact and to know what weight to assign to each. Further, because the subject is in its infancy, instrument quality is still highly variable and, therefore, a confusing extra factor. To wit, the author has seen excellent images obtained at operating fields of 0.15T and 1.5T and conversely, very poor images at both fields.

An obvious starting point in any analysis is the signal-to-noise of the free induction decay (f.i.d.) from the portion of the patient being examined. Any imaging technique effectively allows one to observe the signal originating from any elementary volume of interest

T. Axenrod and G. Ceccarelli (eds.), NMR in Living Systems, 117–122.

in the patient, the size of that volume being dependent upon the desired resolution.   On the other hand, the noise is in no way correlated with the spatial location of interest, being predominantly a function of the receiving coil's geometry and the patient's size. Thus if one knows the f.i.d. signal-to-noise ratio Ψ_t from, say, 1 ml of water in a person's head, it is trivial to scale by volume and to know the ratio pertaining to an elementary volume (voxel) Δv.   Thus Hoult and Lauterbur[1], in their generally accepted analysis of image sensitivity, consider only briefly the signal strength while dwelling at length on the possible sources of noise. They show that while the e.m.f. induced in the receiving coil by the nuclear magnetization increases as the square of Larmor frequency, the Brownian motion of the electrolytes in the human body induces, in the coil, noise which increases linearly with frequency.   Hence, above a few Megahertz, regardless of the coil geometry, the dominant source of noise is the subject, rather than the receiving coil's resistance.   It follows that in most situations, the f.i.d. signal-to-noise ratio rises only linearly with frequency rather than to the customary 7/4 power.

     Such is our starting point, and it, of course, raises expectations that a ten-fold increase in field strength will reward the investigator with a similar increase in image signal-to-noise ratio. However, this is not the case, for an image is a function not only of field strength, but also of chemical shift and relaxation times T_1 and T_2, and therefore we must pursue the matter further.

FROM F.I.D. TO SPECTRUM

The basic premise of the imaging experiment - the zeugmatographic principle, to use Lauterbur's Greek coinage - is a linear relationship between Larmor frequency and spatial position induced by the application of a linear field gradient. Under such conditions, the Fourier transform of the f.i.d. from, say, water becomes a projection - a graph of water content versus distance - for the strength of the signal is, of course, dependent on the amount of water present, while distance, by virtue of the gradient, is synonymous with frequency. However, this basic principle takes no account of field inhomogeneity, transverse relaxation and chemical shift. While inhomogeneity may be removed with the appropriate technology, relaxation and shifts are fundamental phenomena which must not be ignored; regrettably, they often are.   Mathematically, the application of a field gradient convolutes the spatial distribution of protons with their spectrum. If the latter were constant throughout the human body, a deconvolution process could remove the spectrum's influence.   However, T_2 may vary from 30-100ms (and, exceptionally, to over 1s,) while the distribution of protons may lie almost anywhere in a 5 p.p.m. range, the principal components of the spectrum being water and fat.   This being the case, the only obvious way to remove the deleterious effects of the convolution is to impose upon the f.i.d. a filter function whose spectrum is broader than that of the chemical shift range, while increasing the field gradient to the point at which the filter creates negligible error in the projection.   To consider a simple spectroscopic example, (no field gradient applied,) suppose we restrict the data acquisition window Δt from its usual value of $5T_2$ to a considerably smaller value. Upon Fourier transformation, the resolution in the spectrum is no longer $\Delta \nu = 1/\pi T_2$, but rather $\Delta \nu = 1/\Delta t$, and if $\Delta \nu$ is greater than the chemical shift range, individual peaks cannot be resolved - we obtain a single line. Its shape, if we care to observe it with the aid of zero-filling following data acquisition, is a sinc function - the Fourier transform of the rectangular window filter we applied. Application of a sufficiently large field gradient now gives us an accurate measure of the total hydrogen distribution - our desired projection. However, by reducing Δt, we have sacrificed signal-to-noise ratio, for the ratio in the spectrum is (for $\Delta t \ll T_2$) proportional to $\sqrt{\Delta t}$. Now the chemical shift in Hertz is, of course, proportional to the operating frequency. It follows that above about 6MHz - the frequency above which chemical shifts in the body can be resolved - Δt must decrease linearly with increasing frequency. In consequence, the signal-to-noise ratio in the projection or spectrum increases only as the square root of frequency.

The concern over chemical shifts voiced above is no theoretical abstraction. There is a grave danger of inaccurate depiction of anatomical borders in the image, and the potential for mistaking such artifacts for real anatomy or pathology. To remove this danger, we therefore sacrifice sensitivity. However such a course is an anathema, and so we must consider, if at all possible, ways of remedying the situation. Two possibilities occur to one. The first is to saturate unwanted chemical shift species (e.g. fat) leaving only one resonance (e.g. water). The second is to form, and then co-add, multiple images produced from multiple echoes with the aid of a Carr-Purcell, Meiboom-Gill (CPMG) sequence. Both protocols are under investigation in various laboratories, and both present major problems. For the first, a homogeneity of about 0.5 p.p.m. or better is needed over the volume of interest (a sphere of 40 cm diameter for imaging of the torso) in order to saturate selectively. For the second, accurate 180° refocusing pulses are needed, and above 30 MHz, as we shall see, power dissipation in the patient becomes a major problem. Thus, for the time being, we must be content with the modest gains a square root dependence of signal-to-noise ratio upon frequency affords.

FROM SPECTRUM TO IMAGE

To produce an image with acceptable resolution for clinical studies, it is usual to collect 256 f.i.d.s using whatever pulse sequence is deemed the most appropriate for the particular patient being examined. However, no matter what sequence is used, the length of time taken to collect the f.i.d.s is dependent on the longitudinal relaxation time T_1. Relatively few measurements of human T_1 values over the entire medical imaging frequency range (1 - 80 MHz at the time of writing) have been made. Thus some reliance must be placed upon results obtained from animals. Literature searches have been made by Beall et al[2] and Bottomley and colleagues[3], and from their findings one can see that T_1 varies with frequency in the range 1 to 100 MHz approximately as $\omega_0{}^n$, where n $\sim 1/3$ for brain and 1/2 for skeletal muscle. Other tissue types have indices lying between these two values. An immediate and inescapable conclusion to be drawn from these findings is that imaging takes longer at higher frequencies. Thus, one might take on average three times as long to conduct an examination at 64 MHz (1.5T) as one would at 6.4 MHz (0.15T). As a reward, however, one would have over three times ($\sqrt{10}$) the signal-to-noise ratio in the image. It would be appealing to utilize this improvement to increase the spatial resolution of the image, but more f.i.d.s would then have to be collected. In short, chasing higher resolution and/or signal-to-noise ratio by increasing field strength can lead to a reduction in patient throughput, the exact extent being dependent on the efficiency of machine usage.

An easily overlooked point when considering this dilemma is that if we are taking three times longer, perforce, to obtain an image at 64MHz, what would happen if we allowed the same amount of imaging time at 6.4 MHz? The answer, of course, is that we may improve our signal-to-noise ratio, by averaging, by $\sqrt{3}$. In other words, allowing a given time to obtain an image of fixed resolution, signal-to-noise ratio varies only as $\omega_0{}^{(1-n)/2}$. This dependency of sensitivity upon frequency is not great, and in the choice of a field for imaging should therefore carry a correspondingly low weight. Siting factors, price and multiple-slice capability may weigh more heavily.

POWER DISSIPATION

In their paper, Hoult and Lauterbur[1] showed that the power absorbed by a saline sphere in the presence of an alternating magnetic field B_1 was proportional to the squares of the frequency of alternation and of the field strength, and to the fifth power of the sphere's radius r. While a sphere is but a poor model of a portion of a human being, these dependencies do appear to hold and have been approximately confirmed in the author's laboratory with the aid of techniques for measuring the Q factor of the transmitting coil (in the presence and absence of a person,) and the alternating field produced when a known amount of power is applied to the coil. Given the above, we must now ask just how large a B_1 field is needed to form a satisfactory image. In general, echo formation with the aid of a 180° pulse is an essential part of the imaging process, and it is easily shown that it is this pulse which normally dominates the problem of absorbed power. Now the usual criterion concerning the pulse's strength is that $\omega_1 = {}^\gamma B_1$ be ten times larger than the frequency range to be covered. However, such extravagance can not possibly be tolerated in an imaging experiment, for we have seen that the minimum frequency range to be covered is determined by the chemical shift range - say 5 p.p.m. Ten times this value is no mean figure at fields of the order of 1.5T (64 MHz), and leads to instantaneous r.f. powers in excess of 100kW. Thus one must compromise to some extent. However, no matter what compromise is adopted, it is clear that B_1 must increase as ω_0 to cover the chemical shift range, and thus the transmitter's power specification W must increase as ω_0^4, for $W \alpha \; \omega_0^2 B_1^2 r^5$. Note also that at least 30 times as much power is needed for the torso as for the head. When one considers the power absorbed per unit weight of a person (the so-called specific absorption rate or SAR,) one has to multiply the transmitter power by the duty cycle and divide by the weight contained in the volume "seen" by the transmitter coil. Further, it may be shown that most of the power is deposited on the surface of the body, and thus to find the surface SAR, one must multiply the average SAR by a factor of about 2.5. In light of the above, only an estimate of SAR may be made, but for a given pulse sequence, repeated at a rate dependent on T_1 , the SAR varies as $\omega_0^{(3-n)}$, and approximately as r^2. As far as hard numbers are concerned, the Food and Drug Administration of the United States has recommended that an SAR of 2W/kg not be exceeded[5]. Using eight 180° pulses per time T_1 (a multiple-slice sequence,) a B_1 field which barely covers the chemical shift range, ($\gamma B_1 = 2.5\,\omega_0 \delta$) and a head coil suitable for both reception and transmission, we estimate that 2W/kg are dissipated at about 80 MHz. However, for the same protocol on the torso, that limit is reached at about 55 MHz.

CONCLUSION

When we combine the above results with those obtained earlier concerning signal-to-noise ratio, it is quite clear that patient throughput has to suffer as we progress to the highest fields. Not only does it take longer to perform the imaging experiment at higher fields on account of the lengthened T_1 values, but at the highest fields (~ 1.5T) the use of multiple slice techniques (particularly on the torso) must be restricted so as to avoid heating the patient. With regard to improving the signal-to-noise ratio, the obvious strategy to use at high fields is the imaging of one chemical shift species only. This device not only restores the sensitivity, (albeit at the expense of losing information concerning other species,) but also reduces the patient heating, for it is no longer necessary to cover such a large bandwidth with the pulses. However, throughput will be reduced still further if the pathology dictates that both water and fat should be studied, for two image sets will then be required. Neither should the stringent requirements concerning magnet homogeneity (<1 p.p.m. over the torso) be forgotten. Another promising course with regard to clinical imaging (as opposed to basic research) is the exploration of the potential of multiple echoes at medium field strengths (~ 0.7T). If their use could be perfected, sensitivity could be recovered in a normal image (i.e. water and fat) to the extent that the signal-to-noise ratio would be comparable to that obtained from an artifact free, single-echo image obtained at a field of 2T (84 MHz). The power dissipation in the torso would be at about the recommended limit, but the instrument specifications. in terms of homogeneity and transmitter power (1kW) would be eminently reasonable and patient throughput would be acceptable. Thus, in conclusion, the author feels that at the present (but not necessarily in the future) the mid-field range (~ 0.7T) is probably the best compromise for diagnostic imaging, for it holds the greatest prospect of image improvement without the imposition of exceedingly demanding technical constraints, and moreover, should allow a patient throughput approaching that used with X-ray scanning equipment.

REFERENCES

1)   D. I. Hoult and P. C. Lauterbur, J. Magn. Reson. **34**, 425 (1979).

2)   D. I. Hoult and R. E. Richards, J. Magn. Reson. **24**, 71 (1976).

3)   P. T. Beall, S. R. Amtey and S. R. Kasturi, NMR Data Handbook for Biomedical Applications, New York, Pergamon Press, 1984.

4)   P. A. Bottomley, T. H. Foster, R. E. Argersinger and L. M. Pfeifer, General Electric Report No. 84CRD072, Schenectady, New York, April 1984, Also Med. Phys. In Press.

5)   F.D.A. Memorandum, Guidelines for Evaluating Electromagnetic Exposure Risk for Trials of Clinical NMR Systems, F.D.A. Rockville, MD., February 12th, 1982.

THE USE OF MODELS IN THE INTERPRETATION OF NMR IMAGES

Aldo Rescigno and Charles C. Duncan
Section of Neurological Surgery
Yale University School of Medicine
333 Cedar Street
New Haven, CT 06510

1. Introduction

Image analysis has become an extraordinarily powerful tool in a
wide range of fields. Applications of this approach have ranged from
sub-atomic analyses to life sciences. Despite the great differences
in the various disciplines utilizing image analysis, there are
several common problems to the optimal elaboration of the information
obtained. These include construction of analytical models, objective
determinations of hypotheses support, quantitative assessment of the
reliability of the information being examined in terms of regions of
interest, comparative interactions, and analysis of special cases.
With the magnitude of information available from many different
sources, the individual observer continues to form general schemes
from the image which represents perception of only a minute portion
of the data.

While much attention has been recently given to the problem of
image reconstruction, image analysis per se has been limited to
specific applications, most notably to the problem of pattern
recognition. Mathematical concepts to construct intelligent models,
i.e. models that are based on a minimum rather than a maximum number
of hypotheses, are relatively recent in terms of the history of
mathematics but date conceptually to the beginning of this century.

Image analysis is only one facet of a more general problem. In
simple words the problem consists in discovering specific features of
the external world. This is done sequentially by
a) obtaining data from a detector,
b) codifying the data in a convenient form,
c) storing the data in a memory,
d) elaborating the stored data,
e) decoding the data to reveal their specific features.

Each of the above steps presents its own problems, but they are
all strictly connected. For instance step b needs not be separate
from step a; as we shall show below, the data can be collected by the
detector in a form suitable for immediate codification. Similarly
step c is limited by the available storage space; a three-dimensional

123

T. Axenrod and G. Ceccarelli (eds.), NMR in Living Systems, 123–156.
© *1986 by D. Reidel Publishing Company.*

image of 1 dm^3 with a resolution of 1 mm includes 10^6 voxels; if
the image is to be followed kinetically at a rate of 50 sec^{-1}, a
one-minute observation requires the storage of the content of $3x10^9$
voxels; a discrimination of 256 levels for the content of each voxel
requires then the storage of 2.4 x 10^{10} bits/min.

Obviously most of this information is useless, as it represents
unneeded redundancy for contiguous voxels; a convenient codification
of the information collected could considerably reduce the redundancy
without reducing the reliability of the data.

In statistical problems, where a very large amount of data need
to be condensed in a few meaningful parameters, a natural answer is
given by the analysis of moments, like Expected Value, Variance,
Skewness, Kurtosis, etc. In the analysis of images there is an
analogous problem, namely one must try to reveal deviations of the
observed image from a preestablished standard image, viz. "pattern
recognition", or from the most probable pattern as determined by that
part of the observed image bordering the part under observation, viz.
pattern reconstruction". For the study of sequential images the
problem is substantially the same, but in one more dimension.

All these problems have one thing in common; in all cases one is
trying to reduce the amount of information available without at the
same time reducing the value of the information preserved. We shall
not give here a formal definition of these two terms because, to our
knowledge, a mathematical theory dealing with the relations between
information and the observer has not yet been developed. We are using
these terms in a loose sense, but their meaning will become clear in
the following pages through their own use.

These common problems of image analysis may be approached by
measuring the successive moments.

2. The Use of Models

Most experimental workers first define a qualitative model, then
use experimental data to compute the parameters of that model. For
instance the model appropriate for the description of dilution
phenomena is a set of ordinary differential equations with constant
coefficients, while for diffusion phenomena partial differential
equations are to be used, for delay phenomena finite difference
equations, etc. Of course the cognitive value of the parameters
computed in this way depends upon the chosen model. An ideal
situation would be to define parameters that are independent, or
almost independent, of the chosen model.

The compartment model, so often used in nuclear medicine and in
pharmacokinetics (Rescigno and Segre, 1964), is formed by a set of
linear differential equations of order one with constant
coefficients; its validity depends upon the hypotheses that the
system described contains a finite number of components, and that
each component is homogeneous. These hypotheses exclude the presence
of diffusion and of age-dependent processes, or in general of
transport of a non-Markovian nature. The fact that frequently the

experimental data agree with this model does not necessarily prove
the model is appropriate, but only that it is flexible (Beck and
Rescigno, 1970).

In fact any number of classes of functions and an infinity of
functions within each class will fit any contiguous single-valued
correspondence with time to any arbitrary closeness. Among the most
well known demonstrations are those for polynomials (Weierstrass,
1885) and for trigonometric functions (Fourier, 1822). In the
specific case of n compartments, the model is a set of n first order
linear differential equations in n state variables; they contain n^2
parameters. With n large enough, this model can be made consistent
with many experimental data, but at the price of a considerable
complexity of the model itself. Frequently many coefficients of the
differential equations are set equal to zero, thus simplifying the
differential equations of the model and the fitting of the data. The
price paid for this simplification is a reduced flexibility of the
model.

In addition to the consistency with the experimental data, an
obvious conceptual requirement of the model is that its parameters
could be interpreted in terms of perceivable physical properties. The
n^2 parameters describing an n-compartment system are the transfer
rates between compartments and the turnover rates of compartments;
some of these parameters may be more "significant" than others, in
the sense that their information is more "valuable" because they are
better correlated to other important physical properties or because
they are more sensitive to specific treatments; furthermore it may be
possible to describe other parametrizations whose descriptive or
predictive value is superior to the compartmental model.

All this considered, we shall try to show how the experimental
data can be examined in terms of a model making a minimum number of
assumptions and giving the best physical interpretation to the
parameters involved.

3. Stochastic transport

Consider the transport of a particle through a living system as a
stochastic process, i.e. as a phenomenon controlled by probabilistic
rather than deterministic laws. We assume here only that the particle
itself behaves in a way depending on its actual location and
physico-chemical state, but not on its past history.

Many papers have been published on stochastic compartments (for
instance Matis and Hartley, 1971; Thakur, Rescigno and Schafer, 1972;
Purdue, 1974), where the number of particles present in a compartment
is a time-dependent random variable; those models require the same
general assumptions made with the ordinary compartments, and
frequently, but not always, lead to distributions with very small
relative variances (Rescigno and Matis, 1981).

As an alternative model, consider as random variable the time a
given particle reaches a certain state in the system, or the interval
of time it stays in that state (Rescigno, 1973); the probability

distribution of this random variable can be analyzed and compared
with the experimental data available.

Call A(t) and C(t) the probability density functions of the time
a given particle is present in two specified states, called the
precursor and the successor respectively; call B(t) the probability
density function of the interval of time for the transition from the
precursor to the successor. More precisely,

A(t)dt = probability that a given particle is in the precursor state
         at a time between t and t+dt,

B(t)dt = probability that a given particle takes a length of time
         from t to t+dt to move from the precursor to the successor
         state,

C(t)dt = probability that a given particle is in the successor state
         at a time between t and t+dt.

Then, ignoring infinitesimals of order higher than one,
A(u)du.B(t−u)dt is the probability that a given particle in the
precursor state during the interval u,u+du will be in the successor
state during the interval t,t+dt. Integrating the expression above
for all values of u from 0 to t, one gets the probability that that
particle is in the successor state at a time between t and t+dt if it
was in the precursor state at any time from 0 to t,

$$(1) \qquad \int_0^t A(u)B(t-u)\,du = C(t).$$

This is the well known convolution integral representing a
linear, invariant system, without invoking the properties of
homogeneous, well-mixed compartments.

4. Definition of moments

Many properties of the convolution integral in (1) can be
analyzed by first defining the moments of the functions in it.

Given a generic function F(t) defined for all values of t from 0
to $+\infty$, define the moments,

$$(2) \qquad F_i = \int_0^\infty t^i/i!\, F(t)dt, \qquad i=0,1,2,\dots$$

and the relative moments,

$$(3) \qquad f_i = F_i/F_0, \qquad i=1,2,3,\dots$$

provided that the integral in (2) converges.

Observe the factor $1/i!$ in (2); we have introduced it because it
simplifies some of the expressions we shall find later on and many
computations; in particulare the moment generating functions defined
in section 11 actually generate these moments and not the moments
defined in other contexts without the factor $1/i!$. We shall not
discuss the general conditions necessary for the convergence of the
integral in (2), but section 9 shows what can be done when this
integral does not converge.

5. Properties of the convolution

Multiply both sides of equation (1) by $t^i/i!$ and integrate from 0 to $+\infty$,

$$\int_0^\infty t^i/i! \int_0^t A(u)B(t-u)\,du.\,dt = \int_0^\infty t^i/i!\, C(t)dt,$$

where i is any non-negative integer; change the order of integration,

$$\int_0^\infty A(u)\int_t^\infty t^i/i!\, B(t-u)dt.\,du = C_i;$$

change the variable of the inner integral,

$$\int_0^\infty A(u)\int_0^\infty (t+u)^i/i!\, B(t)dt.\,du = C_i,$$

expand the binomial to obtain finally,

(4) $$\sum_{j=0}^i A_{i-j}.B_j = C_i; \qquad i=0,1,2,\dots$$

in particular,

$$A_0B_0 = C_0$$

$$A_1B_0 + A_0B_1 = C_1$$

$$A_2B_0 + A_1B_1 + A_0B_2 = C_2$$

$$A_3B_0 + A_2B_1 + A_1B_2 + A_0B_3 = C_3.$$

Dividing both sides of equation (4) by A_0B_0 we get

(5) $$\sum_{j=0}^i a_{i-j}b_j = c_i, \qquad i=1,2,3,\dots$$

where conventionally we put $a_0 = b_0 = 1$; in particular,

$$a_1 + b_1 = c_1$$

$$a_2 + a_1b_1 + b_2 = c_2$$

$$a_3 + a_2b_1 + a_1b_2 + b_3 = c_3.$$

In general the number of particles in a given state is very large, and if it can be observed as a function of time it is a very good approximation of the probability density function defined in section 3. This means that the functions $A(t)$ and $C(t)$ corresponding to two given observable states can be measured, their moments computed, and finally the moments of the unknown function $B(t)$ obtained using equations (4) or (5).

These last moments can be given a clear physical meaning; for instance B_0 is the fraction of particles leaving the first state that actually reach the second state, a quantity analogous to the

Bioavailability as defined in Pharmacokinetics (Wagner, 1971); b_1 is the expected interval of time for a particle to move from the precursor to the successor; $2b_2-(b_1)^2$ is the variance of the above time, etc. (Rescigno and Michels, 1973).

6. Moments of a compartment

Consider a single compartment, i.e. a well mixed pool of homogeneous particles, all with the same probability m.dt of leaving that state in the interval of time t,t+dt, where m is a constant; in other words the probability of leaving the compartment does not depend on the time when a particle entered it or on the absolute time. If A(t) is the probability density function characteristic of the compartment, i.e., the probability that a particle is in the compartment at time t, then the probability that the same particle is still in that compartment at time t+dt is the product of A(t) by the probability of not leaving in the interval of time t,t+dt, i.e.

$$A(t+dt) = A(t).(1-mdt);$$

rearranging this equation,

$$dA/dt = -mA(t),$$

and integrating,

$$A(t) = A(0).e^{-mt},$$

where the constant of integration A(0) is the probability that a given particle is present in the compartment at the initial time. Using definitions (2) and (3) we get for a simple compartment,

$$A_i = A(0)/m^{i+1}, \qquad i=0,1,2,\ldots$$

$$a_i = 1/m^i. \qquad\qquad i=1,2,3,\ldots$$

7. Synthesis

Consider two systems in series, that is two systems such that all particles entering the second of them are originating from the first; the first system is called the unique precursor of the second (Rescigno and Segre, 1961). If
A(t)dt = probability that a particle present in the first system at
time 0 leaves it in the interval t,t+dt,
B(t)dt = probability that a particle entering the second system at
time 0 leaves it in the interval t,t+dt,
then, ignoring infinitesimals of order higher than one, the probability that a particle present in the first system at time 0 moves to the second in the interval u, u+du and leaves this one in

the interval t, t+dt is given by A(u)du.B(t-u)dt. Taking the integral of the expression above for all values of u from 0 to t, one gets the probability that a particle present in the first system at time 0 leaves the second at a time between t and t+dt, no matter when it moved from the first to the second, i.e. the convolution

$$\int_0^t A(u)B(t-u)\,du$$

is the probability density function characteristic of the system formed by two systems in series.

Obviously the properties of the convolution described in section 5 apply in this case also.

If two systems are in parallel, i.e. a particle can enter either system and be detected when it leaves either of them, then calling A(t) and B(t) the probability density functions of the two separate systems, the probability density function of the two systems taken globally is A(t)+B(t). The moments of the resulting system are

$$A_0 + B_0,$$
$$A_1 + B_1,$$
$$A_2 + B_2,$$
$$\dots\dots\dots$$

For the relative moments we have

(6) $$\frac{A_i+B_i}{A_0+B_0} = \frac{A_i}{A_0}\frac{A_0}{A_0+B_0} + \frac{B_i}{B_0}\frac{B_0}{A_0+B_0}$$

$$= a_i w_a + b_i w_b,$$

where i is any positive integer and

$$w_a = A_0/(A_0+B_0), \qquad w_b = B_0/(A_0+B_0),$$

called the **weights** of the two systems (Rescigno, 1973), are factors representing the probability that a particle goes through one rather than the other system.

If a system forms a loop, i.e. a particle can reenter it after leaving it, put

A(t)dt = probability that a particle present in the system at time 0 leaves it for the first time in the interval t, t+dt,

M(t)dt = probability that a particle present in the system at time 0 leaves it in the interval t, t+dt irrespective of the number of passages through it;

then the convolution of M(t) and A(t) is the probability density function corresponding to a particle going through that system two or more times; by adding to it the probability density function corresponding to just one passage, we should get again the function M(t), i.e.,

$$M(t) = \int_0^t M(u)A(t-u)\,du + A(t);$$

taking the moments of the functions above, using equation (4),

$$M_i = \sum_{j=0}^{i} M_{i-j}A_j + A_i, \quad i=0,1,2,\ldots$$

thence

(7) $M_0 = A_0/(1-A_0)$,

and using definition (3),

(8) $m_i = a_i + M_0 \sum_{j=1}^{i} m_{i-j}a_j; \quad i=1,2,3,\ldots$

from this equation the relative moments m_i can be computed sequentially.

8. Analysis

If the formulae of the previous section are inverted, from the moments of a system the moments of its separate subsystems can be computed. A new notation is necessary here. Call F_n^{ij} the n-moment of the transport of a particle from state i to state j, and F_n^{ii} the n-moment of the transport through a cycle beginning and ending in state i. Also call F_n^{ii*} the n-moment of the one time transport through the cycle around i, and $F_n^{ij}(l,m,\ldots)$ the n-moment of the transport from i to j excluding the particles that are going through the states $l,m,\ldots$, indicated in parenthesis. As a consequence of this last definition, if j is one of the superscripts in parenthesis, then from that moment the transport along a cycle through j is excluded. Lower case letters represent corresponding relative moments.

With this notation equation (7) for instance becomes

(9) $F_0^{jj} = F_0^{jj*}/(1-F_0^{jj*})$

and equation (8),

(10) $f_n^{jj} = f_n^{jj*} + F_0^{jj}\sum_{\ell=1}^{n} f_{n-1}^{jj}f_1^{jj*};$

by inversion,

$$F_0^{jj*} = F_0^{jj}/(1+F_0^{jj}),$$

$$f_n^{jj*} = \frac{f_n^{jj} - F_0^{jj}\sum_{\ell=1}^{n-1} f_{n-1}^{jj}f_1^{jj*}}{1+F_0^{jj}}$$

Suppose now that two states, say i and j, have been observed, and from experimental data the moments F_n^{ij} have been computed for a sufficient number of values of n. From section 7, remembering equation (4),

$$F_0^{ij} = F_0^{ij}(j)F_0^{jj},$$

and remembering equation (5),

$$f_n{}^{ij} = \sum_{\ell=0}^{n} f_{n-1}{}^{ij}(j) f_1{}^{jj}, \quad n=1,2,\dots$$

because the direct transfer of a particle from state i to state j is followed by an indeterminate number of recyclings of that particle around state j. If in the two equations above we substitute the values of $F_0{}^{jj}$ and $f_n{}^{jj}$ given by equations (9) and (10), we have a number of equations representing the relationship between the moments $F_0{}^{ij}(j)$, $f_n{}^{ij}(j)$ of the direct transfer from i to j, and $F_0{}^{jj*}$, $f_n{}^{jj*}$ of a single recycling around j, on one side, and the moments $F_0{}^{ij}$, $f_n{}^{ij}$ of the global transfer from i to j, as observed experimentally. By inversion of those equations, the moments of the subsystems can be computed; they describe the behavior of a particle during transfers not directly observable.

9. Non-converging moments

The definitions given in section 4 require the convergence of the integral

(11)
$$\int_0^{\infty} t^i/i! \, F(t)dt;$$

this requires that function $F(t)$ decreases fast enough when t approaches infinity. It is a known fact (Rescigno and Segre, 1961) that most functions found in biological modeling are of exponential order, i.e. they have the property that a constant a>0 exists such that the product $\exp(-at)F(t)$ is bounded for all values of t larger than some finite value T; for a function of exponential order the integral (11) always converges, no matter how large i is. A different case is presented by a closed system, i.e. by a system from where not all particles are eventually lost; in this case

$$\lim_{t \to \infty} F(t) = 0,$$

and integral (11) does not converge for any non-negative value of i. Obviously the expected time spent by a particle in such a system is infinite. We shall not consider this case here, but the more interesting case when function $B(t)$, as defined in section 3, is of exponential order, while function $A(t)$ is bounded but does not approach zero as t approaches infinity. This corresponds to feeding a "regular" system with an endless stream of particles. Equation (1) shows that function $C(t)$ too will have a non-zero limit, therefore neither the moments of $A(t)$ nor $C(t)$ are defined, while $B(t)$ has defined, but unknown moments.

From the hypothesis that $A(t)$ is bounded, it follows that $\exp(-gt)A(t)$ is of exponential order for any g>0; the convolution integral in (1) can be rewritten as

$$\int_0^t e^{-gu}A(u) \cdot e^{-g(t-u)}B(t-u)du = e^{-gt}C(t),$$

showing that the multiplication of both A(t) and C(t) by e^{-gt} is
equivalent to the multiplication of B(t) by the same exponential
function. The new functions $\exp(-gt)A(t)$ and $\exp(-gt)C(t)$ have finite
moments, and using equations (4) and (5) we can compute the moments
of $\exp(-gt)B(t)$; calling B_i^* the moments of this last function,
then

$$B_i^* = \int_0^\infty t^i/i! \cdot e^{-gt}B(t)dt$$

$$= \sum_{j=0}^\infty \int_0^\infty (-gt)^j/j! \cdot t^i/i! \cdot B(t)dt$$

$$= \sum_{j=0}^\infty (-1)^j g^j (i+j)!/i!j! \cdot B_{i+j}, \qquad i=0,1,2,\ldots$$

and by inversion

$$(12) \qquad B_i = \sum_{j=0}^\infty g^j (i+j)!/i!j! \cdot B_{i+j}^*. \qquad i=0,1,2,\ldots$$

10. Counting the particles

In section 5 we said that the functions A(t) and C(t) can be
measured by counting the number of particles present in a state at a
given time t, and then their moments computed. Two observations are
needed at this point.

First, any particle detector has a finite resolution time,
therefore it does not measure the exact number of particles present
at time t, but the average number of particles present in a certain
interval of time; this implies an error when the number of particles
changes fast enough compared to the resolution time of the detector.

Second, the computation of the moments of A(t) and C(t) is done
with a number of integrations; they introduce some errors that are
added to the errors intrinsic to the detection process.

An alternative method that reduces both kinds of errors to their
theoretical minimum is presented here. In this section we consider
the case where the particles present are counted one by one; if the
particles are detected collectively, for instance by measuring the
intensity of a light source instead of counting the number of
photons, this algorithm needs to be interpreted in a slightly
different way, as shown in section 18.

Let X(t) be the number of particles present in a particular voxel
or a particular pixel; then kX(t) is the probability that a single
particle will be detected in the interval t,t+dt, where k is a
constant depending upon the efficiency of the detector; the
probability of two particles being detected in the same infinitesimal
time interval dt is an infinitesimal of higher order and can be
neglected. The constant k can be determined by measuring for a
sufficiently long interval of time a calibrated phantom.

Define now the random variable N(t) equal to the number of
particles detected in the interval of time 0,t; the probability
distribution of this random variable is

$$p(r,t) = \text{Prob}\{N(t)=r\}.$$

Each time a particle is detected, the value of the random variable increases by one unit; it stays constant when no particles are detected. Therefore

$$p(0,t+dt) = [1-kX(t)dt].p(0,t)$$

$$p(r,t+dt) = kX(t)dt.p(r-1,t) + [1-kX(t)dt].p(r,t), \quad r>0$$

and of course

$$p(0,0) = 1$$

because the particle counter is set to zero at the beginning of the experiment.

Rearranging,

$$\partial p(0,t)/\partial t = -kX(t).p(0,t).$$

$$\partial p(r,t)/\partial t = -kX(t).[p(r,t)-p(r-1,t)], \quad r>0$$

Integrating,

$$p(r,t) = 1/r!.[\int_0^t kX(u)du]^r.\exp[-\int_0^t kX(u)du], \quad r=0,1,2,\ldots$$

i.e. $N(t)$ is a Poisson random variable with intensity

$$f(t) = \int_0^t kX(u)du.$$

It follows that its expected value, variance, and third moment around the mean are

$$E[N(t)] = \text{Var}[N(t)] = M_3[N(t)] = f(t).$$

11. Recording higher moments

We introduce now another random variable, $N_i(t)$, equal to the sum of the i-th power of the times of detection of a particle in the interval 0,t, divided by i!, where $i=1,2,3,\ldots$; in other words, if $t_1, t_2, \ldots$ are the times when the first, second, ... particle are detected, with

$$0 < t_1 < t_2 < \ldots < t_n < t,$$

where n is the number of particles detected in the interval 0,t; then

$$N_i(t) = (t_1^i+t_2^i+\ldots+t_n^i)/i!, \quad i=1,2,\ldots$$

$$p_i(r,t) = \text{Prob}\{r<N_i(t)<r+dr\} ;$$

we can also define

$$N_0(t) = n,$$

a random variable identical to $N(t)$ as described above.

If several registers are used, each time a particle is detected, its instant of detection is read on a clock, this value is raised to the power i, divided by $i!$, and this number is added to the corresponding register. When time t is reached, the different registers will show a particular realization of the random variables $N_0(t)$, $N_1(t)$, $N_2(t)$, ...

When a particle is detected in the interval $t,t+dt$, the value of the random variable $N_i(t)$ increases by an amount $t^i/i!$, while it does not change if no particles are detected, therefore

$$p_i(r,t+dt)dr = [1-kX(t)dt].p_i(r,t)dr, \qquad r<t^i/i!$$

$$= kX(t)dt.p_i(r-t^i/i!,t)dr +$$

$$+ [1-kX(t)dt].p_i(r,t)dr, \qquad r \geq t^i/i!$$

for any positive integer i. Rearranging,

$$(13) \quad \partial p_i/\partial t.dr = -kX(t).p_i(r,t)dr, \qquad\qquad r<t^i/i!$$

$$(14) \quad \partial p_i/\partial t.dr = -kX(t).[p_i(r,t)dr-p_i(r-t^i/i!,t)dr].$$
$$r \geq t^i/i!$$

Define the moment generating function

$$F_i(s,t) = \int_0^\infty e^{rs} p_i(r,t)dr;$$

multiply equations (13) and (14) by e^{rs}, then integrate (13) from 0 to $t^i/i!$ and (14) from $t^i/i!$ to ∞; add the two results together,

$$\partial F_i/\partial t = -kX(t)[1-\exp(st^i/i!)]F_i(s,t);$$

at time 0 no pulses are recorded and by hypothesis all registers read zero, therefore

$$F_i(s,0) = 1;$$

by integration we get

$$F_i(s,t) = \exp\left(-\int_0^t [1-\exp(su^i/i!)]kX(u)du\right), \qquad i=0,1,2,\ldots$$

By taking successive derivatives with respect to s,

$$\partial F_i/\partial s = \int_0^t u^i/i!.\exp(su^i/i!).kX(u)du.F_i,$$

$$\partial^2 F_i/\partial s^2 = \int_0^t (u^i/i!)^2.\exp(su^i/i!).kX(u)du.F_i +$$

$$+ \int_0^t u^i/i!.\exp(su^i/i!).kX(u)du.\partial F_i/\partial s,$$

$$\partial^3 F_i/\partial s^3 = \int_0^t (u^i/i!)^3.\exp(su^i/i!).kX(u)du.F_i +$$
$$+ 2\int_0^t (u^i/i!)^2.\exp(su^i/i!).kX(u)du.\partial F_i/\partial s +$$
$$+ \int_0^t u^i/i!.\exp(su^i/i!).kX(u)du.\partial^2 F_i/\partial s^2;$$

making $s=0$ we get the first three moments of $N_i(t)$ around the origin,

$$E[N_i(t)] = \int_0^t u^i/i!.kX(u)du,$$
$$E[N_i(t)^2] = \int_0^t (u^i/i!)^2.kX(u)du + [\int_0^t u^i/i!.kX(u)du]^2,$$
$$E[N_i(t)^3] = \int_0^t (u^i/i!)^3.kX(u)du +$$
$$+ 3\int_0^t (u^i/i!)^2.kX(u)du.\int_0^t u^i/i!.kX(u)du +$$
$$+ [\int_0^t u^i/i!.kX(u)du]^3,$$

and from these the variance and the third central moment,

$$Var[N_i(t)] = \int_0^t (u^i/i!)^2.kX(u)du =$$
$$= (2i)!/(i!)^2.E[N_{2i}(t)]$$
$$M_3[N_i(t)] = \int_0^t (u^i/i!)^3.kX(u)du =$$
$$= (3i)!/(i!)^3.E[N_{3i}(t)].$$

Observe that while equations (13) and (14) were written only for positive integer values of i, the moments computed here are valid for any non-negative integer i, because for $i=0$ they coincide with the results of the previous section.

The value given by register i is the best estimator of the i-moment of $kX(t)$, while from register $2i$ we compute the best estimator of its variance, and so forth. Of course k can be determined for a particular experimental set-up by measuring N_0 with a calibrated phantom.

In short, by this method the successive moments of function $kX(t)$ are accumulated in separate registers; because no analog transformations are required, the only errors involved are due to the random fluctuations of the detection process, and these are estimated by higher moments.

12. Scaling the counting rate

If the detection rate is too fast for the resolution time of the registers, it may be necessary to scale the detection events before recording their time. Suppose that only every m-th event is recorded, and call $N_i^{(m)}(t)$ the sum of the i-th power divided by $i!$ of the

times of recording every m-th event in the interval 0,t; define, for
any positive integer i,

$$p_i^{(m)}(r,a,t)dr =$$

$$= \text{Prob}\{r<N_i^{(m)}(t)<r+dr.N(t)\equiv a(\bmod\ m)\}, \quad 0\leq a<m;$$

proceeding as in section 10,

$$p_i^{(m)}(r,0,t+dt)dr = [1-kX(t)dt].p_i^{(m)}(r,0,t)dr, \quad r<t^i/i!$$

$$= kX(t)dt.p_i^{(m)}(r-t^i/i!,m-1,t)dr +$$

$$+ [1-kX(t)dt].p_i^{(m)}(r,0,t)dr. \quad r\geq t^i/i!$$

$$p_i^{(m)}(r,a,t+dt)dr = kX(t)dt.p_i^{(m)}(r,a-1,t)dr +$$

$$+ [1-kX(t)dt].p_i^{(m)}(r,a,t)dr. \quad a=1,2,\ldots,m-1$$

Rearranging ,

$$\partial p_i^{(m)}(r,0,t)/\partial t.dr = -kX(t)dt.p_i^{(m)}(r,0,t)dr, \quad r<t^i/i!$$

$$= -kX(t)[p_i^{(m)}(r,0,t)dr -$$

$$-p_i^{(m)}(r-t^i/i!,m-1,t)dr], \quad r\geq t^i/i!$$

$$\partial p_i^{(m)}(r,a,t)/\partial t.dr = -kX(t)[p_i^{(m)}(r,a,t)dr -$$

$$-p_i^{(m)}(r,a-1,t)dr]. \quad a=1,2,\ldots,m-1$$

Adding these equations together,

(15) $$\partial P_i^{(m)}/\partial t.dr = -kX(t).p_i^{(m)}(r,m-1,t)dr, \quad r<t^i/i!$$

(16) $$\partial P_i^{(m)}/\partial t.dr = -kX(t)[p_i^{(m)}(r,m-1,t)dr -$$

$$-p_i^{(m)}(r-t^i/i!,m-1,t)dr], \quad r\geq t^i/i!$$

where

$$P_i^{(m)}(r,t)dr = \sum_{a=0}^{m-1}p_i^{(m)}(r,a,t)dr$$

$$= \text{Prob}\{r<N_i^{(m)}(t)<r+dr\}.$$

Define now the moment generating functions

$$F_i^{(m)}(s,t) = \int_0^\infty e^{rs}P_i^{(m)}(r,t)dr,$$

$$f_i^{(m)}(s,t) = \int_0^\infty e^{rs}p_i^{(m)}(r,m-1,t)dr;$$

multiply equations (15) and (16) by e^{rs}, then integrate equation

(15) from 0 to $t^i/i!$, equation (16) from $t^i/i!$ to ∞, and add the two results together,

$$\partial F_i{}^{(m)}/\partial t = -kX(t)[1-\exp(st^i/i!)]f_i{}^{(m)}(s,t).$$

From this equation, by differentiation, we get

$$\partial^2 F_i{}^{(m)}/\partial s\partial t = kX(t)\Big(t^i/i!.\exp(st^i/i!)f_i{}^{(m)}(s,t) -$$
$$- [1-\exp(st^i/i!)]\partial f_i{}^{(m)}/\partial s\Big)$$

$$\partial^3 F_i{}^{(m)}/\partial s^2\partial t =$$
$$= kX(t)\Big((t^i/i!)^2\exp(st^i/i!)f_i{}^{(m)}(s,t) +$$
$$+ 2t^i/i!.\exp(st^i/i!)\partial f_i{}^{(m)}/\partial s -$$
$$- [1-\exp(st^i/i!)]\partial^2 f_i{}^{(m)}/\partial s^2 ;$$

for s = 0 these two equations become

$$dE[N_i{}^{(m)}(t)]/dt = kX(t).t^i/i!.f_i{}^{(m)}(0,t),$$

$$dE[N_i{}^{(m)}(t)^2]/dt = kX(t).t^i/i![t^i/i!f_i{}^{(m)}(0,t) +$$
$$+ 2\partial f_i{}^{(m)}(0,t)/\partial s].$$

Observe that

$$f_i{}^{(m)}(0,t) = \int_0^\infty p_i{}^{(m)}(r,m-1,t)dr = \mathrm{Prob}\{N(t)\equiv m-1(\mathrm{mod}\ m)\}$$

and

$$\partial f_i{}^{(m)}(0,t)/\partial s = \int_0^\infty r p_i{}^{(m)}(r,m-1,t)dr$$
$$= E[N_i{}^{(m)}(t).N(t)\equiv m-1(\mathrm{mod}\ m)]$$
$$= E[N_i{}^{(m)}(t)/N(t)\equiv m-1(\mathrm{mod}\ m)].\mathrm{Prob}\{N(t)\equiv m-1(\mathrm{mod}\ m)\};$$

from section 9 we have

$$\mathrm{Prob}\{N(t)\equiv m-1(\mathrm{mod}\ m)\} = \sum_{j=1}^\infty p(jm-1,t)$$
$$= \exp[-\int_0^t kX(u)du]\sum_{j=1}^\infty [\int_0^t kX(u)du]^{jm-1}/(jm-1)!;$$

therefore,

(17) $$dE[N_i{}^{(m)}(t)]/dt =$$
$$= kX(t).t^i/i!.\exp[-\int_0^t kX(u)du].\sum_{j=1}^\infty [\int_0^t kX(u)du]^{jm-1}/(jm-1)!$$

$$dE[N_i{}^{(m)}(t)^2]/dt = dE[N_i{}^{(m)}(t)]/dt.$$

$$\cdot \left(t^i/i! + 2E[N_i{}^{(m)}(t)\,|\,N(t)\equiv m-1(\bmod m)]\right),$$

thence

$$dVar[N_i{}^{(m)}(t)]/dt = dE[N_i{}^{(m)}(t)^2]/dt -$$

$$- 2E[N_i{}^{(m)}(t)].dE[N_i{}^{(m)}(t)]/dt$$

(18) $dVar[N_i{}^{(m)}(t)]/dt = dE[N_i{}^{(m)}(t)]/dt.$

$$\cdot \left(t^i/i! + 2E[N_i{}^{(m)}(t)\,|\,N(t)\leq m-1(\bmod m)] - 2E[N_i{}^{(m)}(t)]\right).$$

13. An approximate solution

The two differential equations (17) and (18) must be solved to compute the values of $E[N_i(t)]$ and $Var[N_i(t)]$ from the measured values of $E[N_i{}^{(m)}(t)]$ and $Var[N_i{}^{(m)}(t)]$; we shall consider here only the first of the two.

Equation (17) can be written

(19) $dE[N_i{}^{(m)}(t)]/dt = 1/m.t^i/i!.kX(t).Y(f).\exp(-f),$

where

(20) $$Y(f) = m.\sum_{j=1}^{\infty} f^{jm-1}/(jm-1)!,$$

and

$$f(t) = \int_0^t kX(u)\,du$$

is the intensity of the Poisson random variable $N_0(t)$ as defined in section 9.

The function defined by equation (20) satisfies the differential equation

$$d^m Y/df^m = Y(f)$$

with the initial conditions

$$Y(0) = dY(0)/df = d^2Y(0)/df^2 = \ldots = d^{m-2}Y(0)/df^{m-2} = 0,$$

$$d^{m-1}Y(0)/df^{m-1} = 1.$$

We shall show here only a few particular solutions of the above equation, namely for $m = 2, 4, 8$, since the easiest scaling factors to implement are the powers of two.

$m = 2$: $Y(f) = \exp(f) - \exp(-f)$

$m = 4$: $Y(f) = \exp(f) - \exp(-f) - 2.\sin(f)$

$$m = 8: \quad Y(f) = \exp(f) - \exp(-f) - 2.\sin(f) -$$
$$- 2.\exp[-\sqrt{2}/2)f].\cos(\sqrt{2}/2.f-\pi/4) -$$
$$- 2.\exp[+\sqrt{2}/2)f].\sin(\sqrt{2}/2.f-\pi/4).$$

In all cases the product $Y(f).\exp(-f)$ rapidly approaches 1 when f increses; as a first approximation we can put

$$Y(f).\exp(-f) = 1$$

and equation (19) becomes

$$(21) \qquad dE[N_i^{(m)}(t)]/dt = 1/m.t^i/i!.kX(t),$$

thence

$$(22) \qquad E[N_i(t)] = m.E[N_i^{(m)}(t)];$$

thus the expected value of the random variable $N_i(t)$ is approximately equal to m times the expected value of $N_i^{(m)}(t)$. The goodness of this approximation depends on how fast f(t) increases and how fast $Y(f)$ approaches 1, and these of course depend on the particular function $kX(t)$ one is trying to evaluate.

As an example consider the function

$$kX(t) = 1 - \exp(-a.t);$$

tables I, II, III show the correct expected values of $N_0(t)$, $N_1(t)$, $N_2(t)$ for some selected values of a.t, together with the relative errors of the approximation given by equation (22).

TABLE I

Relative Errors in the
Evaluation of $E[N_0(t)]$ from $E[N_0^{(m)}(t)]$

a.t	Correct value	Error for m=2	Error for m=4	Error for m=8
5	4.007	.125	.381	.897
10	9.000	5.6×10^{-2}	.167	.379
20	19.000	2.6×10^{-2}	7.9×10^{-2}	.184
50	49.000	1.0×10^{-2}	3.1×10^{-2}	7.1×10^{-2}
100	99.000	5.1×10^{-3}	1.5×10^{-3}	3.5×10^{-2}
200	199.000	2.5×10^{-3}	7.5×10^{-3}	1.8×10^{-2}

TABLE II

Relative Errors in the
Evaluation of $E[N_1(t)]$ from $E[N_1^{(m)}(t)]$

a.t	Correct value	Error for m=2	Error for m=4	Error for m=8
5	11.541	4.7×10^{-2}	.216	.845
10	49.001	1.1×10^{-2}	4.8×10^{-2}	.146
20	199.000	2.8×10^{-3}	1.2×10^{-2}	4.1×10^{-2}
50	1249.000	4.4×10^{-4}	1.9×10^{-3}	6.6×10^{-3}
100	4999.000	1.1×10^{-4}	4.8×10^{-4}	1.6×10^{-3}
200	19999.000	2.8×10^{-5}	1.2×10^{-4}	4.1×10^{-4}

TABLE III

Relative Errors in the
Evaluation of $E[N_2(t)]$ from $E[N_2^{(m)}(t)]$

a.t	Correct value	Error for m=2	Error for m=4	Error for m=8
5	19.958	2.1×10^{-2}	.125	.803
10	165.671	2.5×10^{-3}	1.3×10^{-2}	1.2×10^{-2}
20	1332.33	3.1×10^{-4}	1.6×10^{-3}	5.1×10^{-3}
50	20832.33	2.0×10^{-5}	1.0×10^{-4}	4.2×10^{-4}
100	166665.7	5.4×10^{-6}	1.2×10^{-5}	5.2×10^{-5}
200	333332.0	1.5×10^{-6}	3.9×10^{-6}	5.2×10^{-6}

14. Other detection processes

The algorithm described in sections 11 and 12 was based on the
premise that the particles present in a particular location could be
counted individually. This is true for instance when detecting
photons with a photomultiplier; in this case $X(t)$ is the
instantaneous rate of production of photons and k the efficiency of
the detector; alternately one can regard $X(t)$ as the number of
photoemitting particles present and k the probability of detecting a
photon emitted per unit time per particle.

Section 12 shows how to reduce the losses due to the finite
resolving time of the registers when measuring high intensity
sources. Counting losses may be caused also by the finite resolving
time of the detector, even though this last time in general is
considerably shorter than that of the registers; this theory is well
known for the case of sources of constant intensity (Takacs, 1956),
but to our knowledge it has not been extended to the case of sources
of variable intensity yet.

A different interpretation of this algorithm is necessary if the detection process is done by measuring an instantaneous intensity instead of a sequence of separate events. Let Q be the integration time of the detector, i.e. the time necessary for the detector to complete a single measure; this time may depend upon the intensity X(t) of the quantity under observation. The registers corresponding to i=0, i=1, i=2, ..., are set to zero for t=0; then during each successive interval of time Q, not necessarily constant, the detector measures the quantity under observation, whose value varies from X(t) to X(t+Q), obtaining a value $kX(t+\vartheta Q)$, where k is the efficiency of the detector and ϑ is a number between 0 and 1; this value is multiplied by $Q.t^i/i!$ and the product added to the corresponding register; it follows that

$$N_i(0) = 0, \quad i = 0, 1, 2, \ldots$$

$$N_i(t+Q) = N_i(t) + k.X(t+\vartheta Q).Q.t^i/i! + o(Q),$$

where o(Q) is a quantity approaching zero when Q approaches zero. For Q sufficiently small,

$$dN_i(t)/dt = t^i/i!.kX(t),$$

and by integration we get for $N_i(t)$ the expected value found in section 10.

15. Truncated moments

The measurement of the moments with a minimum error requires that the integral in definition (2) converges rapidly enough during the time interval of the experiment; this is not always the case, and the problem of incomplete moments has been studied by many authors in different contexts (see for instance Isenberg, 1973).

One possible method for correcting the error introduced by the finiteness of the limits of integration in described here.

Because part of the information contained in F_i is missing, a reconstruction of the unknown function f(t) is possible only by making some additional hypotheses. For instance assume that

$$(23) \qquad f(t) = \sum_{i=1}^{n} b_i \exp(-a_i t),$$

where the b_i's and the a_i's are unspecified constants, with the only restriction that $a_i > 0$ and $b_i \neq 0$ for all i; this is the case when the system under observation is formed by a finite number of perfect compartments with different turnover times and is fed by an instantaneous injection; in other cases this provides a good approximation if the system is sufficiently "regular" and n is large enough.

There is no loss of generality if we consider all a_i's different. In some special cases it may be appropriate to use complex values for some of the a_i's and polynomials in t for some of the

b_i's; we shall not consider this possibility here, but it is not difficult to expand our treatment to that case.

According to the results of section 6, the moments of function $f(t)$ defined above are

$$F_j = \sum_{i=1}^{m} b_i/a_i^{j+1}; \quad j=0,1,2,\ldots$$

Define the persymmetric matrix (Sylvester, 1853)

$$P\{F\} = \begin{bmatrix} f(0) & F_0 & F_1 & \cdots & F_{j-1} \\ F_0 & F_1 & F_2 & \cdots & F_j \\ F_1 & F_2 & F_3 & \cdots & F_{j+1} \\ \cdots\cdots\cdots\cdots\cdots\cdots\cdots\cdots\cdots \\ F_{j-1} & F_j & F_{j+1} & \cdots & F_{2j-1} \end{bmatrix}$$

formed by the initial value of function $f(t)$ and by its moments F_0, $F_1,\ldots,$ where j is an arbitrary index not smaller than $n-1$. With the coefficients a_i we form the matrix

$$A = \begin{bmatrix} 1 & 1/a_1 & 1/a_1^2 & 1/a_1^3 & \cdots & 1/a_1^j \\ 1 & 1/a_2 & 1/a_2^2 & 1/a_2^3 & \cdots & 1/a_2^j \\ 1 & 1/a_3 & 1/a_3^2 & 1/a_3^3 & \cdots & 1/a_3^j \\ \cdots\cdots\cdots\cdots\cdots\cdots\cdots\cdots\cdots\cdots\cdots \\ 1 & 1/a_n & 1/a_n^2 & 1/a_n^3 & \cdots & 1/a_n^j \end{bmatrix};$$

the rank of A is n; in fact the determinant formed by the first n column of A is a Vandermonde determinant (Vandermonde, 1771; Cauchy, 1841) and is equal to the product of the differences, two by two, of the coefficients a_i, all different by hypothesis.

It is easy to check that

$$P\{F\} = A^{tr}.B.A,$$

where A^{tr} is the transpose of A, and B is the diagonal matrix

$$\begin{bmatrix} b_1 & 0 & 0 & \cdots & 0 \\ 0 & b_2 & 0 & \cdots & 0 \\ 0 & 0 & b_3 & \cdots & 0 \\ 0 & 0 & 0 & \cdots & b_n \end{bmatrix}$$

formed by the coefficients b_i. From the hypothesis on those coefficients this last matrix is non-singular, therefore the rank of $P\{F\}$ is also n.

If we make $j=n$, the kernel of $P\{F\}$ is the vector C formed by the coefficients $c_0, c_1, c_2, \ldots, c_n$ of the polynomial

$$c_0 + c_1 x + c_2 x^2 + \ldots + c_n x^n = (x-1/a_1)\ldots(x-1/a_n);$$

in fact the product of the matrix formed by any $n+1$ consecutive columns of A by vector C is identically zero, therefore

$$A.C = 0$$

thence

$$P\{F\}.\underline{C} = \underline{0}.$$

If the moments of $f(t)$ were known, from vector $\underline{C}$ we could compute the coefficients a_i; in the present situation the moments F_0, F_1, ... are unknown, but the truncated moments

$$G_i = \int_0^T t^i/i! \; f(t)dt \quad i=0,1,2,...$$

are known in their stead, with T a finite value of t such that $f(T)$ is different from zero. The differences

$$F_i - G_i = H_i$$

are the moments of the unknown tail of $f(t)$, i.e.

$$H_i = \int_T^\infty t^i/i! \; f(t)dt.$$

If the tail of $f(t)$ is shifted toward the origin and the moments of this new function are called $H_i{}^*$, then

$$H_i{}^* = \int_0^\infty t^i/i! \; f(t+T)dt;$$

from the previous equation, with a change of variable,

$$H_i = \int_0^\infty (t+T)^i/i! \; f(t+T)dt$$
$$= \sum_{j=0}^i T^j/j! \int_0^\infty t^{i-j}/(i-j)! \; f(t+T)dt$$
$$= H_i{}^* + T.H_{i-1}{}^* + T^2/2!.H_{i-2}{}^* + ... +$$
$$+ T^i/i!.H_0{}^*. \quad i=0,1,2,...$$

According to assumption (23) the moments $H_i{}^*$ are the moments of

$$\sum_{i=1}^m b_i exp[-a_i(t+T)] = \sum_{i=1}^m b_i exp(-a_i T) exp(-a_i t),$$

therefore

$$P\{H^*\} = \underline{A}^{tr}.\underline{B}^*.\underline{A},$$

where $\underline{B}^*$ is the diagonal matrix formed by the coefficients $b_1 exp(-a_1 T)$, $b_2 exp(-a_2 T)$,... It follows that the kernels of $P\{H^*\}$ and of $P\{H\}$ are the same.

The kernel of a matrix does not change if that matrix is multiplied by a non-singular matrix; also in general the difference of two matrices with the same kernel has the same kernel; therefore the kernel of

$$P\{F\} - T.P\{H^*\},$$

where

$$T = \begin{bmatrix} 1 & 0 & 0 & 0 & \cdots \\ T & 1 & 0 & 0 & \cdots \\ T^2/2! & T & 1 & 0 & \cdots \\ T^3/3! & T^2/2! & T & 1 & \cdots \\ \cdots\cdots\cdots\cdots\cdots\cdots\cdots\cdots \end{bmatrix},$$

is always $\underline{C}$.

The element in row i and column j of matrix $P\{F\} - \underline{T}.P\{H^*\}$ is

$$G_{i+j} + \sum_{l=i+1}^{i+j} H_{i+j-1}{}^*T^l/l! \qquad i=0,1,2,\ldots; \; j=1,2,\ldots$$

The kernel of a matrix does not change if from the elements of a row we subtract the corresponding elements of another row multiplied by the same quantity. Now from row i subtract the previous one multiplied by $T/(i+1)$; from row i of the new matrix subtract the previous one multiplied by $iT/(i+1)(i+2)$; from row i of this new matrix subtract the previous one multiplied by $iT/(i+2)(i+3)$, and so forth. All these transformations do not change the kernel of the original persymmetric matrix; the new matrices are not persymmetric any more, but after each transformation one of the unknown moments disappears. By induction we can prove that after m such transformations the element of row i (i>m) and column j (j>0) is

$$\sum_{l=0}^{i+j} (-1)^l \binom{m}{l} \Big/ \binom{i+m}{l} T^l/l! . G_{i+j-1} + \text{terms with } H_0, H_1, \ldots, H_{j-m}.$$

By making m=n the rows from the n down contain only the truncated moments of f(t), which are known.

If enough truncated moments of f(t) have been measured, the transformations above can be repeated until one finds a singular matrix, or one with a determinant sufficiently small to consider it singular within the bounds of the expected experimental errors. The kernel of that matrix is the vector $\underline{C}$, and from it the coefficients a_i can be computed. Using again assumption (23), the truncated moments of f(t) are

$$G_j = \sum_{i=1}^{n} b_i/a_i [1/a_i{}^j - (1/a_i{}^{j+1}/a_i{}^{j-1}.T+$$

$$+ 1/a_i{}^{j-2}.T^2/2!+\ldots+T^j/j!)\exp(-T/a_i)]; \quad j=0,1,2,\ldots$$

these are linear expressions in the b_i's; if the G_j's are measured and the a_i's are computed, the b_i's can be determined from n of those equations.

16. Use of the moments

It is a well known fact that, in general, a function is uniquely determined by its moments (Wald, 1939). Even if only few of its moments are known, a function can be reconstructed with some accuracy using Chebyshev's inequality and its generalizations.

From what said above it should be clear that with this method we can store a maximum amount of information, thence reconstruct the function $kX(t)$; but more important is the fact that this information is already coded for the analysis as described in section 8.

As an example consider the measurement of local blood flow with a tracer; most methods relate back to the original Kety-Schmidt (1948) equation

(24) $$dQ_b/dt = F(C_a-C_v),$$

where
  Q_b = amount of tracer in the organ,
  C_a, C_v = arterial and venous concentrations of the tracer,
  F = flow rate of blood through the organ;
this equation states simply that the amount of tracer circulating through the organ is conserved. An additional assumption is usually made, i.e.

(25) $$Q_b = LWC_v,$$

where
  W = volume of the organ,
  L = partition coefficient between organ and blood.

This assumption implies that the amount of tracer present in the organ is simply proportional to the venous concentration. From this assumption follows

(26) $$dQ_b/dt + F/(LW).Q_b = F.C_a.$$

This is the equation of a single compartment of volume W and turnover rate LW/F. By measuring the arterial concentration C_a of the tracer and the organ concentration Q_b/W of the same tracer, with a simple operation one could compute the partition coefficient L and the blood flow rate per unit volume of organ F/W, provided the hypotheses formalized by equations (24) and (25) are valid.

Calling C_b the concentration of the tracer in the organ, and f the blood flow rate per unit volume of tissue,

$$C_b = Q_b/W,$$

$$f = F/W,$$

the differential equation (26) becomes

$$dC_b/dt + f/L.C_b = fC_a.$$

Supposing $C_b = 0$ at $t = 0$ and f constant, then

(27) $$C_b(t) = f\int_0^t C_a(u)\exp[-f/L.(t-u)]du.$$

Observe now that equation (27) is a special case of equation (1); calling A_0, A_1, ..., B_0, B_1, ... the successive moments of C_a and C_b respectively, then, using the results of section 5,

$B_0 = L.A_0$

$B_1 = L.A_1 + L^2/f.A_0$

$B_2 = L.A_2 + L^2/f.A_1 + L^3/f^2.A_0$

$B_3 = L.A_3 + L^2/f.A_2 + L^3/f^2.A_1 + L^4/f^3.A_0.$

In particular these equations show that L is the zeroth moment, L/f the first relative moment, $(L/f)^2$ the second relative moment,... of the function describing the blood flow through the organ. A check on these last equations can tell whether the assumptions embodied in equations (24) and (25) were warranted. When they are not, then the moments above still have a clearly defined physical meaning: L is the fraction of tracer particles transferred from the arterial blood to the organ, f/L is the average time spent by a tracer particle in the organ, and so forth.

With a non-diffusible tracer, equation (1) still describes the circulation through an organ; more specifically we can write, with Meier and Zierler (1954),

$$V = f.<t>,$$

where V = volume of distribution of the tracer,
      f = volumetric flow rate of the intravascular fluid,
      <t>= mean transit time of the tracer in the organ;
this equation simply states that the tracer is conserved, i.e. that what is perfused into an organ must sooner or later be washed out. Now <t>, the mean transit time, is directly measurable (the First Relative Moment), the volume of distribution V is also directly measurable (the Zeroth Moment), therefore f can be computed. Additionally, the higher moments can be used to describe the distribution of the actual transit times of the tracer through the organ. This last datum may be important because of the possibility that, in some pathological cases, there may be a considerable increase in the variance of those times without a corresponding change in their mean value.

17. Multidimensional moments

The next step is the extention of this algorithm to a larger number of dimensions (Rescigno, 1979). If the function $f(t,x,y,z)$ describes a state variable (concentration of a drug, activity of a tracer, intensity of a light source, etc.) at time t at a point of coordinates x,y,z, then define the moments

$$F_{ijkl} = \iiiint t^i x^j y^k z^l f(t,x,y,z)\, dt\, dx\, dy\, dz \qquad i,j,k,l=0,1,2,\ldots$$

and the relative moments

$$f_{ijkl} = F_{ijkl}/F_{oooo},$$

where the integral above is extended to the whole domain where the function has positive values; obviously the set F_{oooo}, F_{1ooo}, F_{2ooo}, ... coincides with the moments defined before. The values of the four-dimensional moments F_{ijkl} ($i,j,k,l = 0,1,2,\ldots$) can be measured using separate registers that accumulate the instantaneous values of f multiplied by the appropriate powers of the coordinates (both spatial and temporal) of the point under observation; the reconstruction of $f(t,x,y,z)$ from these moments should be made with a method analogous with the one described for fewer dimensions (Rescigno, 1984). But here again the main problem rather than the reconstruction of the function $f(t,x,y,z)$ is the determination of some of its parameters, as described in section 8, and this could be done in a most efficient and direct way by using the moments of the function.

It is impossible to examine here all properties of these moments, but a few examples should give a general idea of their possible uses.

18. Moments of a "box"

Consider for instance the function

$$f(t,x,y,z) = g(t) \quad \text{for } x_1 < x < x_2,\ y_1 < y < y_2,\ z_1 < z < z_2$$
$$= 0 \quad \text{everywhere else;}$$

then the moment F_{ijkl} of this function is

$$\frac{x_2^{j+1}-x_1^{j+1}}{(j+1)!} \cdot \frac{y_2^{k+1}-y_1^{k+1}}{(k+1)!} \cdot \frac{z_2^{l+1}-z_1^{l+1}}{(l+1)!} \cdot G_i,$$

and the relative moment f_{ijkl} is

$$\frac{x_1^p x_2^{j-p}}{(j+1)!} \cdot \frac{y_1^p y_2^{k-p}}{(k+1)!} \cdot \frac{z_1^p z_2^{l-p}}{(l+1)!} \cdot g_i,$$

where G_i and g_i are, respectively, the one-dimensional moment and relative moment of the one-variable function $g(t)$.

Specifically we have

$$F_{oooo} = (x_2-x_1)(y_2-y_1)(z_2-z_1)G_o,$$

$$f_{i000} = g_i, \quad i=1,2,\ldots$$

$$f_{0100} = (x_1+x_2)/2,$$

$$f_{0010} = (y_1+y_2)/2,$$

$$f_{0001} = (z_1+z_2)/2,$$

$$f_{0200} = (x_1^2+x_1x_2+x_2^2)/3!,$$

$$f_{0110} = (x_1+x_2)/2.(y_1+y_2)/2,$$

$$f_{0101} = (x_1+x_2)/2.(z_1+z_2)/2,$$

$$f_{0020} = (y_1^2+y_1y_2+y_2^2)/3!,$$

$$f_{0011} = (y_1+y_2)/2.(z_1+z_2)/2,$$

$$f_{0002} = (z_1^2+z_1z_2+z_2^2)/3!;$$

therefore the relative moments f_{i000} are the relative moments of $g(t)$; the first order relative moments f_{0100}, f_{0010}, f_{0001} are the coordinates of the center of the "box"; from the second order relative moments f_{0200}, f_{0020}, f_{0002} the coordinates x_1, x_2, y_1, y_2, z_1, z_2, can be computed. The second order relative moments f_{0110}, f_{0101}, f_{0011} must be the products of the corresponding first order relative moments, and can be used to verify whether $f(t,x,y,z)$ is the box function hypothesized.

19. Multiple boxes

This problem can easily be extended to the case when $f(t,x,y,z)$ is formed by a number of "boxes", each of them defined by a one-variable state function $g_i(t)$, i.e.

$$f(t,x,y,z) = g_i(t) \quad \text{for } x_{i1}<x<x_{i2}, \; y_{i1}<y<y_{i2},$$
$$z_{i1}<z<z_{i2}, \; i=1,2,\ldots$$
$$= 0 \quad \text{everywhere else.}$$

Without restricting our treatment to a specific number of dimensions, let us first enumerate the different moments of order k of a function of n variables. Each moment of order k in n dimensions is represented by a capital letter with the subscripts i_1, i_2, $\ldots$, i_n, those subscripts being non-negative integers such that

$$i_1 + i_2 + \ldots + i_n = k;$$

the number of different strings of subscripts with these properties is equal to the number of different combinations with repetition of k objects chosen among n objects, i.e.

$$C_k{}^n = \binom{n + k - 1}{k}.$$

To enumerate the moments of order up to k, we construct all possible lists i_0, i_1, i_2, ..., i_n of non-negative integers such that

$$i_0 + i_1 + i_2 + ... + i_n = k,$$

where i_1, i_2, ..., i_n are the actual subscripts of the moment, and i_0 is the difference between the maximum order k and the actual order of the moment; the number of different lists with these properties is equal to the number of different combinations with repetition of k objects chosen among $n+1$ objects, i.e.

$$C_k{}^{n+1} = \binom{n + k}{k}.$$

Tables IV and V show the values of these coefficients for some selected values of n and k.

If the function considered is formed by b different boxes in n dimensions, the unknown data of the system are $2.b.n$ spacial coordinates of the boxes, plus $(k+1).b$ moments of the one-variable functions of the separate boxes, where k is the order of the highest moment considered. The problem is determined if the available moments

TABLE IV

Number of moments of order k in n dimensions

k	n = 1	2	3	4	5
0	1	1	1	1	1
1	1	2	3	4	5
2	1	3	6	10	15
3	1	4	10	20	35
4	1	5	15	35	70
5	1	6	21	56	126
6	1	7	28	84	210
7	1	8	36	120	330
8	1	9	45	165	495
9	1	10	55	220	715
10	1	11	66	286	1001
11	1	12	78	364	1365
12	1	13	91	455	1820

TABLE V

Number of moments of order up to k in n dimensions

k	n = 1	2	3	4	5
0	1	1	1	1	1
1	2	3	4	5	6
2	3	6	10	15	21
3	4	10	20	35	56
4	5	15	35	70	126
5	6	21	56	126	252
6	7	28	84	210	462
7	8	36	120	330	792
8	9	45	165	495	1287
9	10	55	220	715	2002
10	11	66	286	1001	3003
11	12	78	364	1365	4368
12	13	91	455	1820	6188

TABLE VI

Number of boxes identifiable with moments up to order k

k	n = 2	3	4	5
1	<1	<1	<1	<1
2	<1	1+	1+	1+
3	1+	2	2+	4
4	1+	3+	5+	8+
5	2+	4+	9	15+
6	2+	6+	14	27+
7	3	8+	20+	44
8	3+	11	29+	67+
9	3+	13+	39+	100+
10	4+	16+	52+	143
11	4+	20+	68+	198+
12	5+	23+	86+	269+

are not fewer that the unknown parameters, i.e. if

$$\binom{n + k}{k} \geqq 2.b.n + (k+1).b.$$

Table VI shows how many boxes can be identified for different values of n and k.

20. Reconstruction of a function

It is known that under very general conditions a function is uniquely determined by all its moments (Wald, 1939). The reconstruction of a function with any degree of accuracy is therefore possible if enough moments are known.

Suppose that a function can be written in operational form as the ratio of two polynomials in s,

$$(28) \qquad \{f(t)\} = \frac{p_{n-1}s^{n-1}+p_{n-2}s^{n-2}+\ldots+p_1s+p_0}{s^n+q_{n-1}s^{n-1}+\ldots+q_1s+q_0}$$

where s is the differential operator and the p's and the q's are arbitrary constants; then from a well known theorem of the operational calculus (Mikusinsky, 1959),

$$(29) \qquad \{f\} = F_0 - F_1s + F_2s^2 - F_3s^3 + \ldots ;$$

equating expressions (28) and (29) we can write the two sets of equations

$$(30) \quad \begin{cases} F_0q_0 = p_0 \\[4pt] F_0q_1 - F_1q_0 = p_1 \\[4pt] F_0q_2 - F_1q_1 + F_2q_0 = p_2 \\[4pt] \cdots\cdots\cdots\cdots\cdots\cdots\cdots \\[4pt] F_0q_{n-1} - F_1q_{n-2} + F_2q_{n-3} - \cdots \\[2pt] \qquad\qquad \cdots + (-1)^{n-1}F_{n-1}q_0 = p_{n-1} \end{cases}$$

$$\begin{cases} F_0 - F_1q_{n-1} + F_2q_{n-2} - \cdots + (-1)^{n}F_nq_0 = 0 \\[4pt] -F_1 + F_2q_{n-1} - F_3q_{n-2} + \cdots + (-1)^{n+1}F_{n+1}q_0 = 0 \\[4pt] F_2 - F_3q_{n-1} + F_4q_{n-2} - \cdots + (-1)^{n+2}F_{n+2}q_0 = 0. \\[4pt] \cdots\cdots\cdots\cdots\cdots\cdots\cdots\cdots\cdots\cdots \end{cases}$$

This second set of equations has a unique non-trivial solution for the constants $q_0, q_1, \ldots, q_{n-1}$ if the persymmetric matrix (see section 15)

$$P\{F\} = \begin{bmatrix} F_1 & F_2 & F_3 & \cdots & F_n \\ F_2 & F_3 & F_4 & \cdots & F_{n+1} \\ F_3 & F_4 & F_5 & \cdots & F_{n+2} \\ \cdots\cdots\cdots\cdots\cdots\cdots\cdots\cdots\cdots \\ F_n & F_{n+1} & F_{n+2} & \cdots & F_{2n-1} \end{bmatrix}$$

is non-singular. In the unlikely event that this matrix is singular,
it can be made non-singular by reducing n, i.e. by taking a smaller
number of moments. Once the q's have been computed from the second
set of equations, the p's can be computed from the first set
sequentially starting with p_0 and ending with p_{n-1}.

This algorithm is practical only if few moments have been
observed and the function $f(t)$ is very "smooth" and can conveniently
be represented by a sum of exponential functions. The following
section shows a more general method.

21. A more general reconstruction algorithm

The general problem is to determine a function $f(t)$ with the
given moments $F_0, F_1, \ldots, F_{n-1}$.

First, choose a weighting function $g(t)$, then determine a set of
functions $f_0(t), f_1(t), \ldots, f_{n-1}(t)$ such that the zero-moment
of $f_0(t)g(t)$, the first moment of $f_1(t)g(t)$, the second moment of
$f_2(t)g(t), \ldots$, the $(n-1)$-moment of $f_{n-1}(t)g(t)$ are equal to one,
while all other moments up to order $n-1$ of these functions are zero.
It follows that

$$f(t) = \sum_{i=0}^{n-1} F_i . f_i(t) g(t)$$

has the moments $F_0, F_1, F_2, \ldots, F_{n-1}$.

For the functions $f_i(t)$ we can choose polynomials in t of
degree $n-1$, thus

$$f_i(t) = \sum_{l=0}^{n-1} a_{il} t^l / l! \quad i=0,1,\ldots,n-1$$

therefore

$$\int_0^\infty \sum_{l=0}^{n-1} a_{il} t^l / l! \; t^j / j! \; g(t) dt = 1 \text{ for } i=j$$
$$= 0 \text{ for } i=j;$$

this equation can be written

$$\underline{A} \cdot \underline{T} = \underline{I},$$

where

$$A = \begin{bmatrix} a_{00} & a_{01} & \cdots & a_{0,n-1} \\ a_{10} & a_{11} & \cdots & a_{1,n-1} \\ \cdots\cdots\cdots\cdots\cdots\cdots\cdots\cdots\cdots \\ a_{n-1,0} & a_{n-1,1} & \cdots & a_{n-1,n-1} \end{bmatrix}$$

is the n x n matrix of the coefficients of the functions to be
determined,

$$(31) \qquad \underline{T} = \left[\binom{i+j}{i} \int_0^\infty \frac{t^{i+j}}{(i+j)!} g(t) dt \right] \quad i,j=0,1,2,\ldots,n-1$$

is the symmetric matrix of the moments of the weighting function $g(t)$ multiplied by the binomial coefficients, and I is the identity matrix.

Obviously

$$A = T^{-1},$$

but it is not necessary to invert matrix T to determine function $f(t)$. In fact

$$f(t) = \sum_{i=0}^{n-1} F_i f_i(t) g(t)$$

$$= \sum_{i,j=0}^{n-1} F_i a_{ij} t^j / j! \, g(t)$$

$$= F.A.[1 \; t \; t^2/2! \; \ldots \; t^{n-1}/(n-1)!]^{tr}.g(t),$$

where the penultimate factor is a column vector formed with the successive powers of the variable t. The unknown product $F.A$ can be determined by solving equation

(32) $(F.A).T = F,$

where both T and F are given.

The meaning of the weighting function $g(t)$ needs some explanations. The first reason for introducing this function is that otherwise the functions $f_i(t)$, as chosen, would not have finite moments; but there is another reason, less obvious but fundamental, for the presence of $g(t)$. As only a finite number of moments are known, there are infinitely many different functions with those moments; the solution found here is correct in the sense that $f(t)$, as computed, has exactly the moments F_0, F_1, F_2, ..., F_{n-1}, as given. Additionally, we impose on $f(t)$ a condition of "regularity", i.e. we want $f(t)$ to be as close as possible to a "model" function, in this case $g(t)$.

For example, suppose that the following moments are given:

$F_0 = 1.5$
$F_1 = 1.75$
$F_2 = 1.875$
$F_3 = 1.9375$
$F_4 = 1.96875;$

if for the weighting function we choose the exponential function

$$g(t) = \exp(-t),$$

from definition (31) we get

$$T = \begin{bmatrix} 1 & 1 & 1 & 1 & 1 \\ 1 & 2 & 3 & 4 & 5 \\ 1 & 3 & 6 & 10 & 15 \\ 1 & 4 & 10 & 20 & 35 \\ 1 & 5 & 15 & 35 & 70 \end{bmatrix},$$

and from equation (32)

$$\underline{F}.\underline{A} = [1.0312 \quad 0.8125 \quad -0.5000 \quad 0.1875 \quad -0.03125].$$

Suppose now that for $g(t)$ we choose the "gate" function

$$g(t) = 1 \text{ for } 0<t<1$$
$$= 0 \text{ elsewhere;}$$

from definition (31) we get

$$\underline{T} = \begin{bmatrix} 1 & 1/2 & 1/3 & 1/4 & 1/5 \\ 1/2 & 2/3 & 3/4 & 4/5 & 5/6 \\ 1/3 & 3/4 & 6/5 & 5/3 & 15/7 \\ 1/4 & 4/5 & 5/3 & 20/7 & 35/8 \\ 1/5 & 5/6 & 15/7 & 35/8 & 70/9 \end{bmatrix}$$

and from equation (32)

$$\underline{F}.\underline{A} = [0.2669 \quad 2.522 \quad -0.07097 \quad -0.02312 \quad 0.008648].$$

These two solutions lead to the two functions

$$f(t) = (1.0312 + 0.8125.t - 0.25.t^2 + 0.0312.t^3 - 0.00135.t^4).\exp(-t)$$

and

$$f(t) = 0.2669 + 2.522.t - 0.03548.t^2 - 0.00385.t^3 + 0.0003603.t^4 \qquad \text{for } 0\leq t\leq 1$$
$$= 0 \quad \text{for } t>1$$

respectively; both functions have the same moments up to the fourth. Of course the higher the number of moments specified, the closer the solving functions will be, irrespective of the weighting function.

On the other hand, using the algorithm of section 20 we find that the persymmetric matrix of order 3 of the given moments is singular, therefore function $f(t)$ can be represented by operator 28 with $n=2$, and solving equations 30 and the following ones we obtain

$$\{f(t)\} = (s + 3)/(s^2 + 3 s + 2)$$

or

$$f(t) = 2.e^{-t} - e^{-2t}.$$

22. References

J. S. Beck and A. Rescigno, 1970. Calcium Kinetics: The Philosophy and Practice of Science. Phys. Med. Biol. 15:566.

A. L. Cauchy, 1841. Exercices d'Analyse et de Physique Mathématique. Paris. Page 151.

J. B. Fourier, 1822. Théorie Analytique de la Chaleur. Paris. Page 212.

I. Isenberg, R. D. Dyson and R. Hanson, 1973. Studies on the Analysis of Fluorescence Decay Data by the Method of Moments. Biophys. J. 13:1090.

S. S. Kety and C. F. Schmidt, 1948. The Nitrous Oxide Method for the Quantitative Determination of Cerebral Blood Flow in Man. J. Clin. Invest. 27:476.

J. H. Matis and H. O. Hartley, 1971. Stochastic Compartmental Analysis. Biometrics 27:77.

J. Mikusinsky, 1959. Operational Calculus. Pergamon Press, New York.

P. Meier and K. L. Zierler, 1954. On the Theory of Indicator-Dilution Method for Measurement of Blood Flow and Volume. J. Applied Physiol. 6:731.

P. Purdue, 1974. Stochastic Theory of Compartments. Bull. Math. Biol. 36:305.

A. Rescigno, 1973. On Transfer Times in Tracer Experiments. J. Theoret. Biol. 39:9.

A. Rescigno, 1979. The Two-variable Operational Calculus in the Construction of Compartmental Ecological Models. In Compartmental Analysis of Ecosystem Models (Matis, Patten and White editors). International Cooperative Publishing House, Burtonsville, Maryland. Page 335.

A. Rescigno, 1984. Multidimensional Operators for the Construction of Mathematical Models. In Modeling and Analysis in Biomedicine (C. Nicolini editor). World Scientific Publishing Company, Singapore.

A. Rescigno and J. H. Matis, 1981. On the Relevance of Stochastic Compartmental Models to Pharmacokinetic Systems. Bull. Math. Biol. 42:245.

A. Rescigno and L. D. Michels, 1973. On Dispersion in Tracer Experiments. J. Theoret. Biol. 41:451.

A. Rescigno and G. Segre, 1961. The Precursor-Product Relationship. J. Theoret. Biol. 1:498.

A. Rescigno and G. Segre, 1964. Drug and Tracer Kinetics. Blaisdell, Waltham, Massachusetts.

J. J. Sylvester, 1853. Philosophical Transactions of the Royal Society of London 143:424 and 546.

L. Takacs, 1956. On a Probability Problem Arising in the Theory of Counters. Proc. Cambridge Philosophical Society 52:488.

A. K. Thakur, A. Rescigno and D. A. Schafer, 1972. On the Stochastic Theory of Compartments. Bull. Math. Biol. 34:53.

A. T. Vandermonde, 1771. Histoire de l'Académie Royale des Sciences. Paris. Page 369.

J. G. Wagner, 1971. Biopharmaceutics and Relevant Pharmacokinatics. Drug Intelligence, Hamilton, Illinois.

A. Wald, 1939. Limits of a Distribution Function Determined by Absolute Moments and Inequalities Satisfied by Absolute Moments. Trans. Amer. Math. Soc. 46:280.

K. Weierstrass, 1885. Sitzungberichte der preuss. Akademie der Wissenschaften. Berlin.

CHEMICAL SHIFT IMAGING

Derek Shaw
I. G. E. Medical Systems,
260, Bath Road,
Slough,
Berkshire, SL1 4ER.
U.K.

Until the 1980s the main use of nuclear magnetic resonance has been as a chemical analytical technique. The sample was homogenous, usually being a solution of the material of interest in a suitable solvent. The end product was a high resolution spectrum, i.e., one containing many narrow lines exhibiting chemical shift and coupling constant effects, and was used for structural analysis or quantification. In the 70s several groups found that living tissue, if suitably mounted, could give spectra which showed chemical shift effects. Suitable mounting meant that the tissue could be fitted into a conventional NMR tube of 10mm or so diameter and kept alive. Using this approach very elegant results on muscle metabolisms were obtained using ^{31}P.N.M.R. (1).

In 1973 Lauterbur demonstrated (2) that by applying magnetic field gradients spatial information could be encoded onto an N.M.R. signal and an image produced. This led, after a slow start, to the development of the new imaging modality of Magnetic Resonance Imaging, MRI.

As will be discussed later, the pulse sequences used collected data in such a way that chemical shift information was suppressed. The tissue discrimination, or contrast, in an MR imaging coming from differences in nuclear density and relaxation times, not chemical shifts (3). The concepts of spectroscopy and imaging seemed divergent.

The incompatability of imaging and spectroscopy was compounded by their differing instrumental requirements. Spectroscopy required high (> 1T) uniform magnetic fields, while imaging used large low field magnets (~ 0.1 to 0.3T) of limited homogeneity. Furthermore, the nuclei used differed, in vivo spectroscopy utilising mainly ^{31}P while MRI used protons. The former being too insensitive for imaging of metalites in a reasonable time, the latter having the sensitivity and hence speed of data collection appropriate for imaging, but showing no chemical shift effects with the fields used for imaging.

In the late 1970s superconducting magnets became available which could produce fields in the 1.5 - 2T region of sufficient homogeneity for NMR spectroscopy and large enough to contain a whole animal, not just a small excised part. Clearly, in order to obtain meaningful spectroscopic results from what was now an inhomogenous sample, localisation of the signal had to be achieved. Localisation was

T. Axenrod and G. Ceccarelli (eds.), NMR in Living Systems, 157–168.
© *1986 by D. Reidel Publishing Company.*

was initially achieved by restricting the volume of the sample from which
signal can be obtained. This was done by means of surface coils with
their restricted field of view (4) and by limiting the volume of field
within the magnet which was sufficiently homogenous to produce a signal,
Topical Magnetic Resonance (TMR) (5). Both these methods are effective,
essentially simple but suffer from physical inconvenience, e.g., the
sensitive volume for TMR must be at the magnet centre.

Despite early pessimism, it has become clear in recent years that
proton imaging is not only possible at fields in the region of 1.5T, but
in many aspects is superior in performance to imaging at lower fields
(6). The techniques of spectroscopy and imaging thus become magnet
compatible, and the combining of the two techniques becomes possible.
This chapter is concerned with methods of combining the two techniques,
especially from the view point of studying in vivo chemistry. The
approach will be to discuss how chemical shift information can be
encoded onto image data, rather than how can gradient be used to define
a sensitive volume, or what is the clinical relevance of the data.

A.   BASIC MAGNETIC RESONANCE IMAGING

The basic pulse sequence used in most MRI systems is shown for the case
of 2D or planar imaging in Figure 1. The first part of the sequence
selects a plane (x, y) by using a selective 90° pulse, i.e., one with a
narrow frequency band-width, in the presence of a field gradient (g_z).
x and y information has now to be superimposed onto the signal.

The necessary presence of a gradient during the slice selection
period produces unwanted spin dephasing and a consequent loss of signal.
This dephasing can be recovered by applying a gradient of the opposite
sign and about $\frac{1}{2}$ the value (or duration) which causes refocussing (7).
Such a gradient is termed a time reversal gradient, since it can be
considered as reversing time for the dephasing caused by the gradient.

In the **original** method of Lauterbur (2) this x,y encoding was
achieved by collecting the data in the presence of two gradients, g_x
cos θ and g_y sin θ and obtaining, after Fourier transformation, a
projection of the sample on an axis at θ with respect to the x axis.
By varying θ a series of projection were produced and an image produced
by method of filtered back projection. This approach is no longer much
used as it is more susceptible to instrumental imperfections such as
magnet inhomogeneity than the 2D method (8). The 2D FT imaging
technique arose as an extension of R. Ernst's work on 2D NMR described
elsewhere (9, 10). In the original Ernst 2D imaging concept (11) the
spins were allowed to precess in different gradients g_y and g_x for the
two time periods t_1 and t_2 of a 2D NMR experiment. Following a 2D
transform with respect to t_1 and t_2 a data array, which is a function
of two frequencies, W_1 and W_2, is produced. Since the data was
collected in the presence of a gradient, to a first approximation, (see
later) these frequencies are a function of spatial position and hence
this data is in effect an image of nuclear magnetisation in the x y
plane.

Data is only collected during the time t_2; information concerning

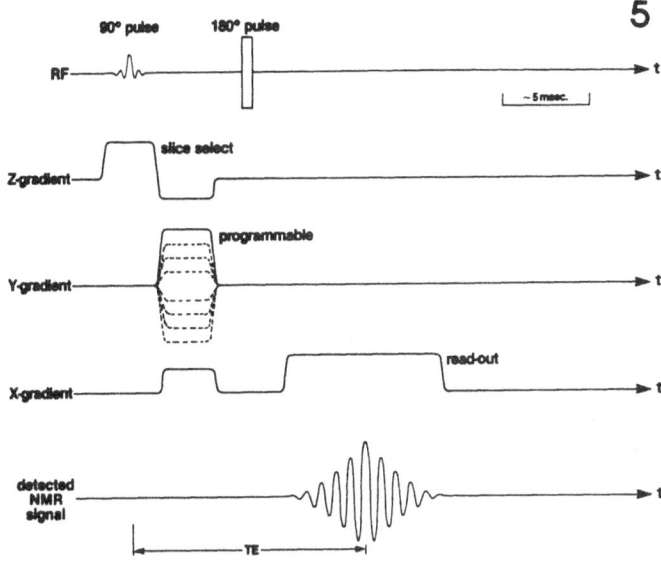

Fig. 1.   The Spin Warp imaging Sequence

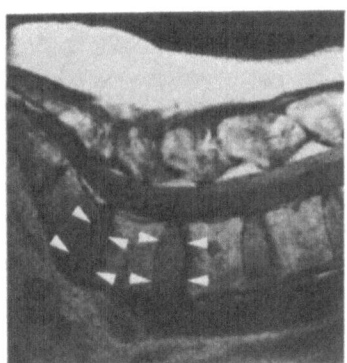

Fig. 2. 1.5T sagittal image of the lumbar spine. Note chemical shift
         effects in the readout direction (x) causing artifactural voids
         (arrows). (Reproduced by permission of G. E. Medical Systems).

the behaviour of the spins in the time period t_1 is phase encoded onto
the data collected during t_2. Phase encoding can also be achieved by
keeping t_2 constant and varying g_y, since it is the product of $t_2 \times g_y$
which defines the phase change introduced. This is the so called spin
warp method (12) which is illustrated in Figure 1. Fixing t_1 and
varying g_y has many practical advantages and the spin warp variation of
2D FT imaging is the one most frequently used.

The pulse sequence shown in Figure 1 contains two further very
important features from a practical viewpoint. Gradients and receivers
do not switch instantaneously, it is therefore advantageous to collect
data array parts of the sequence involving switching.. This is achieved
by generating a field echo which produces the signal some time after the
application of the read gradient. In the period following slice
selection when the time reversal and phase encoding gradients are being
applied (t_1) the third, i.e., read, gradient is also applied; this
causes dephaing with respect to the x axis. At the end of this period,
when g_y and g_z are switched off, the polarity of g_x is reversed (by a
180° pulse applied to the spins for reasons discussed below) and a field
echo is produced. The reason for using a 180° pulse instead of simply
reversing the sign of g_x is that it generates a spin echo which
refocusses magnet inhomogeneity effects. The timings and values of the
gradient used are such that the spin and field echoes occur
simultaneously and this is the data collected.

The full procedure for obtaining an image with m x n points, i.e.,
m rows of n points (columns) is

1. Select slice.

2. Phase encode y information with g_y.
    Refocus slice selection gradient, etc. $\Big\}$——— t_1

3. Collect n data points in presence g_x.   ------- t_2

4. Increment g_y.

5. Wait until time TR and repeat steps 1 to 4 m times.

The waiting time TR is determined by the degree of saturation, i.e.
T_1 weighting required in the image and is typically in the second region
(3). Steps 1 through 4 take only 10s of msec.. The time t_2 required
for data collection is by Niquest theory the signal bandwidth/2 number
of x points (19). As discussed below, bandwidths are in the 10s of KHz
range and n typically being 256; t_2 is thus t_2 is a few msecs. It
follows therefore that total imaging time is insensitive to the number
of x data points but directly related to the number of y points, i.e.,
total imaging time, ignoring any averaging, is m x TR.

B. THE EFFECT OF THE CHEMICAL SHIFT

The effect of the chemical shift on an image obtained by the spin warp method described above depends on three things. The magnitude of the chemical shift itself measured in Hz, magnet homogeneity and the strength of the read gradient used.

The gradient strength is determined by the homogeneity of the magnet. The gradient has to be sufficiently large to dominate inhomogeneity otherwise spatially distorted images would be produced. On the other hand, the larger the gradient, the larger the receiver bandwidth and the lower the signal to noise of the system; hence the move to more homogenous magnets for the sake of imaging performance as well as to permit spectroscopy. Typically field gradients used are in the order of 0.5 gauss/cm (5mT/M) which, over a field of view of say 50cms, typical for a body image, corresponds to $\pm$ 12.5 gauss or about 50KHz. If the image has 256 points, the frequency between each pixel is about 200 Hz.

It is important to note frequency shift between pixels is expressed in Hz, hence the significance of chemical shift effects increases with magnetic field. The proton signal from human tissue can be considered to a first approximation as consisting of two signals, those from the protons in water and CH_2 resonances of mobile triglycerides (13). These signals are separated by about 3 ~ 3.5 ppm, which at 1.5T corresponds to 200 ~ 250 Hz or between 1 and 2 pixels using the values given above. The result is that ghost, or false edges, can be seen in images at interfaces between tissues of very different fat/water ratios as is shown in Figure 2. Such interfaces occur in the lower abdomen, e.g., kidney region, but are not frequently found in the head, where little CH_2 signal is found.

It should be noted that using the scheme shown, chemical shift effects only appear in the read direction, i.e., along the x axis using the conversion used in this chapter. This is a consequence of the y information being phase encoded or modulated onto the signal and spin echoes being used. The y information is contained in the phase of the signal at the origin of the data in the t_2 domain. If, as is the case for practical reasons discussed above, the origin is the mid point of spin echo, then at this point chemical shift effects are refocussed and thus are not encoded onto the data (10). We will return to this point in Section D.

C.   CHEMICAL SHIFT IMAGING

The straight forward approach to combining imaging and spectroscopy is to use a sequence where data could be collected in the absence of a gradient (15). The pulse sequence is illustrated in Figure 3. Spatial information for both the x and y axis is phase encoded during the t_1 period using 1 and m incremented steps and n data points are collected during t_2 in the absence of a field gradient. The 3D set (1 m n) is subjected to a 3D transform to produce $M(x,y,\delta)$. This imaging sequence is called the chemical shift imaging, CSI, sequence and produces a 3D data set which is formally equivalent to that produced by a full 3D imaging sequence where the data is collected during t_2 in the presence of g_z and a simple non-selective 90° pulse used for excitation (16).

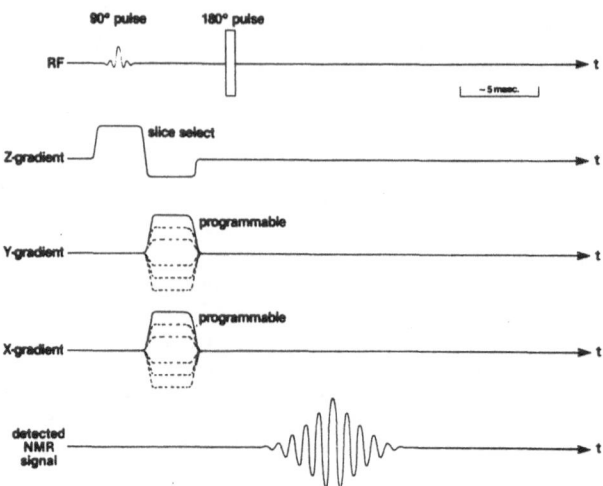

Fig. 3.   The Chemical Shift imaging sequence.

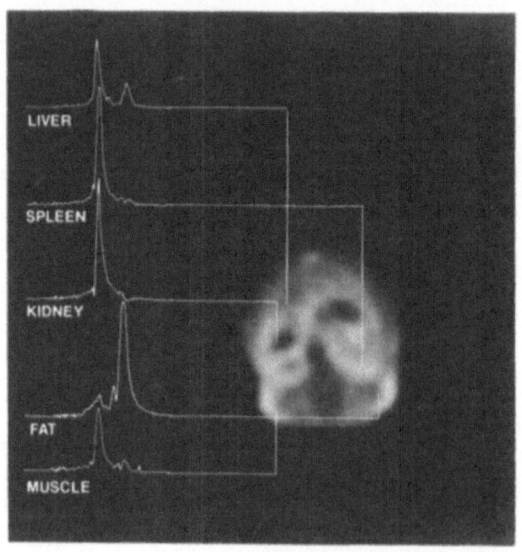

Fig. 4. Summation of 25 acquired chemical shift images of a normal dog
        abdomen. Spectra, derived from one-pixel areas in regions-of-
        interest, are indicative of fat and water distribution in liver,
        kidney, spleen, muscle and fat. Study performed on a 1.5T whole-
        body research system at the General Electric MR Development Center
        in Milwaukee.

The CSI sequence has the advantage of allowing n to be chosen to be large enough to fully represent the chemical shift spectrum without any time penalty. The disadvantage of the sequence is it takes 1 times longer than a normal imaging sequence, i.e., 1 x m x TR, as both x and y are phase encoded onto the data. Consequently compromises on spatial resolution are required to keep the total time within reasonable limits. As illustrated in Figure 4, this data set can be displayed either as an image of a specific chemical shift, i.e., $M_\delta(x,y)$ or a spectrum of each pixel $M_{x,y}(\delta)$.

Spectra produced by this sequence have a complex dependance on magnet homogeneity, which can be considered in two parts, firstly the intra voxel homogeneity and secondly the inter-voxel homogeneity. The former has to be sufficient so as not to cause significant line broadening, while the latter has to be adequate to prevent ambiguity across the image. Achieving sufficient inter-voxel homogeneity is usually not a problem, except at the periphery of the field of view where significant high order gradients can be found. The inter-voxel inhomogeneity, is amenable to software corrections (17). A CSI of a uniform single component phantom provides a map of field uniformity which can be used for frequency corrections across an image or as the basis for shimming the magnet.

1.   CSI Compared with Spectral Localisation

At this stage it is profitable to consider the differences between spectra obtained by chemical shift imaging techniques and other forms of localised spectroscopy. A full review of this complex topic is outside the scope of this article, but some generalisations are informative.

A major difference lies in the size of the volume from which the spectrum originates. The voxels of a chemical shift image tend to be small, since the number of them has to be fairly large in order to overcome problems of under sampling associated with small digital Fourier transforms (18). Cross pixel mixing occurs to approximately 1/n of the pixel size where n is the number of points in the transform. Smaller voxel size in general means lower signal to noise and hence chemical shift imaging techniques are probably only applicable to proton studies (in in vivo studies at least). Other forms of localisation, such as surface coils, with and without defect tubes (19), appear a better approach for nuclei like ^{31}P and ^{13}C, where large sensitive volumes are required on grounds of low sensitivity.

The other major difference between CSI and other techniques is that the former use gradients. The need for gradients has two ramifications. First and most obvious is that the "spectrometer" has to have gradient coils and the electronics to control them, i.e., it has to be more complex. Secondly, and less obvious, is that the time between excitation and data collection must in general be longer when using gradients than can be achieved without their use. This is because of the time necessary for gradient stabilisation following the eddy currents induced by gradient switching in the magnet cryostat. This extra time can be very significant when studying spectra containing lines with a short T_2, e.g., ATP. Significant relaxation can occur, leading to the under-estimation, or in extreme cases, the total loss, of signal.

The major strength of chemical shift imaging is the obvious one that an image is produced. The exact location of the nuclei producing the spectrum can therefore be demonstrated. All non "image technique" based on methods of localisation suffer from a significant uncertainty on the question of signal origin. Finally, CSI can produce an image, or map, of metabolic concentration; this form of presentation may be critical in getting spectroscopy techniques accepted in clinical practice.

D. CHEMICAL SHIFT SELECTIVE IMAGES

To date it has been assumed that a complete NMR spectrum is required. This is of course the case when there are many lines which may or may not be present, as is the case for ^{31}P or ^{13}C. For protons, however, with the signal to noise ratios found in images which are only about 20:1 or less (above about 20:1 the eye perceives little improvement in image quality) the signal can be considered as consisting of only two signals. All minor components are lost in the noise and dynamic range problems. This gross simplification wastes important information, but as discussed below can provide significant time saving. The signals from minor components can be detected using water suppression techniques, etc., to overcome dynamic range problems, and time averaging techniques to improve signal to noise (20). This is an active area of research, but will not be discussed further.

Given that we are prepared to accept the limitation that we will consider the proton signal as consisting of only two components, then, as pointed out by Dixon (21), we can rethink our pulse sequence. If there are only two points required on the chemical shift axis, as opposed to the 1K or so required to produce a spectrum, then it is more time effective to phase encode this information and use a gradient, again during the data collection period. Using this approach to resolve separate images for two chemically shifted components would require only twice the time for a normal image.

Chemical shift information can be encoded onto the signal by arranging for data collection not to coincide with the spin echo as it normally does. The timing of data collection is dictated by timing of the field echo. If the time between the 90° and 180° pulses is shortened by τ then the spin echo occurs 2τ early. The time of the spin echo is the time when chemical shift effects are refoccused and all vectors are in phase. During the time period between the spin echo and data collection zero, i.e., $2T$, the water and CH_2 vector will dephase at a rate dependant on their chemical shift difference Δ. If the time 2τ is set such that the vectors get 180° out of place, i.e., $2\tau = \frac{1}{2}\Delta$, then the signal detected will be the difference between the water and fat signals.

The procedure to produce a 2 component chemically selective image is thus to collect one data set with the spin and field echo coinciding, i.e., $\tau = 0$, which is the sum of the water and **fat** signals, and a second

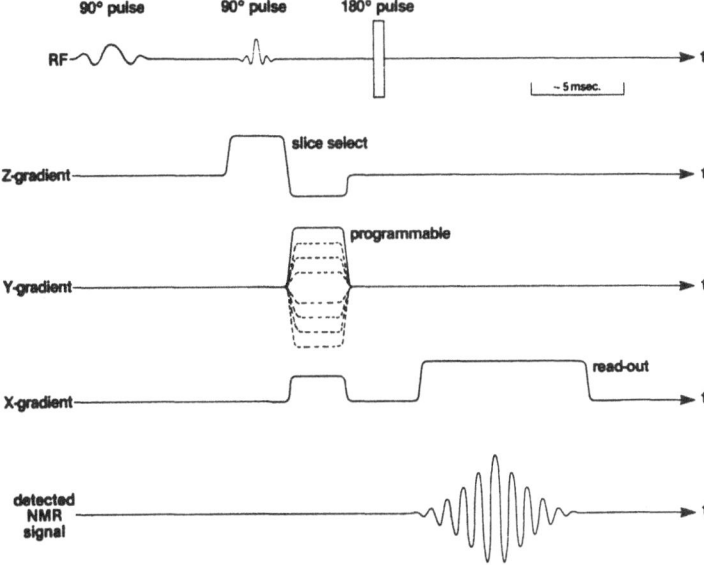

Fig. 5.   The Chemical Shift Specific Sequence.

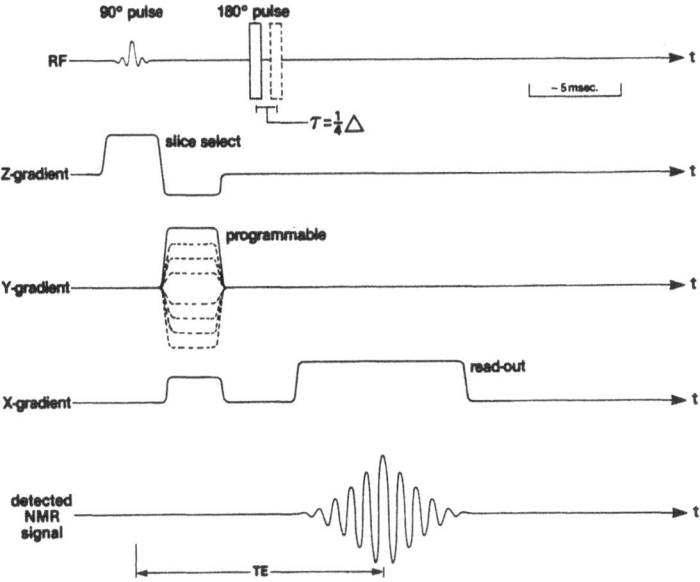

Fig. 6.   The Chemical Shift Selective Sequence.

data set with $\tau = \frac{1}{4}\Delta$, which is the difference image of the resonances separated by a chemical shift of Δ. For water and fat Δ is about 3.5ppm, therefore at 1.5T τ should be about 1.12 msec. Having data sets which are the sum and difference, it is trivial to generate the separate images. An example of 2 such images is shown in Figure 5. Also, a chemical shift corrected image (see Section B) can be produced by shifting one image, e.g., the water image, by the appropriate number of pixels and then adding it to the fat image to produce a "sum" image.

The procedure outlined above is simply a special case of a general 3D FT sequence. τ could be incremented 1 times over a range and the data set transformed to produce a $M(\delta,x,y)$ set. For small values of 1, digital Fourier transforms produce problems due to undersampling (18), hence for 1 = 2 it is more efficient to operate as described above. Specific phase encoding of spectra information is only possible where the chemical shifts are known in advance, since specific values of τ have to be chosen. The procedure is also only suitable for cases where the components are of roughly equal concentration, since it relies on subtractions.

A completely different approach to obtaining chemical selective images is to selectively saturate specific chemical shifts (22). In this method, as shown in Figure 6 a highly selective pulse is applied to, say, the water resonance prior to a conversional spin warp sequence. The resultant image contains no signal from the saturated species.

E.   CONCLUSION

This article has not set out to be a comprehensive review of all the methods of adding chemical information to magnetic resonance images. There are many other variations, e.g., to use pure projection reconstruction techniques (23) or phase encode chemical shift information prior to a normal projection reconstruction imaging scheme (24). The field is rapidly developing, and with the availability of dedicated chemical shift imaging systems and of spectroscopy accessories for imaging systems should continue to do so. It is hoped that this article has provided a brief overview of the principles of the techniques employed. The long term value of chemical shift imaging and related techniques will only become apparent when it has been established as to whether they produce any information which is unique and useful.

REFERENCES

1.   D. G. Gadian 'Nuclear Magnetic Resonance and its applications to living systems', Oxford University (1982).

2.   P. L. Lauterbur, Nature, 242, 190 (1973).

3.   F. W. Wehrli, J. R. McFall, G. H. Glover et al, Magnetic Resonance Imaging, 2, 3 (1983)

4. J. J. Ackerman, T. H. Grove, G. G. Wong et al, Nature, 283 167 (1980).

5. R. E. Gordon, P. E. Harley, D. Shaw, 'Prog. NMR Spectras' 15, 1 (1983).

6. W. A. Edlestien, Proceeding 3rd Meeting Soc. Magnetic Resoance in Medicine, 202 New York (1984).

7. J. M. S. Hutchinson, R. J. Sutherland, R. J. Mallard, J. Phys. E. 11, 217 (1978).

8. K. Sikipara, M. Kuroda, H. Kohno, Phys. Med. Biol., 29, 15 (1984).

9. A. Bax, 'Two Dimensional Nuclear Magnetic Resonance in Liquids', Delft University Press (1981).

10. D. Shaw, Fourier Transform NMR Spectroscopy, Elsivier, (1984).

11. A. Kumar, D. Welte, R. R. Ernst., J. Magn Res, 18, 69 (1975).

12. W. A. Edlestien, J. M. S. Hutchinson, G. Johnson, T. Redpath, Phys. Med. Biol, 25, 751 (1980).

13. D. Shaw, in 'NMR Imaging', Ed. C. L. partain et al W. B. Saunders Co. (1983) 166.

14. H. Hricak, R. D. Williams, K. L. Moon et al Radiology, 147, 765, (1983).

15. I. C. Pybettar, B. R. Posen, Radiology, 149, 197 (1983).

16. C. M. Lai, P. C. Lauterbur, Phys. Med. Biol., 26, 851 (1981).

17. A. A. Maudsley, H. E. Simon, S. K. Hilal, J. Phys. E., 17, 216 (1984).

18. R. Bracewell, 'The Fourier Transform and its Physical Applications' Mc Graw-Hill (1983).

19. R. Bendall in 'Biomedical Magnetic Resonance', Eds A. R. Magulis and E. James, Radiology Research and Education Foundation, (1984).

20. K. L. Behar. J. A. Den Hollander, M. E. Stromski et al, Proc. Matl. Acad. Sci. USA, 80, 4945, (1983).

21. J. K. T. Lee, W. T. Dixon, D. Ling et al, Radiology, 153, 195, (1984).

22. P. A. Bottomley, T. H. Foster, W. M. Lene, Lancet, 1120 (1984).

23. P. C. Lauterbur, D. M. Kramer, W. V. House Jr., C. N. Chen,
     J. Amer. Chem. Soc., 97, 6866 (1975).

24. Z. H. Xho, H. W. Park, J. B. R. etal, Proc. 3rd Meeting Society
     Magnetic Resonance in Medicine 155 New York. (1984)

MEDICAL ASPECTS OF MAGNETIC RESONANCE

L.D Hall and W.A. Stewart
Department of Chemistry
University of British Columbia
Vancouver, B.C.
Canada V6T 1W5

ABSTRACT. Nuclear magnetic resonance has already been used clinically in two distinctive ways. The first, proton tomography, is a valuable new method for imaging the anatomy of the intact human body. Its advantages include the fact that it can produce slice-images, either transverse or sagittal or coronal. Furthermore, the variations in spin-lattice and spin-spin relaxation rates of water in different tissues provide not only a powerful new means for detecting aberrant pathology but also for heightening the perceived contrast in the final image. Independently of the above, methods have been developed for producing high resolution NMR spectra from intact human tissues. Most attention has been directed to ^{31}P NMR studies, which provide a quantitative measure of biochemical transformation in-vivo. More recently, methods have been developed which combine tomography with spectroscopy.

Although, as yet, NMR has not been universally recognised by the appropriate medical authorities as a generally applicable diagnostic tool, that situation is approaching rapidly, and effectively has already been reached for studies of brain. One of the main attractions to those who are involved with clinical diagnosis is the fact that the NMR method does not use ionising radiation and, as a result, it is possible to make numerous follow-up studies at no risk to the patient.

As with other medical procedures, NMR does have its disadvantages, the main one being its inherent insensitivity; as a result, it can take a substantial time to obtain either an image, or a spectrum, of suitable quality. This has prompted the various medical imaging companies to expend a great deal of effort pursuing methods for reducing the total time required for data acquisition. At present, the most widely used of these involves "multi-slice scanning". This technique makes use of the "dead-time" required for the nuclei in one particular slice to relax back to their equilibrium state, to sample the spins of a second, third, or even twentieth slice. As a result, it is possible to obtain numerous parallel slice images almost as rapidly as the time required to measure a single slice-image.

The choice of optimum parameters for measuring images and/or

169

spectra, will clearly be dependent on the particular instrument used, and the clinical diagnosis required. For example, as a result of detailed studies it is now well known that a spin-echo pulse sequence can be used to heighten the image contrast between multiple sclerosis (1) plaques and normal brain tissue. Nevertheless, it is still necessary to optimise the choice of imaging parameters, and to decide which slice and from which direction the brain should be viewed. At the present time, most magnetic resonance imaging groups are still collecting data in order establish the best diagnostic protocols for evaluation of essentially all of the organs of the body, and for most disease states which result in aberrant pathology, such as multiple sclerosis and posterior fossa tumours, to name just two examples from the brain, and for pancreatic and colonic tumours, to name two examples from the abdominal cavity. For such protocols to be accepted, it must be shown that the NMR method can provide a more efficient means of identifying the particular pathology than other methods which are already available, such as x-ray CT. The latter technique, which is already highly developed, provides images with excellent spatial resolution, very rapidly; in that sense it can be regarded as being more cost-effective than MRI, which is invariably slower using most existing methods. Nevertheless, the NMR method has the undoubted advantage in that it has a far wider array of measurable parameters such as the spin-lattice, and spin-spin relaxation rates, and the proton density. If it proves possible to measure those parameters quantitatively and to relate the resultant data with specific aberrant pathology, then this would undoubtedly swing the balance of opinion of MRI.

The early signs, based on qualitative studies are indeed very encouraging, but it remains to be seen if unequivocal tissue characterization can be achieved.

There are numerous problems associated with the accurate measurement of the NMR parameters of water in human tissue, using imaging methods. Briefly, these include the following:
1. Even in a volume of tissue which can be considered to be homogeneous, the cell water which provides the basis for the MRI measurement may exist in more than one state. Furthermore, additional signal may come from any "fat" in a mobile environment.
2. The above problem is further compounded by the fact that the environment within any cell is not static, so that the measured parameters may vary over a period of time; for example, the tissue of a tumour may have completely different properties at its onset compared with those of the same tumour at maturity. Indeed, given the fact that the pathological status of a particular cell may only involve changes in the concentration of a chemical species present at millimolar concentrations, it is in some ways remarkable that such changes can have an effect on the properties of water, which is present to a concentration of approximately 50 molar.
3. To the complications associated with the above classes of chemical averaging, must be added an impressive array of uncertainties in the precise location of the volume of tissue which produces the magnetic resonance signal. For example, depending on

the thickness of the slice which is measured, both normal and abnormal tissue may simultaneously contribute to the perceived signal, thereby leading to a measured value which is intermediate between the values corresponding to the two types of tissue. Such volume-averaging effects clearly depend on the spatial resolution which can be achieved. Most whole body scanners in current clinical use can produced spatial resolution of the order of a few millimeters within the imaging plane, with a slice thickness of 1 or 2 centimeters. Instruments operating at higher field strengths however have the advantage of higher signal-to-noise per volume element and, as a result, can produce an in-plane resolution of better than 0.5 millimeters with a slice thickness of approximately 5 millimeters or less.

4. It is usually the tacit assumption that the various fields which are used to elicit the NMR responses from the nuclei are themselves linear; thus, it is assumed that the static magnetic field is completely homogeneous over the volume of interest, that the linear gradients used to encode the image are themselves linear, and that the radiofrequency field influences all of the magnetic spins evenly over the entire volume of interest. The very fact that modern instruments produce such high quality images is a clear indication that these assumptions concerning instrument linearity and homogeneity are in fact reasonable.

It is now appropriate to direct attention to the clinical viability of NMR spectroscopy. In many ways, the technical choices are simpler than those for conventional imaging; however, this is largely because the technical requirements are more exacting. Thus the requirement to obtain a separate resonance signal from individual chemical species can only be satisfied by working at high field strengths; most whole-body devices currently available have magnets which operate at 1.5 or 2.0 Tesla. The further requirement, namely that the homogeneity of the field be sufficiently high to enable the individual resonances to be resolved, is still a major limitation. In practice, the necessary homogeneity, one part in 10^7 can only be achieved generally over a diameter of approximately 10 centimeters.

Given access to a magnet with the above specifications it is then necessary to both restrict, and define, the precise volume of tissue which is to be examined. Most studies reported so far make use of the surface coil technique which was developed at Oxford University in the joint laboratories of Sir Rex Richards and George Radda (2). This technique makes use of a small coil of copper wire typically 4 centimeters in diameter, which is placed on the surface of the tissue of interest. The assumption is made that the radiofrequency from that coil can penetrate into the tissues to a depth equivalent to the radius of the coil; thus providing a crude, yet simple, means for volume localisation.

The spectra shown in Figure 1 illustrate the use of this approach for the measurement of both proton and phosphorus high resolution NMR spectra. The latter in particular encodes (3) a remarkable amount of useful information. Most importantly, the relative intensities of the peaks from ATP, phosphocreatine, and

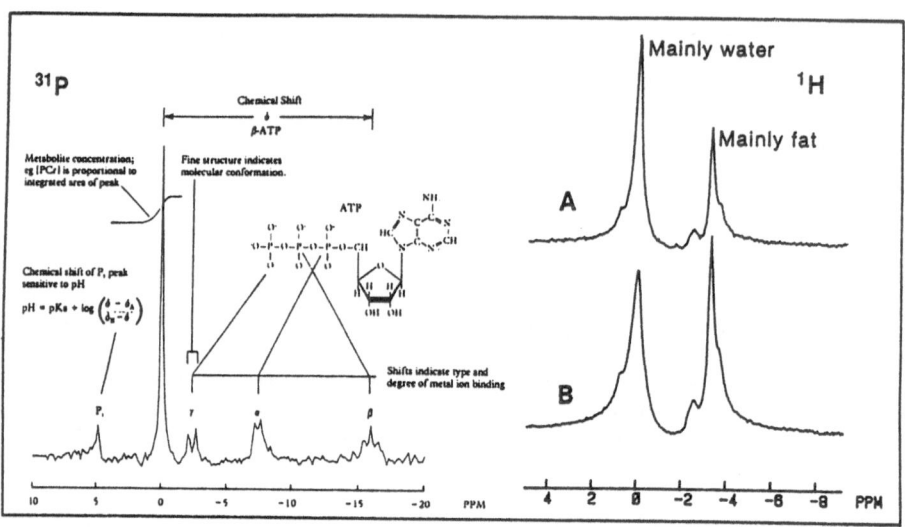

Figure 1. On the left: information available from a phosphorus spectrum of a human forearm. On the right: the proton spectrum of the forearm of a normal 13 year old boy (A) and that of a boy of similar age suffering from muscular dystrophy (B). {The Lancet i, 725 (1982)}.

inorganic phosphates provide a direct measure of the metabolic status of the tissues under investigation. In particular, the relative intensities of the phosphocreatine peak versus the inorganic phosphate peak has been used to follow the depletion of the phospho-creatine energy reservoir. Although much work has been done using human forearm muscle the most dramatic results have come from studies of neonate brain. The neonate in an incubator, is inserted in the bore of the magnet such that the head is positioned above a surface coil and then the NMR spectrum of the brain tissues is recorded in the usual way. This approach is currently being explored at University College Hospital in London in the Neonate Unit supervised by Professor Reynolds, to monitor the recovery of neonates which have suffered trauma at birth (4).

All of the initial in-vivo spectroscopic studies were made using a magnet operating 1.9 Tesla and with a room temperature bore of 30 centimeters. More recently, a development of magnets with a room temperature bore of 100 centimeters has made feasible equivalent studies in adult man. These studies have revealed the inadequacies of the surface coil approach since the use of a relatively small coil diameter to restrict the region of interest automatically limits the depth of radiofrequency penetration into the tissues. This has prompted the development of a number of different procedures. The simplest (5) referred to as "depth pulses" effectively nulls the signal produced by nucleus spins near the surface of the coil and enhances that from the nuclei which are deeper within the sample. A more versatile procedure developed by Bottomley and colleagues (6) at General Electric, uses a linear field gradient perpendicular to the surface to induce a depth dependent dispersion of resonance frequencies, together with radiofrequency pulses which have a defined bandwidth. The precise frequency at which the radiofrequency is applied then defines the depth at which the nucleus spins are sampled, and the bandwidth of the radiofrequency pulse defines the thickness of the slice. This is certainly going to be one of the major methods for measuring localised spectra in the future, either in its own right, or in its extensions to produce point-specific spectra. In this latter area, magnetisation of the spins within a slice is first defined as described above; then an orthogonal gradient is used to define a further slice through the original one; finally a third orthogonal gradient cuts a section from the resultant column; the net result of these three operations in close sequence is to define a point within the volume of the object from which the high resolution NMR spectrum is obtained (7). Notwithstanding the technical elegance of these methods for obtaining high resolution spectra from any defined volume of tissue within a patient, it is still not clear where the resultant data can be used for clinical diagnosis of disease in man. The results from human muscle metabolism are of course important, but not sufficiently so to justify the development of an entire diagnostic instrument. The results obtained from neonates is inspirational, but here too the global patient flow is marginal. It is clear then that for this modality to justify the substantial costs which it involves, it must be relevant to one or more of the major classes of disease in man; these are, neurological disorders especially those of the aged such as Alzheimers disease, cardiac problems, and of course cancers of various forms.

Considerable interest has been shown in the development of other combinations of imaging and spectroscopy; in particular, chemical shift resolved tomography has been evaluated in a number of different laboratories (8-15). The purpose here is to produce a series of tomographic slice images each corresponding to the same physical slice through the object, but showing the distribution within that volume of individual chemical species. Simplistically, the process is somewhat akin to taking a pack of cards, moving one of them (this corresponds to slice selection), and then splitting that card into a series of separate slices each corresponding to a different colour. Although this is certainly technically feasible, it must be realised that the addition of a chemical shift dimension further increases the time required for data acquisition. Nevertheless, separate images for the water and fat in mammalian tissues have been described (16) and attempts are in progress to establish the clinical utility of such displays. In passing, it is worth noting that other methods exist which can be used to obtain images in which the contributions of water are displayed separately from those of fat (17). This is an area which certainly merits a great deal of further attention, both from the clinical standpoint as well as from the basic science.

Another area still in its infancy, but which shows considerable promise for detecting aberrant pathology, is imaging based on sodium-23. The first clinical results using this nucleus were recently reported from Halal's laboratory (18).

Although one of the major advantages of clinical magnetic resonance is that the technique is, to the best of available knowledge, non-invasive, it remains that some diagnoses cannot be made solely on the basis of the responses from the water in the tissues. In such circumstances it may be feasible to administer to the patient a chemical species which can influence the NMR properties of the water in the tissue of interest. There is ample precedent for this approach in CT x-ray procedures where barium gels or iodinated substances are used. So far, most attention to the use of "image contrast" agents for MRI have centered around some complexes of paramagnetic species, such as gadolinium (19-22). Although some small degree of additional invasiveness may be clinically acceptable, it is obvious that this approach will only become clinically acceptable after the development of contrast medium which are biochemically inert. This is difficult, but not impossible.

Undoubtedly the most important issue in the entire area of clinical magnetic resonance concerns the correct choice of field strength for the imaging or spectroscopic device. It is an unfortunate fact that many of the discussions on this topic during the past four years appear to have been deliberately intended to "create more heat than light", and to protect those companies which have chosen to concentrate all of their efforts at one particular field-strength. Nevertheless, the delivered base of equipment in clinical environment is now so substantial that the true merits of the various alternative forms of clinical magnetic resonance must surely be revealed by experience. Essentially all of the clinical magnetic resonance devices which are currently on the market were designed in the very early stages of this area, and as a result most have the flexibility of an instrument intended for research, rather than the simplicity of "turnkey-device" intended for routine clinical practice. Undoubtedly this situation which will change in the not remote future; this will decrease the capital costs of the equipment and increase the ease of use.

REFERENCES

1. Young, I.R., Randell, C.P., Kaplan, P.W., James, A., Bydder, G.M., Steiner, R.E. J. Comput. Assist. Tomogr. 7(2) 290-294 (1983).
2. Ackerman, J.J.H., Grove, T.H., Wong, G.G., Gadian, D.G. and Radda, G.K. Nature (London) 283 167 (1980).
3. Hoult, D.I., Bushy, S.J.W., Gadian, D.G, Radda, G.K., Richards, R.E. and Seeley, P.J. Nature (London) 252 285 (1974).
4. Cady, E.B., Dawson, M.J., Hope, P.L., Tofts, P.S., Costello, A.M. deL., Delpy, D.T., Reynolds, E.O.R., Wilkie, D.R. Lancet, 1059 (1983).
5. Bendall, M.R. and Gordon, R.E. J. Magn. Reson. 53 365-385 (1983).

6. Bottomley, P.A., Foster, T.B. and Dorrow, R.D. J. Magn. Reson. **59** 338-342 (1984).

7. Hinshaw, W.S. J. Appl. Phys. **47** 3709 (1976).

8. Lauterbur,P.C., Kramer, D.M., House, W.V. and Chen, C.N. J. Am. Chem. Soc. **97** 6866 (1975).

9. Bendell, P. Lai, C.M. and Lauterbur, P.C. J. Magn. Reson. **38** 343 (1980).

10. Maudsley, A.A., Hilal, S.K., Perman, W.H. and Simon H.E. J. Magn. Reson. **51** 147 (1983).

11. Mansfield P. J. Phys. D. **16** L235 (1983).

12. Cox, S.J. and Styles, P. J. Magn. Reson. **56** 314 (1984).

13. Brown, T.R., Kincaid, B.M. and Ugurbil, K. Proc. Nat. Acad. Sci. U.S.A. **79** 3525 (1982)/

14. Hall, L.D. and Sukumar, S. J. Magn. Reson. **56** 179 (1984). 14.

15. Pykett, I.L. and Rosen, B.R. Radiology **149** 197 (1983).

16. Rosen, B.R., Wedeen, V.J. and Brady, T.J. J. Comput. Assist. Tomogr. 8(5) 813-818 (1984).

17. Hall, L.D., Sukumar, S. and Talagala, S.L. J. Magn. Reson. **56** 275-278 (1984).

18. Hilal, S.K., Maudsley, A.A., Ra, J.B., Simon, H.E. et al. J. Comput. Assist. Tomogr. 9(1) 1-7 (1985).

19. Weimann, H.J., Brasch, R.C., Press, W.R. et al. Am. J. Roentgenol. **142** 619 (1984).

20. Brasch, R.C., Weimann, H.J., Wesbey, G.E. Am. J. Roentgenol. **142** 625 (1984).

21. Huberty, J., Engelstad, B., Wesbey, G. et al. NMR contrast enhancement of the kidneys and liver with paramagnetic metal complexes. Proc. Soc. Magnet. Reson. Med. 1983 pp. 175-176.

22. Wesbey, G.E., Engelstad, B.L., Huberty, J.P. et al. Radiology **149** 98P (1983).

MR-IMAGING AND SPECTROSCOPY OFFERING NEW POSSIBILITIES IN MEDICAL DIAGNOSES

A. GANSSEN, PH.D.
ERLANGEN, SIEMENS U.B. MED.
W. GERMANY

ABSTRACT

The first clinical applications of magnetic resonance imaging have been in existence for two to three years. Medical applications of magnetic resonance spectroscopy have been clinically tested only in a few instances. It is too early to evaluate the diagnostic value of these new modalities in comparison with other well established methods. In order to make such a judgement, the diagnostic potential and limitations have to be taken into consideration. •

In this survey some of the more important technical possibilities with present day equipment are discussed and some possible future developments are suggested.

INTRODUCTION:

The information provided by Nuclear Magnetic Resonance (NMR: in medicine, only MR) in living organisms is basically different from the information obtainable from the well known conventional diagnostic modalities. It also exceeds the amount of information available from any other noninvasive method. With the competing procedures, only one parameter per volume element can be obtained, while with MR normally several characteristic parameters are available.
Analytical MR has been around and applied in analytial chemistry since the discovery of the chemical shift in 1951 (1) just 5 years after the discovery of NMR in early spring 1946 by the two independent groups under E. Purcell at Harvard and F. Bloch, at Stanford (2)(3). It has since developed into an extremely valuable tool for the in vitro analysis in chemistry, and chemical physics, and since the late 60's, also in biophysics. The magnetic field dependent "chemical" shift is caused by the spatial distribution of the field compensating intramolecular electron currents. It is characteristic for each molecular

T. Axenrod and G. Ceccarelli (eds.), NMR in Living Systems, 177–191.
© *1986 by D. Reidel Publishing Company.*

configuration. The field independent MR-line splitting is caused by spin-spin interaction providing additional information on the molecular constitution. The particular line amplitudes are proportional to the numbers of isotopic nuclei involved in similar steric positions.

Basically, the same information which is being extracted from small samples in vitro should also be available from living tissue, and organisms. A serious difficulty arises from the usually rather small molecular concentrations i.e., of body metabolites, and also from the poor sensitivity of MR to other nuclear species which might occur only in small isotopic concentrations.

In compensation for the low molecular concentrations, usually larger volume elements have to be investigated, thus excluding the spatial resolution available in proton MR-imaging. But even in cases where the spectral information cannot be obtained, the relaxation times T_1 and T_2 are always measurable providing information on the average molecular mobility of the molecules involved. The relaxation times T_1 and T_2 have been shown to be most sensitively affected by tissue pathology.

For the medical application it is also of interest that MR lends itself to the measurement of time dependent parameters like blood flow and perfusion.

A basic difference of MR-imaging as compared to other modalities is the way image generation allows data collection independently from an exteriorly located point source or detector array: thus, two and three dimensional images can be produced under any desired angle and at any location within the homogenous magnetic field volume of a whole body magnet.

An outline of some possibilities offered by present day MR-imaging and spectroscopy to medical diagnostics should demonstrate the state of the art in the following.

MR-IMAGING

Basically MR can be excited in all nuclei consisting of an odd number of protons or neutrons or an odd number of both. This means that MR-detectable isotopes exist in basically all elements. However, these isotopes are often hard to detect because of their low natural abundance or broad line width.

It is fortunate that the most abundant nuclei in living nature, the hydrogen nuclei or protons, can be measured most easily. This can be seen in Table 1, in which the more important MR-parameters of some isotopes normally existing in living systems are listed. In practice, the relative MR-sensitivity for each element has to be modified not only for the natural isotope abundance but also for the tissue concentration which is often in the order

TABLE 1. MR-data on stable isotopes, which are more abundant
in living tissue.

Isotope	Spin Unit $\frac{h}{2\pi}$	MR Frequency in MHz $/_T$	Relative Sensitivity at Constant B_O	Natural Abundance in %
^1H	½	42.577	1.00	99.985
^2H	1	6.536	0.0096	0.015
^7Li	3/2	16.547	0.294	92.57
^{13}C	½	10.705	0.0150	1.106
^{14}N	1	3.075	0.001	99.63
^{19}F	½	40.055	0.834	100
^{23}Na	3/2	11.262	0.0927	100
^{31}P	·½	17.235	0.066	100

of μ-Mol so that the practical sensitivity is often by a factor of 10^{-6} and less further down as listed.

Most of the medical MR applications are therefore concerned with proton magnetic resonance, especially MR-imaging. The most exciting feature of proton MR-imaging is the extremely high soft tissue contrast obtainable without the application of contrast media. Three parameters can always be used for tissue differentiation. These are the proton density and the magnetic proton relaxation times T_1 and T_2. The MR-signal in the case of the mostly used spin echo sequence is determined by the well known formula:

$$S = \mathcal{G} \cdot \exp(-TE/T_2) \ (1-\exp(-TR/T_1))$$

Where TE is the spin echo time and TR is the repetition time between two successive individual pulse series applied.

Two parameters like i.e., the proton density $\mathcal{G}$ and the relaxation time T_2 can be simultaneously obtained in one scan by observing more than one spin echo.

It is above all the biologically important water concentration in tissues which is being recorded with the proton density parameters. In healthy soft tissue, this parameter might not vary too much. In pathologic cases, however, like edema or bone tumor, considerable changes can be observed. More contrast can most frequently be detected by looking at the relaxation times, which are influenced by the chemical bonding conditions and the mobility of the molecules involved.

In pure liquids T_1 and T_2 change proportionally while T_2 is nearly always shorter than T_1. Both relaxation times become shorter with increasing viscosity. Approaching the solid state, there can be a reversal for T_1 becoming longer again while T_2 continues to decrease. In the mixed composition of living tissues containing within the detected volume element low viscous liquids, highly viscous macromolecular protein suspensions, close to solid state membranes and fat, etc., the effective relaxation rates $(1/T_{1,2})$ eff, are given by the sum of the fractional contributions:

$$(1/T_1)_{eff.} = \sum_{k=1}^{n} (f)_k/(T_1)_k \ , \ (1/T_2)_{eff.} = \sum_{k=1}^{n} (f)_k/(T_2)_k$$

where $(T_1)_k$ and $(T_2)_k$ represent the relaxation times T_1 and T_2 for the corresponding material within the fraction of $(f)_k$ of the total number of contributing protons. In present day MR-imaging however, mainly the long relaxation time contributions are being considered because of the comparatively long spin echo times i.e., $TE \geq 20ms$ applied for the signal readout. A finer tissue discrimination can

be expected if the shorter relaxation time contributions
could also be measured.

As far as the visualization of fast growing neoplasms
is concerned however, present day apparatus seems to be already highly sensitive. Since in these cases considerably
enhanced relaxation times can be measured because of increased vascularization, edema or increased intracellular
water. The figures 1 and 2 give examples of the contrast
easily obtainable with a 0.5 T-MR imager. Figure 1 represents frontal spin echo scans which have been simultaneously
obtained from a healthy volunteer. Sagital and transaxial
inversion recovery scans of the brain of a healthy person
are shown in Figure 2.

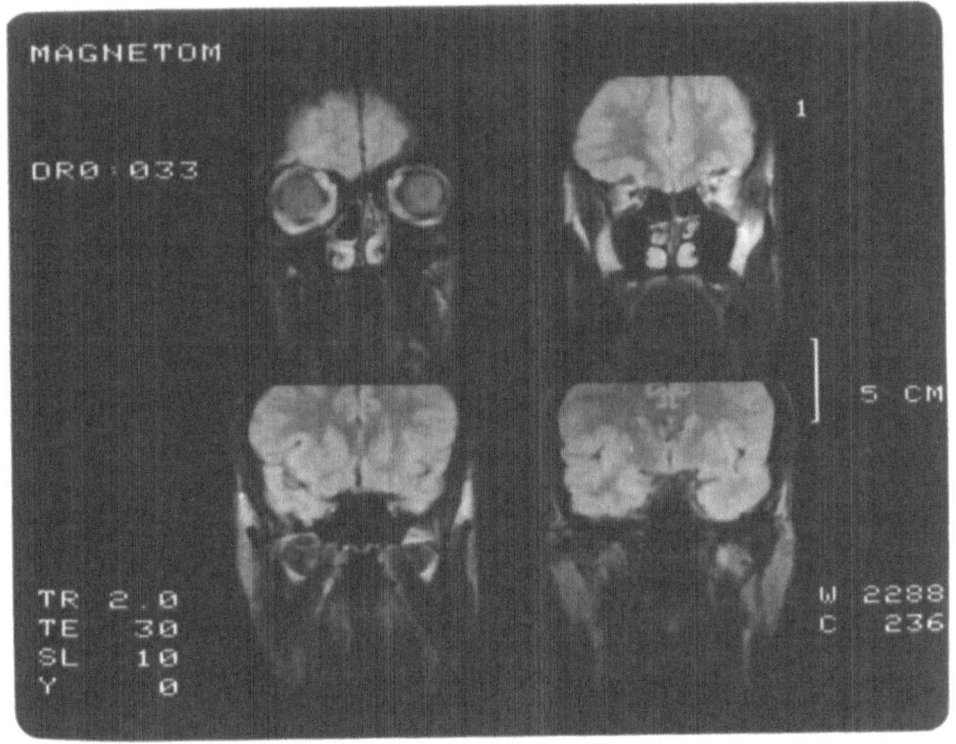

Figure 1: Four simultaneously scanned coronal spin echo
           images.

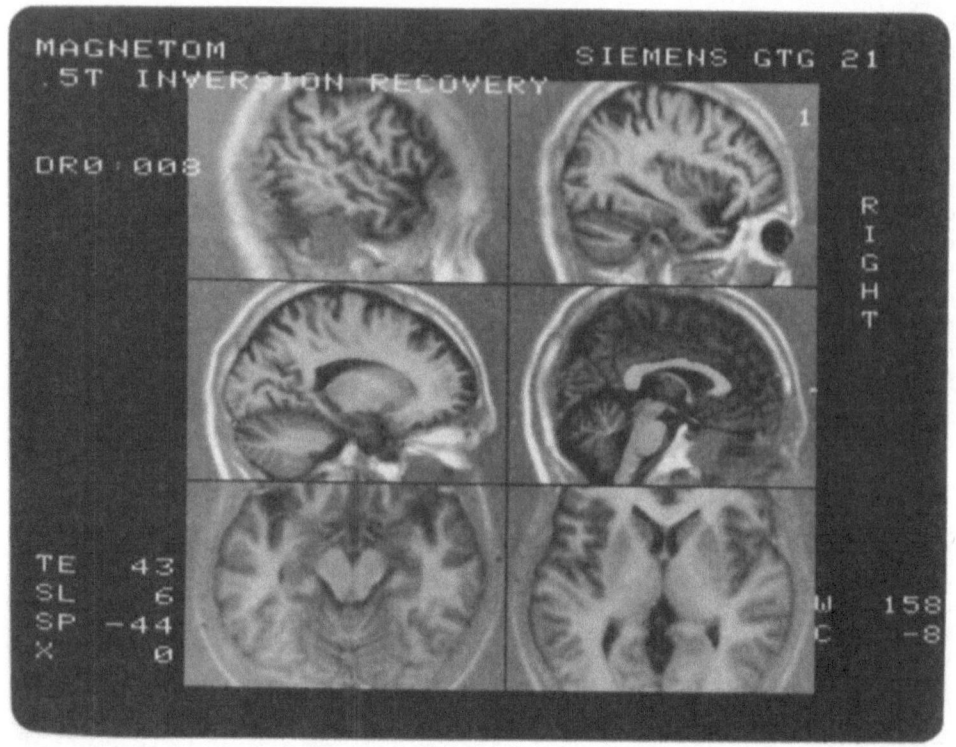

Figure 2:   Four simultaneously scanned sagital inversion
            recovery, and two transaxial head images. The
            slice thickness is 6 mm.

       A definite advantage of MR-imaging in comparison to
x-ray CT is the arbitrary choice of slice orientation which
can be obtained instantaneously without moving the patient;
thus enabling, in most cases, the anatomically optimal display of pathology without the loss of spatial resolution.
The slice thickness can be arbitrarily chosen within certain
limits: thus it becomes possible to survey a body area
first with a larger slice thickness and then to obtain
thinner slices with a higher spatial resolution of the region of interest.   Since the signal to noise ratio is directly proportional to the volume from which the signal is
derived the survey scan with increased slice thickness can
be done faster without averaging being necessary.   Survey
images with a slice thickness of 8mm and a 64x64 voxel
image matrix have been obtained in about 12 seconds in contrast to images with a 256x256 matrix which usually take
several minutes.
       The comparatively long scan time of MR-imaging as com-

pared to other imaging modalities is being compensated to
a certain extent by the simultaneous multi-slicing capability enabling modern MR-imaging to generate 15 slices and
more in a time hardly longer than the time required for
one single slice.

Even more economical with respect to time are three
dimensional scans of more or less extended body volumes
containing the suspected pathology. In this case, projection and image plane selection can be done afterwards using
the image data matrix. Image choice and evaluation can be
so completely separated from the patient scan that the total
patient scanning time will be significantly reduced. Figure
3 gives a fraction of the sagital images obtained from a
human knee with 64x64 image elements per slice.

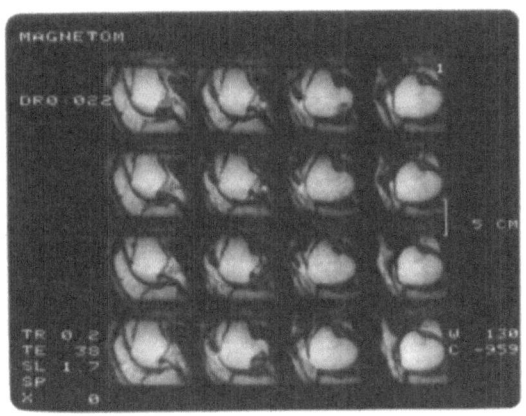

Figure 3:   Eight sagital and eight transaxial images
             recovered from a three dimensional scan of a
             human knee with 64x64 pixels per slice.

The absence of bone artifacts and beam hardening effects can give MR a definite advantage over x-ray CT especially in the exploration of the posterior fossa of the skull
and of the spine.

Contrast media like in CT do not seem to be necessary
in most cases because of the high natural soft tissue contrast. For special problems and procedures however, paramagnetic contrast media are presently being developed. Important applications of these contrast media are suspected
in body areas in which improved tissue discrimination between adjacent organs of similar tissue is desirable and in
cases where complicated anatomical structures have to be
resolved. Problem areas in which contrast media could be
of considerable help are, for instance, the upper abdominal
area including the pancreas, and the lungs. Additional
applications can be expected in functional tests like clear-

ance investigations of kidneys and liver.

Because of the comparatively long scan times in MR-
imaging, body motion is still one of the greatest problems.
Periodic motion can be overcome by synchronized triggering
as it is done in the case of the heart and lung.   An ECG
triggered heart is shown for instance on a scan obtained
with a 0.5T system in coronary projection (Fig 4)   In dependence of ECG phasing considerable details can be seen in
the myocardium.   By monitoring the signal of a respiratory
transducer the MR-imager can also be gated to any phase of
the respiratory cycle.   Motion unsharpness can thus be reduced in the thorax and in the upper abdomen, especially if
respiratory gating is being used in conjunction with ECG
triggering.

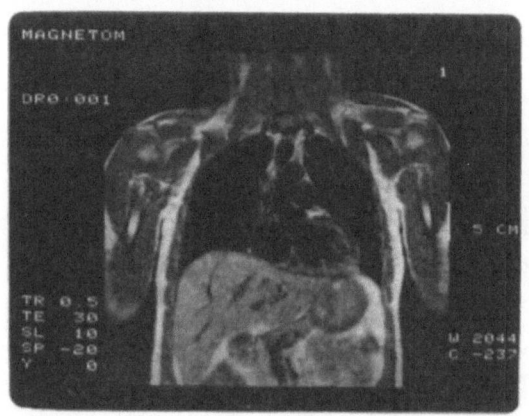

Figure 4:   Coronal spin echo image of the human heart
            scanned with ECG triggering.   TR=500 ms,
            TE-30 ms, slice thickness 10 mm.

True region of interest scans become possible in MR-imaging
by increasing the spatially selective gradients.   The size
of the sensitive volume, the voxel is thus reduced.   As a
compensation for the decreased signal to noise ratio, the
scanning time has to be correnspondingly increased.

Improved spatial resolution with increased signal to
noise ratio can be obtained with special surface coils.
The surface coil should be chosen according to the size of
the area which should be imaged.   While the MR-excitation
usually is still being achieved with the whole body radio
frequency coil, the surface coil is applied as a sensitive
pick-up coil.   The depth of the volume which can be imaged
with a cylindrical loop arrangement corresponds about to
the radius of the loop.

Several reports have been published recently on the
localized application of surface coils in different areas
of the human body.   One example of a surface coil image of

a human ear with a glomus tumor is seen (Figure 5). Good
results were obtained so far with female breasts and seg-
ments of the spine. The mamma image (Figure 6) showing a
solid carcinoma was taken at 0.5T within 50 seconds. The
scan was performed at a field of 0.5T with a slice thickness
of 0.5cm. Much development can still be expected in the
field of various applications of dedicated coils for signal
pick up in MR-imaging.

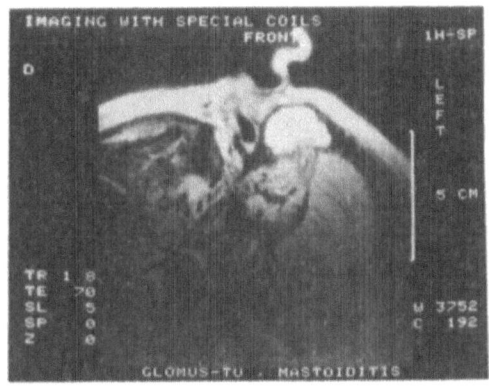

Figure 5:   Surface coil spin echo-image of a human ear with
             glomus tumor TR =1.8 s, TE = 70 ms, slice thick-
             ness 5 mm.

    There is a high sensitivity to nuclear motion built in
to MR which can be used for blood flow measurements. Blood
flow measurements were probably the first medical applications of MR, proposed in 1959 by J. Singer (4). Comparatively little has been done in this field in connection with
MR-imaging yet. Flow effects can always qualitively be observed in larger vessels. In this case a vessel is cut
perpendicular to it's axis, the MR signal values will be
diminishing the faster the flow value, since only the spins
which have been exposed to the whole 90°-180° pulsing will
contribute to the signal. If the blood volume within the
imaged slice is being replaced by new blood before the sequence is completed, the whole signal will decrease in dependence of the flow velocity. Quantitative values can be
obtained by simultaneous ECG-triggering and by the adequate
choice of the imaged slice thickness. Additional possibilities are given by the application of "time of flight"
methods where a proton preparation is done in one slice in
which the protons are tagged by a 90° or 180° flip. In a
successive parallel slice, this tagging can then be detected with a corresponding time delay from which the flow
velocity can be derived.

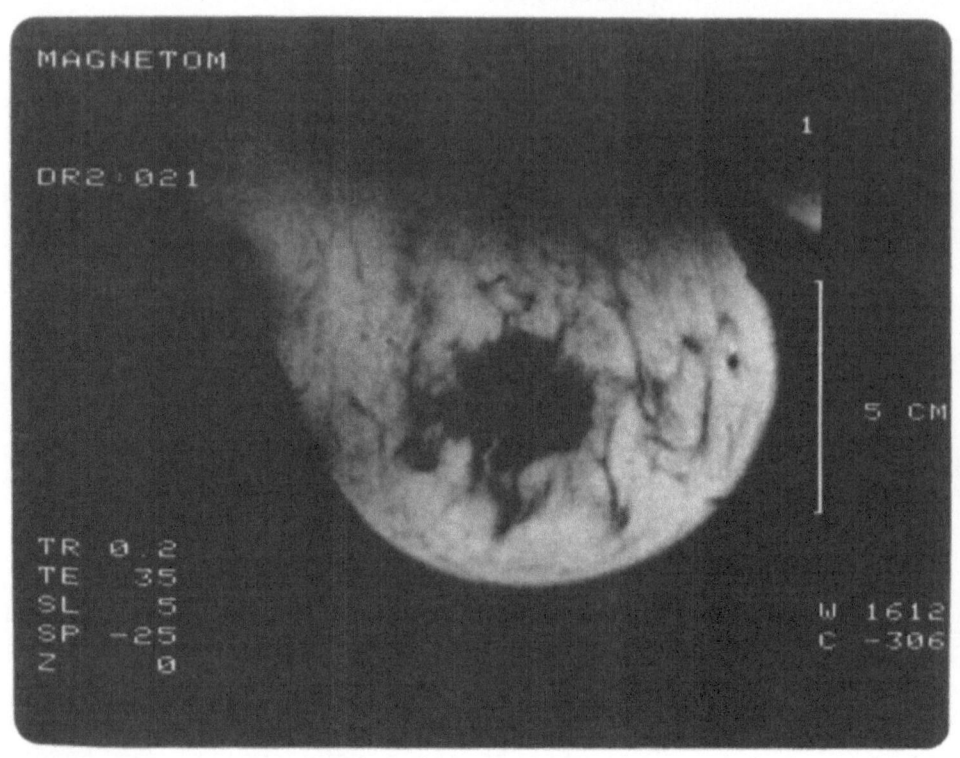

Figure 6:   Sagital spin-echo mammascan with solid carcinoma
            visible.   TR =200 ms, TE=35 ms, slice thickness
            5 mm.   Total scan time about 1 1/2 min.

If the flow takes place within the imaged slice, it is seen as a dark area because the signals of the moving protons are imaged spatially remote from the site where the flow occurs. The resulting artifact consists normally of a diffuse shadow spread over an extended area within the image plane so that it is hardly discernable for smaller flow volumina. Where a resolution is sufficient, plaques on the intima of the vessel should become visible because of the high-fat and fat-water contrast. Figure 7 gives an example of a fast, low resolution 0.35T head and neck scan with a slice thickness of 20 mm. The carotis bifurcation is well recognizable.

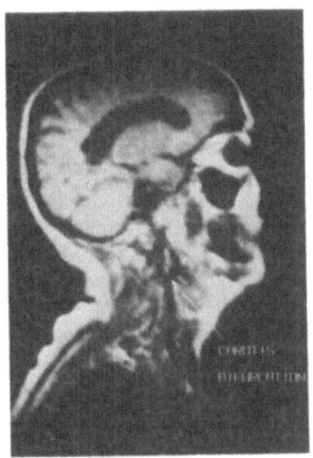

Figure 7: Low resolution sagital head scan (slice thickness 20 mm). The carotis bifurcation is clearly visible.

IN VIVO MR-SPECTROSCOPY

Hardly exploited is still the clinical applications of MR-spectroscopy for the in vivo-diagnosis of body chemistry and the follow-up of metabolic processes. The main problems are the rather low concentrations of the metabolites which are in the micromolar to millimolar range, and the limited sensitivity of MR towards nuclei other than protons. These difficulties can only be overcome by increasing the magnetic field for increased nuclear magnetization and reduced spatial resolution.

Since the seventies, considerable work has been done in the use of high resolution phosphorus-NMR for the investigation of the energy delivering adenosine triphosphate (ATP) phospho-creatine (PC), sugar phosphates (SP) and inorganic phosphates (P_1)which have narrow resonant lines with a chemical shift within a frequency range of 30 ppm which can be assigned and measured easily. Valuable information on

the cellular energy status can be obtained by quantitative
evaluation of the relative metabolite concentrations (11).
     The acidity or ph dependent chemical shift of the in-
organic phosphate line with respect to the PCr-line can provide diagnostically useful information on the degree of
oxygen perfusion within tissue. It can also be expected
that this possibility of ph-measurement together with the
MR-spectral analysis will eventually contribute to noninvasive differential diagnostic procedures (12). The
ischemic effect in a ligated arm muscle in comparison to the
normally perfused muscle can be seen in Figure 8, which represents the corresponding ^{31}P spectra obtained at 1.5T in
a time of approximately 6 minutes within a muscle volume of
about 27 ml. First clinical applications of ^{31}P-MR spectroscopy for the diagnosis of metabolic disorders were done at
Oxford University by G.K. Radda et al (13). Noninvasive
metabolic studies on babies are presently performed at the
University College in London (14). The same groups used
also ^{31}P-spectroscopy on kidney transplants for viability
assurance before transplantation. ^{13}C-lines show a much
bigger chemical shift of up to 200 ppm. The minute natural
abundance of ^{13}C renders it more difficult in its application in natural concentrations. For special purposes this
could be bypassed by the use of ^{13}C-enriched compounds, i.e.,
for metabolic studies in liver and kidneys.

SIEMENS   P-31 SPECTRUM

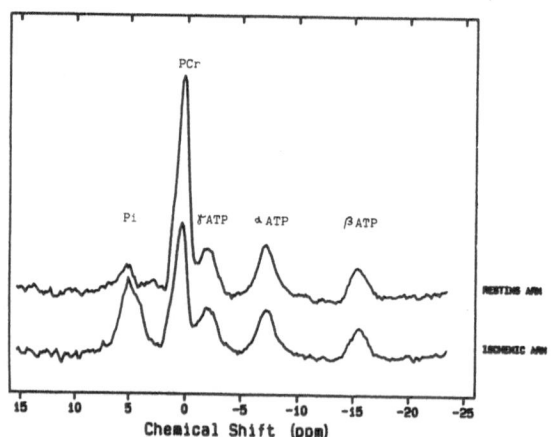

Figure 8:   The decrease in phospho-creatine (PCr) and the
            build up of inorganic phosphates (Pi) can
            clearly be seen in the ^{31}P-spectral lines ob-
            tained with a surface coil on the arm muscle
            before and after exercise under ischemic condi-
            tions.

Comparatively easily detectable is the Na-MR within the body. Only one larger line is detectable from the sodium dissolved in body liquids like i.e., CSF. Na-MR-images have been obtained at magnetic fields above 1T. According to S.K. Hilal, Na-MR would give an earlier detection of brain stroke then a proton resonance imaging (15).

The high MR sensitivity for fluourine and lithium in the normal human body could show existence of these only in very small quantities. This suggests the application of biologically acceptable compounds in which these isotopes could be incorporated acting as MR acceptable labels. Such substances exist already i.e., in the form of fluorine containing blood substitues which hav e been tested mainly in animals.

Practically all organic substances within the human body contain protons which should give rise to discrete proton MR lines. These lines can however, not be seen under normal conditions because of the dominating contributions of the water and fat (lipid) which are about 3 to 4 ppm apart, exceeding all other proton MR-lines by many orders of magnitude. By corresponding modification of spin echo imaging pulse sequences, these two separate contributions can be used for the generation of distinguished water and lipid images of the human body (16).

Analytical MR-spectroscopic methods with waterline suppression are already well known. It is expected that such schemes, which have already been tested on animals, will also be applicable for biochemical in vitro analysis of more prevailing substances like glucosis or lactic acid (17). The high MR-sensitivity for protons makes this type of spectroscopy especially attractive.

Presently the medical application of MR spectroscopy seems still to be in its infancy. With the availability of high field, high homogeneity whole body magnet systems, it is likely that MR spectroscopic procedures will become more and more important in some fields of human biochemical diagnosis.

CONCLUSION

In spite of the short time of existence of MR-imaging and spectroscopy, a considerable number of new techniques and new applications has been developed. The pace of the first most exciting years might slow down eventually. It exists however, no doubt that there is still a lot to come. The most important objective for further development is probably the finding that the exposure to the magnetic resonance fields seems to be harmless to the chromosomes, cells, and whole organisms. An extended exposure study must certainly investigate whether long term effects exist.

The harmless application of MR, according to our present knowledge, seems to make it a suitable tool for repeated therapy control; especially in cases of benign
diseases where possible ionizing radiation hazards would be
a concern. Similar considerations hold true especially for
exploration of the lower pelvis area even in cases of preg-
nancy and the diagnosis of babies, where body motion seems
to pose some problems. Another application could be the
exploration of apparently healthy people in a screening
procedure for diseases like cancer. What stands against it
is the comparatively long investigation time per patient
which is presently in the order of an hour and the high
cost involved. Further development might change this
drastically.

ACKNOWLEDGEMENTS:

The contribution of Johanne Brooks in the completion of
this paper is gratefully acknowledged.

REFERENCES

1.   Arnold J.T., Dharmatti S.S., Packard M.E.: J. Chem
     Phys. 19: 507 (1951
2.   Purcell E.M., Torrey H.C., Pound R.V.: Phys Rev. 69,
     37 (1946)
3.   Bloch F., Hansen W.W., Packard M.: Phys. Review 70,
     474 (1946)
4.   Lauterbur P.C.: Nature 242, 190 (1973)
5.   Bloembergen N., Purcell E.M., Pound R.V.: Phys. Rev.
     73, 679 (1948)
6.   Bakker C.J.G., Vriend J: Phys. Med. Biol. 28, 331
     (1983)
7.   Sauter R., Mueller E., Fritschy P.:" Design of Special
     (Surface) Coils for MR Imaging." Radiology 153 (p)
     175 (1984)
8.   Stelling C.B. et al.: "MR Imaging of the female Breast
     Using a Prototype Breast Coil." Radiol. 154. 457 (1985)
9.   Singer J.R.: Blood Flow Rates by NMR Measurements.
     Science 180, 1652 (1959)
10. Deimling M., et al.: "Description and Quantification
     of Flow Phenomena Seen on MR Images", Radiol. 153 (p)
     64 (1984)
11. Gadian D.G., Hoult D.I., Radda G.K. et al.: "Phosphorus
     NMR Studies on Normoxic and Ischemic Cardiac Tissue."
     Proc. Acad. Sci., USA 73, 4446 (1946)

12. Ng, T.C., Evanochko, W.T. and Glickson, J.D.:" Faraday
    Shield for Surface-Coil Studies on Subcutaneous Tumors."
    Journ. of Magr. Res. 49, 526 (1982)
13. Ross, B.D., Radda, G.K., Gadian, D.G., et al: "Exam-
    ination of a Suspected Case of McArdell's Syndrome"
    by 31-P-NMR. N. Engl. J. Med. 304, 1338 (1981)
14. Cady, E.B. et al.: "Non-invasive Investigation of
    Cerebral Metabolism in Newborn Infants by Phosphorus
    NMR-Spectroscopy." Lancet 1: 1059 (1983) ·
15. Hilal S.K. et al., "Proton and Sodium MRi-Stroke."
    Radiol. 153 (p), 165 (1984)
16. Dixon, W. Th., "Simple Proton Spectroscopic Imaging".
    Radiol 153, 189 (1984)
17. Hore, P.J., "Solvent Suppression in Fourier Transform-MNR."
    Journ. of Magn. Res. 55, 283, (1983).

COST AND AVAILABILITY OF COMMERCIAL NMR EQUIPMENT; AND REQUIREMENTS FOR HOUSING, INSTALLATION AND OPERATION

L.D. Hall
Department of Chemistry
University of British Columbia
Vancouver, B.C.
Canada V6T 1W5

ABSTRACT. A brief overview is given of some of the factors which are pertinent to the installation of a large NMR instrument. Specific details of the actual installation and operating costs are not given because they vary so widely. Attention is drawn to the fact that all the major suppliers provide a detailed planning service and subsequent maintenance contracts.

The depth of commercial interest in the development of clinical magnetic resonance devices is immense, indeed almost unmanageable at present. All the major manufacturers of medical imaging devices have a substantial commitment; these include, Diasonics, Elscint, General Electric, Phillips, Picker, Siemens, Technicare. Other companies which have a major stake in the area include Bruker, Fonar, M. and D. Enterprises, Oxford Research Systems, Thompson-C.G.A. However, in virtually all countries, groups have already made their own imaging systems and some of these have taken the opportunity to commercialise their knowledge. These include groups in Italy, Korea, Scandinavia, U.S.A. There are also innumerable initiatives in Japan, many of which will be public knowledge by the publication date of this article. Given the immense capital investments required to pursue an active research and development programme in such a rapidly moving area, and the subsequent demands for very rapid field service, it seems highly improbable that all those companies will be able to survive commerically. Nevertheless, the speciality research market is probably sufficient to sustain a number of small, highly innovative companies, especially those which will price their equipment for science based groups.

In the early days of clinical NMR, the two main techniques, tomography and spectroscopy, were pursued by completely separate companies, generally with no overlap of interest. Fortunately, a more rational attitude now prevails and much emphasis is now centred on a broader, more integrated approach. Machines strictly developed for proton tomography are available at field strengths for 0.1 - 2.0

193

T. Axenrod and G. Ceccarelli (eds.), NMR in Living Systems, 193–197.
© 1986 by D. Reidel Publishing Company.

Tesla. All systems now available for spectroscopy, automatically include all facilities necessary for imaging, and operate in the range 1.5 - 2.0 Tesla for whole body sized instruments. Systems based on smaller sized magnets are available at substantially higher operating fields.

The approximate cost for purchasing various systems are summarised in the Table below. It must be emphasised that these can only be regarded as approximate, because most of the systems which have been sold so far have included a research agreement and a concommittant reduction in original price.

Table. Price ranges ($ American) for NMR devices suitable for imaging and spectroscopy.

Purpose	Magnet Bore (cm)	Magnet Field (Tesla)	Price (millions)
Proton Tomography	100	0.1 - 0.5	1 -1.5
Tomography/Spectroscopy	100	1.5 - 2.0	1.5-2.5
Tomography/Spectroscopy	30	ca. 2	0.65
Tomography/Spectroscopy	30	ca. 4.7	0.8
Spectroscopy	10	ca. 6.2	0.3

Until very recently essentially all the magnets used for imaging systems have come from one source, Oxford Instruments, in England. That company has recently expanded its manufacturing base into the U.S.A. and Japan. However, several other manufacturers have now sold magnets including Bruker (Germany), Fonar (U.S.A.), Intermagnetic General (U.S.A.), Nalorac (U.S.A.), Walker Magnets (U.K.) and Wang (U.S.A.). It seems likely that this diversification will increase in the future; futhermore, it seems inconceivable that the larger companies such as General Electric, Phillips, Siemens and Technicare will long refrain from manufacturing their own magnets.

The requirements for housing, installing and operating an NMR imaging device are dominated at present by the fringing field of the magnet itself. This field, which extends for a substantial volume surrounding the magnet, can have a major effect on field-sensitive objects in its vicinity; and, in turn, the overall quality of the field produced within the bore of the magnet can be seriously degraded by iron objects, both stationary, or moving. Thus, the presence of large masses of structural iron near to the magnet can pose serious problems for magnet shimming; large masses which move with respect to the magnet, such as elevators or trucks, can result in field shifts and subsequent variable distortions of the images.

Obviously the magnitude and extent of the fringing field depends critically on the strength of the magnet; thus the size of the suite used to house the instrument is generally substantially larger for the higher field systems. Self-shielding magnets have now been developed which minimise this problem.

The most important additional features of the fringing field, concern safety. Although there is no indication that static magnetic fields are injurious to man, the pumping rate of most heart pacemakers is set to its base level when exposed to a field of 5-20 gauss. Although an accidental change of pumping rate is not a lethal experience, it is clearly unacceptable and hence access within the volume enclosed by the 3 gauss line must be stringently controlled to exclude this possibility. Access by persons who have any implanted prosthetic device is similarly restricted, especially when that device is made from magnetic materials. The most important in this context are metallic surgical clips used to seal internal incisions. Given that ferromagnetic objects in the near vicinity of the magnet will experience a strong attractive force, it is absolutely mandatory that they be rigorously excluded from the suite. This is especially important when a patient is to be examined! Installation of a metal detector at the outer access to the suite is strongly recommended.

Three considerations are pertinent to the choice of access routes of which patient access is of dominant concern. Ideally, the NMR suite should be directly connected by a corridor to the Hospital itself. And, given that for a single instrument the patient flow will almost certainly not exceed 15 per working day, which is small compared with the total flow through a Radiology Department, it is economically desireable that patient management be controlled by the same staff which operates the tomograph itself. This very ease of access for patients places stringent demands on the system devised for keeping unauthorised personnel from entry near to the magnet itself. Besides the metal detector referred to earlier, it is desireable to have to have automatic visual and audible warning systems to alert persons who are either deaf, or blind, that they have accidently penetrated into a restricted area.

Physical access for the installation of the original equipment, and for subsequent delivery of the cryogens necessary for a superconducting magnet, are not normally difficult. Yet, here too, careful planning is obviously mandatory. Fortunately all the instrument companies can provide detailed advice, and in some instances planning and construction as well. Depending on the particular system chosen, a part of, or often the entire, imaging suite will require radiofrequency screening. Achievement of an attenuation factor of 100 decibels is not trivial. The suite has to be lined with copper foil and all doors fitted with grounded, brass-fingering along their edges. More difficult, all cables must themselves be connected to the outside world via appropriate isolation connectors.

Given these constraints, the ideal location for an instrument is in a wooden hut, copper lined, and located in the middle of a green field, connected to the hospital via a long corridor! Given the reality that many instruments must be installed into an existing hospital, often located in a metal framed building in a city area, much attention is now being directed to magnetic shielding. One approach is to line the suite with soft iron sheets, about 2 cm thick. A more sophisticated solution is to locate the magnet inside a soft iron tube. The ultimate expression of this approach is to include this iron cladding into the magnet itself, and it seems probable that this will become the approach of choice. Resistive magnets based on this concept already have fringing fields of as little as 5 gauss/cm as close as 2 metres to the ends of the magnet.

Both cryo- and resistive- systems require routine maintenance which can be achieved either <u>via</u> a service contract or by in-house personnel. Likewise, all systems will require competent radiologic technicians. For a proton tomograph operating at a daily-throughput of 8 patients per day, one dedicated person can barely manage the combined demands of instrument operation and image work-up and archiving. For a daily throughput of 12 persons two persons will suffice. However, this throughput can only be sustained if access is available to a separate station for data processing, display and archiving. It is the author's view that this facility is not only desirable, and financially prudent, but is mandatory for the efficient functioning of the imaging facility.

For resistive magnets, the main source of maintenance will be the water cooling system and the high current power supplies. For superconducting magnets the regular replenishment of the cryogens takes this place. Liquid nitrogen can be transferred economically through insulated transfer tubes over distances of tens of metres. This is advisable since conventional, iron dewars can then be used. In contrast, liquid helium transfer tubes must be as short as is physically feasible; hence access must be provided for non-magnetic dewars to be positioned immediately adjacent to the superconducting magnet. Although the unit cost of liquid nitrogen is not high, the relatively large volumes used have prompted the development of heat exchange pumps which can take the place of the large nitrogen reservoir. And although liquid helium boil-off rates are now remarkably low, typically less than 400 ml/hour for a 1 metre bore magnet, the high cost of liquid helium, coupled with concern as to its regular supply, have both resulted in the development of cryopumps. It seems highly probable that future generations of superconducting magnets will require rather infrequent, perhaps annual, delivery of cryogens. Those developments will certainly increase the already favourably low operating costs of a cryo- versus resistive-magnet. A further, interesting possibility involves the development of permanent magnets. It is improbable that these will be suitable for spectroscopy, but low field proton tomography is assuredly within the range of fields that can be generated.

Although most of the above technical discussion is also pertinent to instruments which are to be used for research, the demands for personnel are likely to be very different indeed. At present, it is desirable to have a science-based team since software and hardware developments are both likely to be necessary.

It is appropriate to note here that the large regional variations which exist worldwide may have a dominant effect on the selection of instrumentation. Difficult access to cryogens will be an obvious factor until such time as efficient cryo pumping is established. Yet frequently those same regions also have erratic supplies of electricity and water, both inimicable to the efficient operation of an electromagnet. These factors, coupled with the high capital costs, will undoubtedly restrict access to these instruments to many who might otherwise find use for NMR. Populous nations such as China and India along with those in South America are obviously in this category.

Finally, I wish to end this article by noting that interest in non-medical applications of both NMR imaging and spectroscopy is, at long last, burgeoning in both university and industrial laboratories. A number of groups have already assembled their own devices and several companies worldwide have already offered suitable instrumentation. This is a welcome, albeit overdue, development which should help to establish a very necessary balance to what has thus far been a somewhat lopsided initiative. Quite apart from the intrinsic importance and merit of the numerous applications which are possible, it is only with access to less expensive and more versatile instrumentation that many university groups will be able to participate in the development of new spin physics for future imaging and spectroscopic methods in a timely way.

PRACTICAL ASPECTS OF "IN VITRO" AND "IN VIVO" T_1 AND T_2 MEASUREMENTS

C.A.BOICELLI, A.M.BALDASSARRI
C.N.R., Istituto di Anatomia Umana Normale - Bologna
IRCCS H.San Raffaele - Milano (Italy)

ABSTRACT. The determination of relaxation times is one of the most critical NMR experiments and needs careful instrumental adjustment and the use of proper models for the interpretation. This is particularly important for relaxation measurements in tissues, both "in vitro" and "in vivo", where the Bloch equations are not valid and the experimental conditions are quite far from ideal.

INTRODUCTION

The relaxation times T_1 and T_2, which have already been introduced and discussed in a preceding chapter, are generally evaluated by following the time behaviour of the magnetization, $\bar{M}$, after the application of a sequence of 90° and/or 180° pulses, appropriately chosen and spaced. The recovery of the equilibrium value of the magnetization is described by the Bloch equations (1). These equations, which describe the behaviour of nuclear magnetic moments in a variable magnetic field, are based on the following assumptions:
1) the macroscopic magnetization vector in a homogeneous magnetic field, $\bar{B}$, behaves as the individual magnetic moment, $\bar{\mu}$, and its motion is described by the equation:

$$d\bar{M}/dt = \bar{M} \times \gamma\bar{B} \qquad (1)$$

This implies that the nuclei have permament magnetic moments whose magnitude is unaffected by any interaction.
2) in a static magnetic field $(B_z = B_o)$ the magnetization of a popula-

199

tion of free spins evolves towards the equilibrium according to:

$$dM_z/dt = - (M_z - M_0)/T_1 \qquad (2)$$

where the rate constant, $1/T_1$, is the longitudinal or spin-lattice relaxation rate.
3) when, by some means (for instance, by applying a radio-frequency
field B_1), a component $M_{x,y}$ of the magnetization is induced perpendicular to M, it decays according to:

$$dM_{x,y}/dt = - M_{x,y}/T_2 \qquad (3)$$

where the rate constant $1/T_2$ is the transverse or spin-spin relaxation
rate.
Assumptions 2 and 3 imply that individual nuclei relax independently
from one another, i.e. they hold for a system of non-interacting spins.
4) when a static magnetic field $\bar{B}_0 = B_0\hat{k} = -(\omega/\gamma)\hat{k}$ is applied to an
ensemble of spins simultaneously with a field, $\bar{B}_1$, rotating at an angular velocity ω and $\bar{B}_0$ and perpendicular to it, the time dependence
of $\bar{M}$ is described by the equation:

$$d\bar{M}/dt = M \times \gamma\bar{B} = (M_x\hat{i} + M_y\hat{j})/T_2 - (M_z - M_0)\hat{k}/T_1 \qquad (4)$$

defined in the laboratory frame of reference. In a frame S', rotating
at an angular velocity ω around $\bar{B}_0$, and where $\bar{B}_1$ lies along the x'
axis, the resultant of $\bar{B}_0$ and $\bar{B}_1$ is an effective field. $\bar{B}_{eff} =$
$(B_0 + \omega/\gamma)\hat{k} + B_1\hat{i}$ static in S'. At resonance, i.e. when $\omega = -\gamma B_0 = \omega_0$
$_0$, the effective field becomes $B_1\hat{i}$ and the magnetization precesses at
a frequency $-\gamma B_{eff} = -\gamma B_1$ around it.
        The phenomenon of nuclear magnetic relaxation described by the
Bloch equations can occur through many mechanisms - interaction between
nuclear spins and local magnetic fields arising from the thermal
motions of the lattice, intramolecular motions, exchange processes,
paramagnetic interactions and so on - which are related to the mobility
of the molecules in the sample (2). The parameter that can be used to

evaluate the molecular mobility is the correlation time τ_c; and as many correlation times can be defined as there are molecular motions (e/g: translation, rotation, diffusion, etc.). Different τ_c values generally correspond to different phases of the system under study. The actual τ_c is therefore the resultant of all the individual τ_c's, each weighted according to its partition function. This means that the motional frequencies in the sample, namely its spectrum, are all those comprised between 0 and $1/\tau_c$ Hz. The correct sampling of a spectrum, therefore, requires a passband of the measuring apparatus wide enough to cover the whole spectrum (for instance, tissue samples where the correlation times can vary between 10^{-12} and 10^{-6} s need a passband of the order of the MHz) and a transmitter power high enough to invert all the spins when a 180° pulse is applied. When dealing with long correlation times, as in the case of tissues, the linewidth $(1/\pi\ T_2)$ and B_0 are comparable; B_1 needs to be fairly intense and becomes to a certain extent comparable to B_0 and the value of M_0 is then given by $x_0 [\ B_0 + B_1(t)]$. In this case, the effective field differs from $B_1\hat{i}$ and the M_z component has a non-zero stationary state value (3). Consequently, T_1 and T_2 are modified and are no more the time constants for the recovery of the equilibrium values of M_z and $M_{x,y}$. Therefore, high resolution NMR spectrometers are not suited for measuring relaxation rates in tissues, since the ideal instrument must feature wide passband, intense radio-frequency field and dead time and pulse length much shorter than the shortest T_2 (in the order of μs) so that the measured values (I) of M_z, $M_{x,y}$ and especially M_0 are not appreciably smaller than the true values. The nature of the sample is also of crucial importance, since the receiver response is modified by the dielectric in which the antenna is immersed. A correct evaluation of the signal intensity (I) is only obtained if the filling factor of the receiver coil is good and, in the ideal instrument, it should therefore be possible to match the coil to the shape of the sample. The problem of the sample shape is critical in the case of bioptic specimens.

We have described the instrumental requirements for a correct determination of the signal intensity I, which is the parameter to be measured for the evaluation of the relaxation rates. We will now discuss the pulse sequences most frequently used for such measurements. Obviously, the results of the experiments are only valid for systems fulfilling the requirements for the validity of the Bloch equations.

The inversion-recovery (I.R.), the saturation-recovery (S.R.), and the progressive saturation (P.S.) sequences are generally used for the determination of the longitudinal relaxation times. The main characteristics of the sequences as described in the literature (4), are summarized in Table I. The advantages and disadvantages of these different pulse sequences for measuring T_1 are compared in Table II.

The pulse sequences generally used for the determination of T_2 as described in standard textbooks (4), and their principle features are shown in Table III. The relative advantages and disadvantages of these sequences are compared in Table IV.

Under ideal conditions, i.e. for a spin system obeying the Bloch equations, with all the spins on resonance and subject to an effective r.f. $\bar{B}_{eff} = \bar{B}_1$, the macroscopic magnetization nutates by 90° or 180° by application of the appropriate pulse. In this ideal case, the magnetization behaves as described in Table V.

Table I. Pulse Sequences for the Determination of Longitudinal Relaxation Times.

SEQUENCE	FUNCTIONS
I.R. $180° - \tau - 90° - T_D^*$	$I_\tau^{\div} = I_0^{\dagger}\ 1 - 2 \exp (-\tau/T_1)$
S.R. $90°-(HSP)-\tau-90°-A_t-(HSP)_n$	$I_\tau = I_0\ 1 - \exp\ (-\tau/T_1)$
P.S. $(90°-\tau)_3\ or\ 4-(90°)-\tau)_n$	$I_\tau = I_0\ 1 - \exp\ (-\tau/T_1)$

* $T_D \sim 5T_1$

$\div$ measured signal intensity

$\dagger$ measured signal intensity after a 90° pulse

Table II. Advantages and Disadvantages of the Different Pulse Sequences for the Determination of T_1.

SEQUENCE	ADVANTAGES	DISADVANTAGES
P.S.	- Very simple - Relatively rapid	- Restricted to long relaxation times - Lower sensitivity than I.R.$_*$ - Applicable only when $T_2 \ll T_1$
I.R.	- Dynamic range twice that of P.S. $(2\ I_0)$ - More general - Most accurate	- More time consuming than P.S. $(T_D \sim 5T_1)$ - I_0 should be determined two or three times - A set of different τ values in the range $0.3\ T_1$-$1.5\ T_1$ is needed
S.R.	- Time saving - Not limited to the measurement of long $T_1's$ as P.S.	- Dynamic range lower than I.R. (I_0) - Extra hardware needed - Non-negligible time (100 ms) required to restore field homogeneity

Table III. Pulse Sequences for the Determination of Transverse Relaxation Times, T_2.

	SEQUENCE	FUNCTIONS
	90°-FID (Free Induction Decay)	$FID = FID\ \exp\ (-\ \tau/T_2)$
S.E.	90°-τ-180°-2τ-echo	$I_{2\tau} = I_0\ \exp\ (-\ 2\ \tau/T_2)$
C.P.	90°-τ-180°-2τ-180°-2τ....	$I_{2\tau} = I_0\ \exp\ (-\ 2\ \tau/T_2)$
C.P.M.G.	$90°_x$-τ-$180°_y$-2τ -$180°_y$-2τ-$180°_y$	$I_{2\tau} = I_0\ \exp\ (-\ 2\ \tau/T_2)$

Table IV. Advantages and Disadvantages of the Different Pulse Sequences for the Determination of T_2.

SEQUENCES	ADVANTAGES	DISADVANTAGES
S.E.	- Very simple - Error in pulse angle not cumulative	- Time Consuming - Sensitive to diffusion - Sensitive to error in the 180° pulse
C.P.	- Refocusing eliminates field inhomogeneity effects - Successive echoes expected to decay exponentially with relaxation rate $1/T_2$	- τ assumed to be so short that spin diffusion is negligible - Missetting of pulse angle introduces cumulative errors - Consequent imperfect refocusing for higher order echoes
C.P.M.G.	- Eliminates cumulative errors due to missetting of pulse angle - Compensates for inhomogeneity of $\bar{B}_1$ field - Compensates for off-resonance effects	- Phase shifter needed - Careful calibration of pulse width recommended - Good field homogenity advisable to prevent diffusion contribution at large τ values

Table V. Behaviour of the Macroscopic Magnetization ($\bar{M}$) in the Rotating Frame.

$\bar{M}$ Component	At Equilibrium	After a 90° Pulse	After a 180° Pulse
M_x, M_y	0	$\pm M_z(\pm M_0)^*$	0
M_z	M_0	0	$-M_z(= -M_0)^*$

$^*\pm$ refers to the phase relationship between Trx and Rcx.

It is obvious that in the NMR experiment the 90° and 180° pulses are optionally defined as those inducing in the receiver coil the maximum signal intensity ($I = 0$; 90° pulse) and the first minimum signal intensity ($I = 0$; 180° pulse), respectively. In a real experiment there are several sources of error in the determination of the relaxation times, which we will discuss now. In this respect, the measurement of T_2 is more critical than that of T_1, since transverse relaxation is more sensitive to the motional components of low frequency and the instrumental requirements for the correct determination of T_2 are very severe.

A - Sources of error attributable to the transmitter.

    1. Inhomogeneity of the r.f. field $(\overline{B}_1)$: the excitation is not uniform over the sample and the tilt angle corresponds to the nominal value in certain regions of the sample, while it deviates from it in others.

    2. The transmitter power, or its passband, is inadequate to uniformly excite the spins over the whole spectral width. This may often happen with tissues, where τ_c's larger than 10^{-7} and linewidths of the order of MHz are frequently encountered. This situation can be similar to A-1, in certain respects.

    3. The carrier of the r.f. field $\overline{B}_1$ is out of resonance: only a fraction of the spins is excited and the excitation is not uniform even if the transmitter power is sufficient. The effect is the same as in cases A-1 and A-2.

B - Sources of error attributable to the receiver.

    1. The passband does not match the spectralwidth: the measured signal intensity is lower than actual. This situation is similar to A-2.

    2. The receiver dead-time is too long: the signal can be sampled only after a time non-negligible compared to T_2 from the beginning of the FID. The measured signal intensity is therefore found to be lower than it really is. This point is particularly crucial for samples with a very short T_2 ($\sim$ms), namely for spin systems with $\tau_c > 10^{-8}$s.

    3. The non-linearity of the receiver influences the relaxation time determination in a way similar to the inhomogeneity of the r.f. field (A-1).

C - Sources of error attributable to incorrect choice of measuring parameters.

    1. Delay time (T_D) between pulse sequences is too short: not

enough time is allowed for the equilibrium magnetization to be restored and erroneous values, I_0 and I of M_0 and M respectively are measured (Table VI).

Table VI. Error Introduced in the Determination of T_1 by I.R. Method When the Delay is too Short.

T_D	$T_1(\%)$
$2.T_1$	-31
$3.T_1$	-11
$4.T_1$	-4
$5.T_1$	-1.5

2. An erroneous evaluation of M_0 (or better I_0) can result not only from a value of T_D that is too short, but also wrong values of the 90° and/or 180° pulses. The use of an incorrect value of I_0 seriously affects the determination of T_1 (Table VII). Since T_2 is calculated by means of the equation $I_{2\tau} = I_0 \exp(-2 \tau/T_2)$, only the intercept at the origin is altered in the evaluation of T_2.

Table VII. Effect of an Erroneous Value of I_0 on the Calculated T_1 Values Determined by the Inversion-Recovery Method.

$I_0(\%)$	$T_1(\%)$
-20	-22
-10	-11
0	0
+10	-11
+20	+22

3. Wrong, or incomplete, information on the relaxation rates might be obtained if the number of experimental points (τ values) is too small, namely when the range of τ explored does not cover the full range of rates of the dynamic events controlling the relaxation or when

the experimental points are not close enough to one another. In this case a multi-exponential decay, that is the existence of more than one relaxation time, may be overlooked (5,6).

The reliability of the measured relaxation rates, under optimum experimental conditions, is obviously based on the presumption that the length of the 90° and 180° pulses has been correctly determined. A wrong value for the 90° pulse is not critical for the determination of T_2, since the equation for the time evolution of the magnetization becomes

$$M_{2\tau} = M_0 \cos\alpha \ \exp(-2\tau/T_2) \qquad (5)$$

where α is the angle between the magnetization vector after the 90° pulse and the axis along which the receiver is placed. Only the inter-cept at the origin of the logarithmic plot is modified, but not the slope.

On the other hand, when the 90° pulse is wrong, correct T_1 values (Table II) cannot be obtained by either SR or IR sequences, since accurate I_0 measurements are essential.

An error in the 180° pulse is instead detrimental to the accurate measurement of T_2: the magnetization in the x', y' plane decays accor-ding to the law:

$$M_\tau = M_0 \exp[-2\tau/T_2 (1-\sin\delta)] \qquad (6)$$

where δ is the deviation of the tilt angle from 180°. The effect of an incorrect 180° pulse on the calculated T_2 value is shown in Table VIII for a spin-echo sequence.

Table VIII. Dependence of the Calculated T_2 on the Deviation in Values of the 180° Pulse Angle Used in a Spin-Echo Sequence.

δ	-30	-20	-10	0	+10	+20	+30
$T_2(\%)$	50	34	17	0	-17	-34	-50

The other sequences for measuring T_2 minimize the effects of the inhomogeneity of B_0 and B_1, but make the errors in the $180°$ pulse cumulative and gross errors in the calculated T_2 may result for a deviation of δ degrees from the nominal $180°$ pulse. With the Carr-Purcell pulse sequence, after n pulses the error in the pulse angle is $n\delta$ and this leads to an underestimation of $I_{2\tau}$. For example, if $\delta = 1°$ an underestimation of 44.7% is obtained after ten echoes.

All the factors so far described contribute to the departure of the actual situation from the ideal one in a real experiment. The deviation may be described by the factor k, which relates the true and the experimental values:

$$M_z = k \, M_0 \qquad \begin{array}{l} k = 0 \text{ for an ideal } 90° \text{ pulse} \\ k = k' = -1 \text{ for an ideal } 180° \text{ pulse} \end{array} \qquad (7)$$

Obviously, also the transverse components, $M_{x,y}$, are affected and the deviation in the experimental conditions can be described by the factor β:

$$M_x = M_y = \beta M_0 \qquad \beta = 1 \text{ for an ideal } 90° \text{ pulse} \qquad (8)$$

Making use of the parameters just introduced, the equations describing the time dependence of the signal intensity for the various pulse sequences becomes:

INVERSION-RECOVERY
$$I = \beta I_0 [\, 1-(1-k')e^{-\tau/T_1}\,] \quad \text{for } T_D {\sim} 5T_1 \qquad (9)$$

SATURATION RECOVERY
$$I = \beta I_0 \frac{1 - [1 - k(1 - e^{-T_D/T_1})] \, e^{-\tau/T_1}}{1 - k^2 \, e^{-T_D/T_1} \quad e^{-\tau/T_1}} \qquad (10)$$

PROGRESSIVE SATURATION
$$I = \beta I_0 \frac{1 - e^{-\tau/T_1}}{1 - k \, e^{-\tau/T_1}} \qquad (11)$$

The β parameter may be ignored in the T_1 measurements, which are an evaluation of the time evolution of the z component of the magnetization vector; the reliability of the measure depends only on k (k') (4). The influence of k (k') on the measured value of T_1 is shown in Table IX.

Table IX. Deviation of the Experimental T_1 Value from the Ideal One as a Function of k in Different Pulse Sequences.

	I.R.		S.R.		P.S.
k(k')	T_1(%)	k	T_1(%)	k	T_1(%)
-0.66	12	0.34	-19	0.34	-18
-0.83	5	0.17	- 9	0.17	-10
-1.0	0	0.0	0	0.0	0

Clearly, the I.R. sequence suffers less than the others from the effects of the k factor. It must be pointed out that departure from ideality is extremely significant when measuring the relaxation times in tissues, since an r.f. perturbing field ($\bar{B}_1$) is needed comparable in magnitude with the static magnetic field ($\bar{B}_0$) and with the spectral width (ΔB_0) because of the τ_c dispersion (from 10^{-12} up to 10^{-6}s or more). In this case, the fundamental requirement $B_1 >> \Delta B_0$ is violated and the effective field $\bar{B}_{eff}$ is titled at an angle $\phi = \text{atang} \frac{\Delta \bar{B}}{\bar{B}_1}$ relative to $\bar{B}_1$. Thus, after the application of a r.f. pulse of nominal flip angle α (90° or 180°, for instance), the magnetization rotates about $\bar{B}_{eff}$ by and angle $\psi = \alpha / \cos\phi$ and its z-component, if the pulse is applied at the equilibrium, will be

$$M_z = k M_0 = (\text{sen}^2 \phi + \cos\psi \cos^2 \phi) M_0 \qquad (12)$$

Moreover, it must be stressed that the relaxation process in tissues does not fulfill at all the basic requirements of the Bloch equations.

Since in tissues liquid-like and solid-like phases coexist, the resulting spin system cannot any longer be described as the resultant of an
assembly of non-interacting magnetic moments and the magnetization decay is no longer a single-exponential (7). Therefore, the application
of models based on the Bloch equations is of little use and somewhat
incorrect. It must be borne in mind that the time constants extracted
from the magnetization time evolution profiles are not the true T_1 and
T_2 but only time parameters related to them even if their names are
still improperly retained.

The experimental check of the points discussed above have been
carried out on a sample of rabbit myocardium. This tissues is stable
for several hours (5-6 h) and can therefore be used without problems.
A cyclindrical, visually homogeneous sample was fitted perfectly into
an NMR tube and a Bruker Minispec p20, operating at MHz was used for
the measurements.

We have systematically modified the instrumental parameters on
which the correct measure of the relaxation times depends: 180° pulse
length, transmitter phase, delay time T_D between pulse sequences. The
results are collected in the following tables where all the data have
been normalized using as reference the magnetization decay after an
inversion-recovery and a spin-echo sequence under optimum instrumental
and measuring conditions. The data are therefore dimensionless, the
magnetization being in I_τ/I_0 units and the time in τ/T_1 or $2\tau/T_2$ units.

Table X. Effect of Erroneous Experimental Parameters on the Determination of T_1.

PARAMETER	T_1	$T_1(\%)$
NONE	1	-
δ = +15°	0.86	-14
δ = -10°	0.95	- 5
ϕ_{trx} =±25°	MEANINGLESS BEHAVIOR OF THE MAGNETIZATION	
T_D = $2T_1$	0.76	-24

Table XI. Effect of Erroneous Experimental Parameters on the Determination of T_2.

	PARAMETER	T_2	$T_2(\%)$
	NONE	1	-
δ	$= +15°$	1.16	+16
δ	$= -10°$	0.86	-14
ϕ_{trx}	$= \pm 25°$	0.88/1.12	$\|12\|$
T_D	$= 2T_1$	0.85	-15
T_D	$= 0.5T_1$	0.50	-50

Another important parameter is the shape of the sample, since it can modify the filling factor of the coil. To study the influence of this parameter on the relaxation time measurements, we have chosen paraffin (m.p. 52-54°C), which can be molded in various geometric shapes because of its malleability and which eliminates the problems connected with vapour pressure. The shape of the samples and their geometrical characteristics are shown in Table XII.

Table XII. Characteristics of the Different Samples of Paraffin.

Shape		Radius (mm)	Height (mm)	Volume (mm^3)
Cylinder	(I)	4.0	14	703
Ellipsoid	(II)	3.5 (Max)	18	924
Sector of Cyl.	(III)	8.0	15	535
Chips	(IV)	1.5 (Av)	16	600

T_1 values have been determined using the inversion-recovery pulse sequence and T_2 values using the spin-echo sequence; the measurements were performed at 30.0±0.2°C under optimum experimental conditions. The magnetization values, in the I.R. sequence, have been determined using both a phase-sensitive detector (PSD) and a diode for linearization to compare the quality of the results (Table XIII).

Table XIII. Relaxation Times T_1 and T_2 Determined for Paraffin Specimens of Different Shapes.

SAMPLE	PDS T_1 (s)	DIODE T_1 (s)	$T_{2(s \times 10^3)}$
(I)	0.16	0.14	0.06
	0.23	0.33	0.44
	0.42	0.71	
(II)	0.14	0.14	0.25
	0.31	0.31	
(III)	0.16	0.13	0.08
	0.32	0.21	0.42
	0.69	0.83	
(IV)	0.15	0.13	0.06
	0.26	0.21	0.36
	0.50	0.55	

It is easily observed that the shape of the specimen is critical, both T_1 and T_2, and particularly for the slow components when the coil is not filled. Different relaxation components are observed depending on the shape: this points out how difficult it is to evaluate the relative weight of the various components of the total magnetization.

A correct evaluation of the relaxation times depends strongly also on the sample handling (8), as is shown in the following tables.

Table XIV. Effect of Long Term Refrigeration at 5°C on Measured T_1(s) Values (from 8).

TIME	MUSCLE	NORMAL BREAST	BREAST CARCINOMA
FRESH	0.748	0.730	0.650
24h	0.710	-	-
48h	0.688	0.673	0.420

Table XV. Effect of Holding the Tissue at 25°C on Measured T$_1$(s) Values (from 8).

TIME	BREAST CARCINOMA	MUSCLE
0	0.375	0.608
2 h	-	0.620
6 h	0.380	0.660

Table XVI. Effect of Keeping the Tissue at -70°C on Measured T$_1$(s) Values.

TIME	RAT LIVER
0	0.210
24 h	0.295
48 h	0.302

The data in these tables clearly show that placing the tissues on ice or in the freezer should be avoided as much as possible. Moreover, it is highly advisable to send to the pathologist the exact piece of tissue used for NMR work (8).

The preceding discussion can be summarized as follows (8):

1. Know the instrument and understand its limitations.

2. Plan the experiment to include control measurements for the calculation of error.

3. Use an adequate number of samples to be clearly significant.

4. Handle the sample appropriately.

To show how critical is the determination of relaxation times in tissues, we report here the results obtained "in vitro" and "in vivo" for different tissues (Tables XVII to XIX). In Table XVII are reported the relaxation times of myocardium of rats treated with different amounts of isoproterenol, together with the fraction of samples for which the various relaxation components have been observed.

In this case, it is possible, at least on a statistical basis, to characterize the control tissue and the tissue treated with isoprotere-

nol. In Table XVIII are collected the relaxation data obtained for
human pacreatic tissue: the healthy tissue can be differentiated from
the tumorous tissue.

Table XVII . Comparison of Sample Fractions and T_1 and T_2 Values in Rat
Myocardium Treated with Isoproterenol.

	%($\pm$5)		
$T_1(s)$	a	b	c
0.30 - 0.45	40	50	10
0.50 - 0.60	75	80	100
> 0.7	45	55	0
$T_1(s)$			
0.01 - 0.22	55	10	60
0.040 - 0.045	35	10	100
> 0.05	85	80	10

(a) 3 mg/kg of isoproterenol twice per day. (b) 80 mg/kg of isoproterenol twice per day. (c) untreated specimen.

Table XVIII. Relaxation Times of Human Pancreatic Tissue (6 specimens
from the same patient suffering from Werner-Morrison syndrome; samples
a to f come from a tumor at the head of pancreas).

Specimen	$T_1(s)$	$T_2(s)$
a (tumor)	0.475 ± 0.008 0.350 ± 0.008	0.070 ± 0.003
b	0.185 ± 0.008	0.041 ± 0.003
c	0.113 ± 0.008	0.042 ± 0.003
d	0.324 ± 0.008 0.113 ± 0.008	0.038 ± 0.003
e	0.196 ± 0.008 0.133 ± 0.008	0.039 ± 0.003
f	0.162 ± 0.008	0.035 ± 0.003

It is interesting that the tumorous specimen shows the presence of a second kind of tissue, characterized by a shorter T_1, which could be lipoid or amyloid in origin and is histologically similar to the infiltrating tissue (T_1 = 0.324s) in sample d.

The comparison between these relaxation parameters, determined "in vitro", implies that in some cases it is possible to give a diagnostic meaning to a specific T_1 or T_2 value; however, very often the relaxation times values are meaningful only on statistical and not on individual basis. This point is crucial, since claims have been made that diagnosis is possible based on the relaxation parameters obtained "in vivo" by means of NMR imaging techniques. Clearly "in vivo", the whole-body NMR scanners do not allow a precise setting and definition of the instrumental parameters because the r.f. phase, the r.f. power and the pulse width are not known and, besides, the gradients play a critical role in the experimental conditions (9). It is fanciful and hasty to claim that the relaxation parameters T_1 and T_2 allow a differential diagnosis of the diseases, not only because T_1 ans T_2 values measured "in vivo" with different experimental settings are essentially not comparable, but also because no real correlation has yet been found with histological findings and pathological conditions. As an example, we report the result obtained "in vivo", with a whole body FONAR 80 scanner (Table XIX). This instrument, in principle, should afford the most accurate determination of the relaxation parameters, since the focalization of $\bar{B}_0$ allows a direct measurement of the magnetization profile and therefore a direct calculation of "T_1".

Table XIX. Comparison of "T_1" Values in the Liver of Diseased Patients[a] and Normal Healthy Volunteers[b] Measured at 0.05 Tesla.

Liver	"T_1"(s)	SD(s)	SD(%)	Range
NORMAL	0.140	0.040	29	0.075 - 0.215
ABNORMAL	0.215	0.084	39	0.070 - 0.485

[a]46 patients. [b]25 volunteers

The abnormal liver includes a set of pathologies, ranging from steatosis to metastasis, and it is clear that, even if, on statistical bases, the relaxation time value is indicative of the presence of pathological conditions, on an individual basis it cannot be of diagnostic relevance, because of the superposition of the range of the measured values.

In conclusion, the determination of the relaxation times T_1 and T_2 is one of the most critical experiments in NMR spectroscopy, even in an ideal situation. In the cases of tissues, "in vitro" or "in vivo", the evaluation of time constants resembling the theoretical T_1 and T_2, is even more critical for instrumental and theoretical reasons and the calculated parameters might even be meaningless. However, careful measurements carried out bearing in mind the limitations of the procedure and an interpretation of the results based on suitable models, will be extremely helpful in predicting the appearance of the NMR images and, consequently in determining their significance for the diagnosis of disease.

ACKNOWLEDGMENTS.We thank Dr. R.Toni, M.D. for his skillful assistance and Dr. A.M.Giuliani, Ph.D. for stimulating discussions and insightful suggestions.

REFERENCES

1.   A.Abragam: Principles of Nuclear Magnetism, Clarendon Press, Oxford 1983, Ch. III.
2.   Ref. (1): Ch. VIII, Ch. X.
3.   G.Withfield, A.G.Redfield: Phys.Rev., 106, 918 (1957).
4.   M.L.Martin J., J.Delpuech, G.J.Martin : Practical NMR Spectroscopy, Heyden and Son Ltd., 1980, Ch. 7.
5.   I.D.Weisman, L.H.Bennertt, L.R.Maxwell, Sr., D.E.Henson: 'Cancer Detection by NMR in Living Animal' in NMR in Medicine, R.Damadian, Editor, Springer Verlag, 1981.
6.   P.A.Bottomley, T.M.Foster, R.E.Argersinger, L.M.Pfeifer: Med. Phys., 11, 425 (1984).
7.   Ref. (1): Ch. IX, Ch. XII.
8.   P.T.Beall: Magn.Res.Imaging, 1, 165 (1982).
9.   B.R.Rosen, I.L.Pykett, T.J.Brady: J.Comp.Ass.Tomogr., 8, 195 (1984).

CONSTRUCTION OF A COMBINED HIGH RESOLUTION NMR SPECTROMETER-TOMOGRAPH

L.D. Hall, H. Chow, S. Luck, T. Marcus, C. Neale, B. Powell, J. Sallos, S. Sukumar and L. Talagala, V. Rajanayagam
Department of Chemistry,
University of British Columbia,
Vancouver, B.C.
Canada V6T 1W5

ABSTRACT. Many research groups will have been frustrated by the fact that the high cost of commercially available nmr instrumentation appears to be a barrier which prevents them from being able to participate in NMR imaging. The purpose of this article is to encourage others to follow the example already described by a number of other laboratories, and to adapt an existing high resolution NMR spectrometer for imaging measurements. Besides providing an inexpensive starting point, this approach can provide access to an imaging system capable of producing very high spatial resolution (<0.1 mm) from small objects (1 - 10 mm), and also chemical shift resolved measurements. A brief overview is given of other pertinent aspects, especially of probe design.

The purpose of this article is threefold. First, it is intended to encourage others who are interested in starting studies associated with NMR imaging, but who lack sufficient funds to purchase a purpose built system, to modify an existing Fourier transform spectrometer for imaging measurements. Second, we wish to note that such a modified spectrometer is not merely a "poor-man's-imager" but is, rather, a device ideally suited to studies of small objects, and hence of interest in its own right. Third, it is to point out that it is technically feasible to perform a simple experiment which combines the spatial localisation of tomography with the analytical chemical function of spectroscopy. It is necessary to note at the outset that each of these objectives has been independently investigated in a number of other laboratories and, in emphasising the work of my own laboratory, I intend no disrespect to those other workers.

1. MODIFICATION OF A HIGH RESOLUTION SPECTROMETER

Most conventional high resolution Fourier transform NMR spectrometers have a pulse programmer which can be used to execute essentially any two dimensional NMR experiment, and the requisite

T. Axenrod and G. Ceccarelli (eds.), NMR in Living Systems, 217–230.
© 1986 by D. Reidel Publishing Company.

software to process and display the resultant two dimensional
spectrum. Those same functions can be used directly for two
dimensional imaging. All that is required in addition is a means for
providing, and controlling, two, or three, linear field gradients.

For most superconducting magnet systems, the x-, y-, and z-shim
coils and power supplies are capable of providing a linear field
gradient of ca 0.1 gauss/cm, with a gradient rise time of ca 1 msec.
These are sufficient for imaging measurements of the liquid filled
phantoms suitable for spin-physics developments. It is necessary to
develop some means whereby the magnitude of these gradients can be
set, and the timing of their on-off periods controlled. In the case
of the systems assembled at U.B.C. we have used three of the spare
control lines which were already available from the Nicolet 293B (or
293C) pulse programmer of our spectrometer. These were connected to
a set of purpose built switches to turn the three shim sets on/off.
The magnitude of each gradient is proportional to the current passing
through each coil, which is in turn set by applying an appropriate
voltage, to the voltage-summing point of the appropriate Oxford
Instruments shim power supply. The magnitude of each of those drive
voltages is set by a digital-to-analog convertor, programmed directly
from the Nicolet computer. As a result, it is trivial to write any
pulse programme which includes in addition to the usual chain of
radiofrequency pulses, any required combination of gradient pulses.

The efficacy of this approach for imaging a phantom is shown (1)
in Fig. 1 below. It should be noted, first that this measurement was
made using an unmodified, high resolution nmr probe, and second that
no slice selection was used because of the axial symmetry of the
phantom; for the same reason, the image could be displayed using
either the contour plot, or the stack plot routines already available
in the standard NMR software. As will be seen later, it is possible
to use a colour or black/white display unit, but that adds to the
cost and to the overall complexity of the conversion, and is not
necessary for studies which are confined to phantoms.

I alluded earlier to the fact that this simple modified
instrument could be used to investigate new pulse sequences, and that
point is illustrated in Fig. 2 which shows (2) the use of selective
pulses to selectively elicit images from different chemical species.
In like fashion, Fig. 3 illustrates the use of the inversion recovery
pulse sequence to measure spatial distribution of spin-lattice
relaxation times of different solutions (3). Note that use of a
phase-sensitive calculation of the image intensity eliminates the
ambiguities which would otherwise prevent distinction between the
initial and final stages of the relaxation curve. This is an
important point since some whole-body proton tomographs only use the
absolute-mode display.

The obvious extension of water tomography to the task of
providing images showing the distribution of each individual species
within a heterogeneously distributed mixture was first alluded to by
Lauterbur (4). Although, as we shall see later, this approach has at
present some formidable limitations, especially in studies of man, it
has attracted substantial attention (5), and is certainly technically

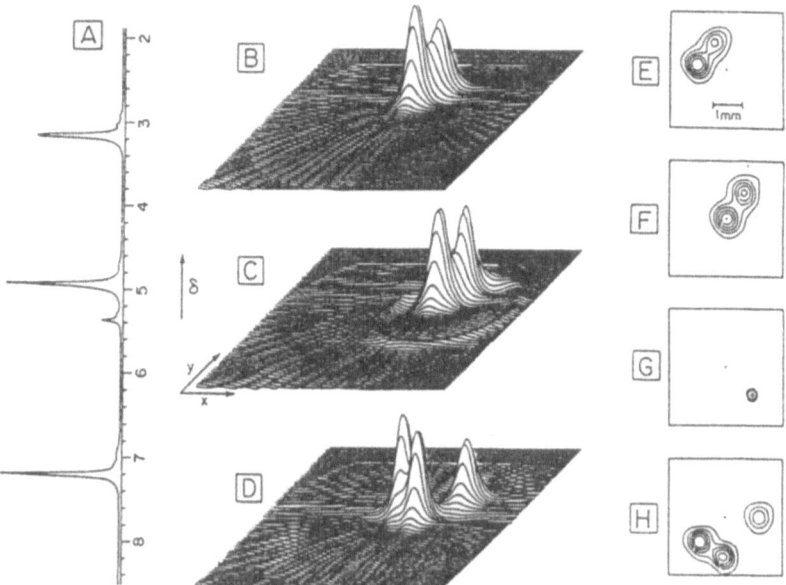

Figure 1. (A) The 270 MHz proton spectrum of a set of capillaries
containing benzene, water, methylene chloride and acetone (ref.
benzene 7.28) surrounded by D_2O in a 10 mm NMR tube. B, C and D are
the reconstructed images of acetone, water and benzene respectively.
Artifacts caused by the back projection procedure, can be seen as
streaks radiating from the base of each peak. The effect of the
overlapping methylene chloride signal (5.188) on the water region is
noticeable in C. The contour plots E-H correspond to the cross
sectional images of acetone, water, methylene chloride and benzene
respectively. Experimental parameters: spectral width (quadrature
detection), 2000 Hz; block size, 1024 points; number of scans, 2;
relaxation delay, 2s; total data acquisition time, 5.5 min; gradient
current, 800mA (500Hz/cm); number of projections, 72; increment
angle of the gradient, 5 ; image digitization, 128 x 128 (1.95
Hz/point).

feasible. Fig. 1 shows (1) what appears to be a chemical shift
resolved tomographic image of a series of 1 mm outer diameter glass
capillary tubes contained inside a convention 5 mm NMR tube. This is
misleading. Separate images have been obtained for each species only

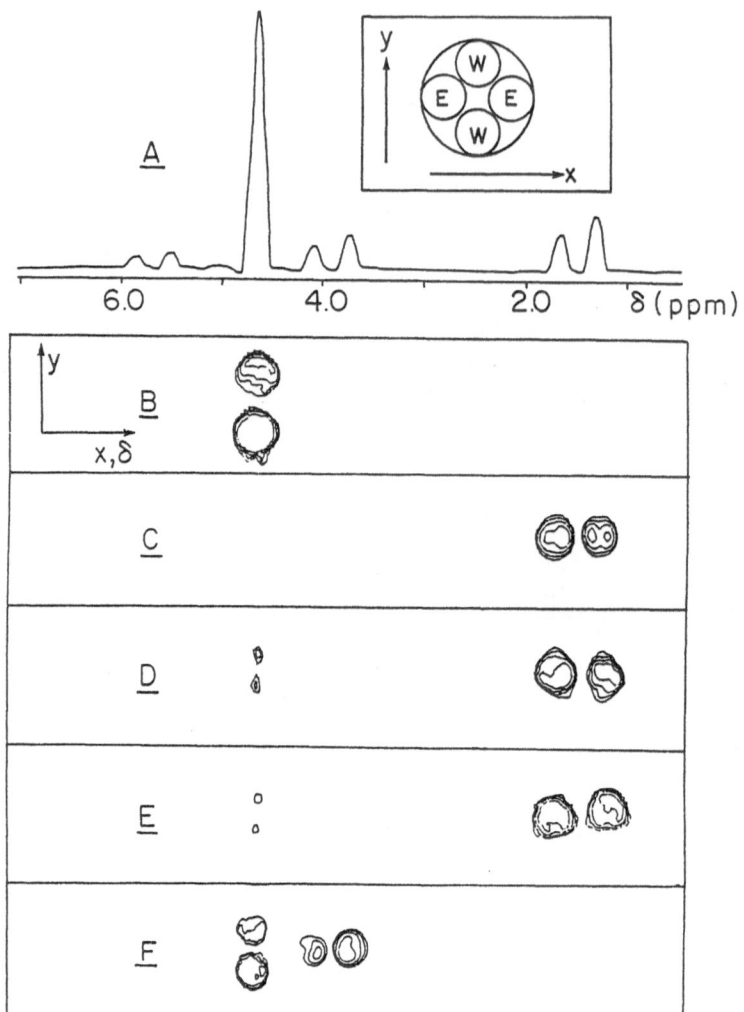

Figure 2. Inset - Orientation of the phantom (W - water, E - ethanol). (A) ^{1}H spectrum of the phantom in the presence of a gradient of 446 Hz/cm. (B) Reconstructed proton 2D image of the phantom. (Maximum y-gradient = $\pm$446 Hz/cm; y-gradient increment = 14 Hz/cm; number of G_y increments = 64; T = 50 msec. (see Fig. 1); Acquisition time = 310 msec.; scans = 2, Relaxation delay = 20 sec., total experimental time = 45 mins.). (C) Water saturated image (saturation time = 1.0 sec). (D) Image with a 90 selective pulse of 20 msec duration through the decoupler at the ethanol-CH$_3$ resonance frequency. (E) and (F) Images with selective 90 DANTE pulse trains on the ethanol-CH$_3$ and -CH$_2$ resonance respectively. DANTE pulses are as described in Figure captions 2(E) and (F).

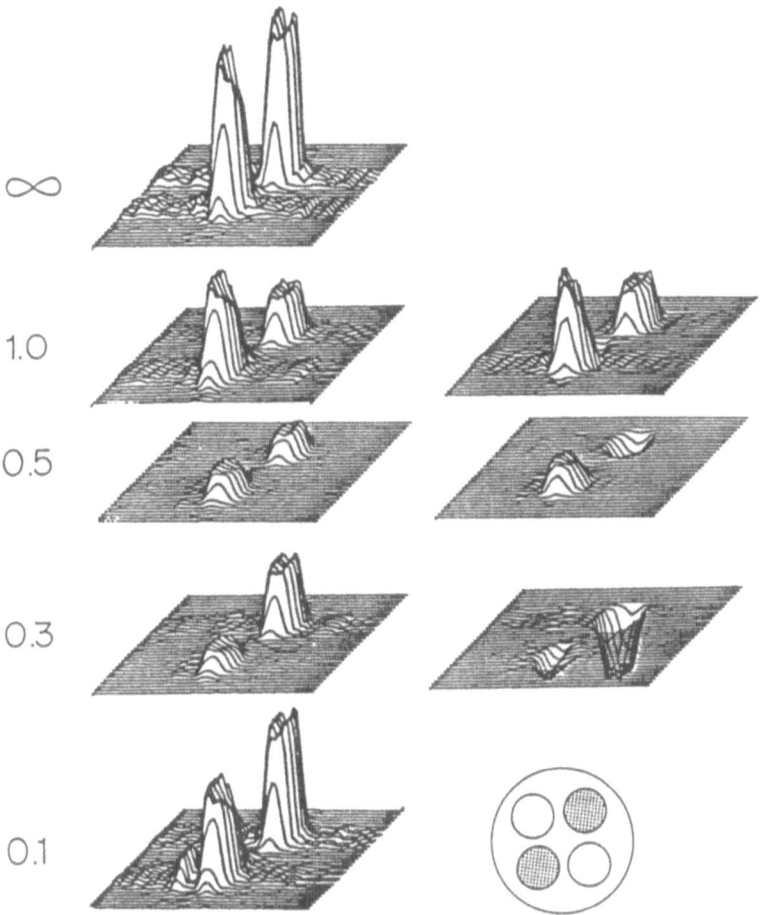

Figure 3. Images of a two-tube phantom containing aqueous solutions
of Mn(EDTA) produced by the two-dimensional spin-warp method (10),
modified to include the two-pulse inversion recovery method (5).
The delay-times (sec) are given to the left of each image. The
images in the left-hand column have all been phased to give a
positive displacement to the largest peak, and with absolute mode
display. The three images in right-hand column were phased using
identical correction-values.

because the "swing" of resonance frequency about the chemical shift, induced by the applied gradients, is smaller than the chemical shift separation. Clearly this is not a widely applicable technique; for example, it would not be compatible with the more complex phantom used (6) for the measurement of Figs. 4 and 5, which are based on a single data set. The underlying concept is as follows; it is known that the applied gradients used in the Lauterbur back projection experiment to define a position within a plane, result in a sinusoidal variation in the resonance frequency of every species in the sample, the amplitude and frequency of which is solely dependent on where within the sample the particular species is physically located. Thus it is possible to acquire experimentally a full data set, to define any arbitrary position with that set, and then, knowing the spatial coordinates and the gradient magnitudes, to search for the species which have the appropriate frequency dependence. The resulting point spectra for the phantom are shown in Fig. 4. It is clear that this procedure is not failsafe because there is inevitably some overlap in the frequency trajectories, which the computer programme cannot decipher. However, a second iteration of the data can cleanly eliminate the artifactual components and give clean, point spectra. The same data set can also be interrogated to produce a series of tomographic images which show the spatial distribution of the different chemical species, as shown in Fig. 5.

Although the above procedure works well with discrete samples, the spatial ambiguities associated with the more typical continuous sample often exceed the ability of even a third spatial iteration.

The only truly general procedure for such measurements involves the acquisition of a three dimensional data set as indicated in Fig. 6. The magnetisation of the nuclear spins is first excited by application of a 90° pulse which, if it is applied selectively and with a z gradient on, can define a slice; it is then allowed to evolve whilst the two gradients Gx and Gy are applied; finally the data are acquired with both gradients off, which ensures that there is no loss of chemical shift resolution in the final image. This procedure produces (7) a single, three dimensional data set S, which in a typical measurement will have dimensions (128 x 128 x 1024). Fourier transformation of that matrix with respect to the acquisition of t produces 512 "slices", $S(tx,ty)$, along the z direction, which is the chemical shift dimension. In practice, only those slices which correspond to a discrete chemical shift are subjected to Fourier transformation to produce $S(fx,fy)$ the required image. The example given in Fig. 6, illustrates how closely lines can be spaced, yet separate images be obtained.

The logical extension of this method is to increase the dimensionality to four, by allowing the magnetisation to evolve during the selective application of all three linear gradients. We have successfully obtained (8) such data sets. The main drawback is the length of time which is required and the method will not be generally applicable until a fast imaging version (9,10) is available; this is being actively pursued at U.B.C.

A major advantage of the measurements described above is that

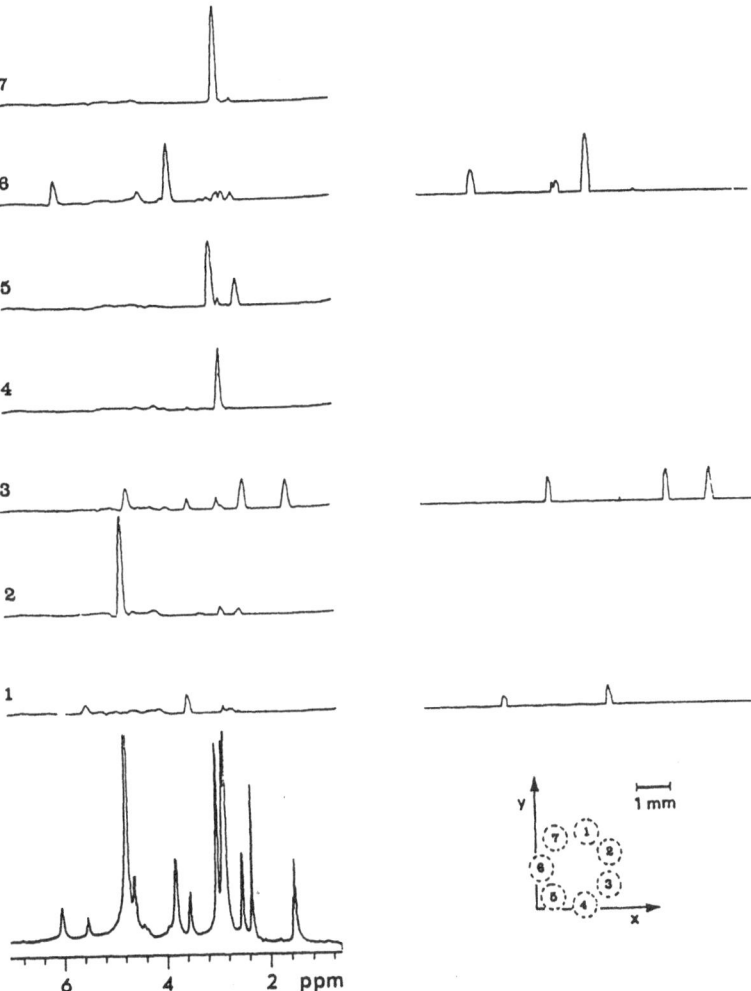

Figure 4. The bottom trace is the high-resolution NMR spectrum of
the test phantom comprising 7 capillary tubes, each containing
different compounds (See Fig.5). 1-7 are the "point-spectra", taken
from an area 0.2 x 0.2 mm at the centre of each tube and represent
the NMR spectrum of the sample in that area. The traces to the right
of 1,3 and 6 show the point-spectra after a second stage of iteration
and show the suppression of artifacts. Experimental Parameters:
spectral width = ± 500 Hz; block size = 512 points; number of
acquisitions = 4; pulse width = 4 s; sampling time = 257 ms;
relaxation delay 15s; field gradients = 0.1 G/cm.

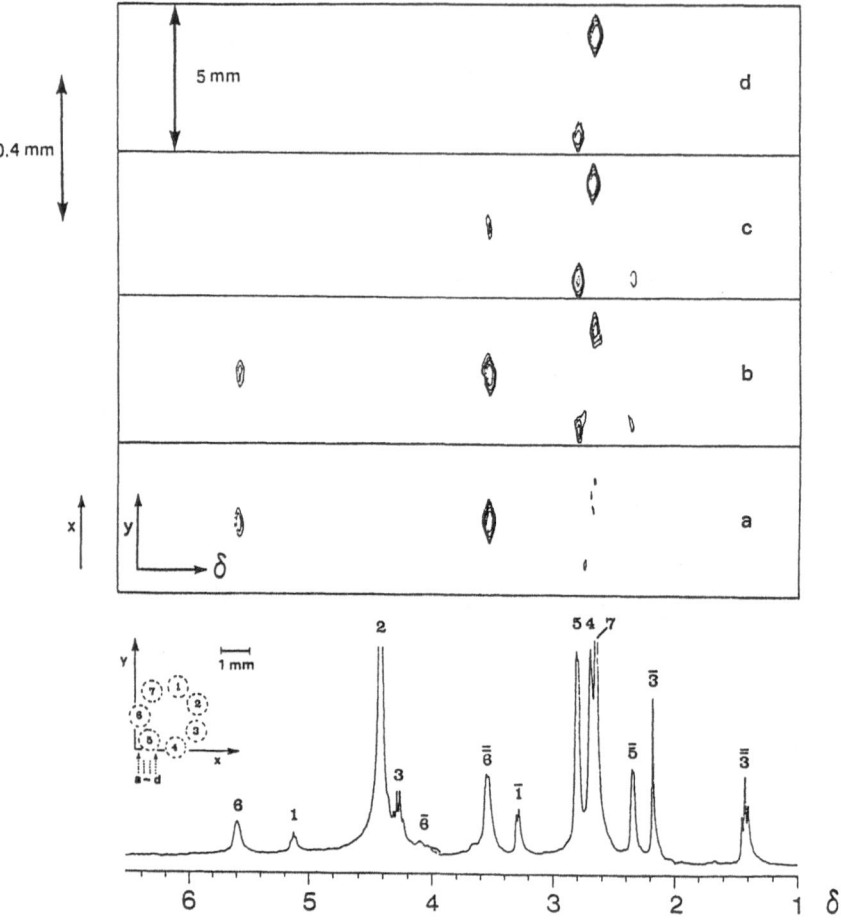

Figure 5.   The bottom trace shows the high-resolution NMR spectrum
of the test sample shown in the figure. Assignments: 1 - 1,1,2-Tri-
chloroethane; 2 - Water; 3 - Ethyl acetate; 4 - Acetone; 5 - Acetone
(5) and Dimethyl sulphoxide (5); 6 - p-Dioxane (6) and impurities (6,
6); 7 - Dimethyl sulphoxide.
                    The contour plots a-d represent the "line-spectra"
(along y). each 0.4mm in thickness (along x) taken at intervals as
shown in the figure below. The contour plots thus correspond to an
NMR spectrum representing four dimensions - x and y spatial
coordinates, chemical shifts and intensities.

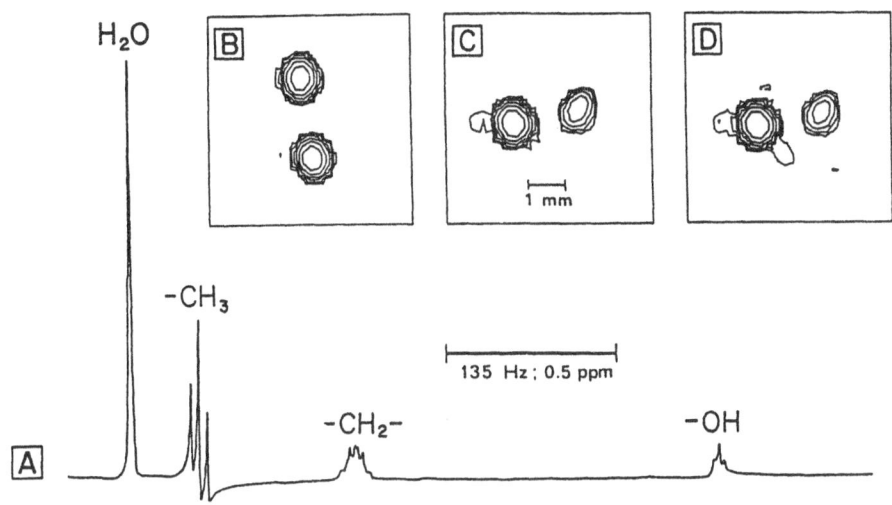

Figure 6. (A) shows the conventional high-resolution NMR spectrum of a phantom comprising two capillary tubes with water and another two with ethanol. The -OH and -CH$_3$ signals were deliberately folded over to decrease the spectral width in the -dimension (which causes the phase distortion in the spectrum). 1024 signals were acquired for each of the combinations G$_x$ and G$_y$ values, which after 3-D Fourier transformation gave the interpolated 64 x 64 images (see text). The images (B), (C) and (D) were processed from the signal corresponding to the water and the two high-field components of the methyl triplet respectively; the latter demonstrates the chemical shift resolution achievable by the above procedure. Experimental parameters: spectral width (f) = +/-400 Hz; Block size ( ) = 512 points; N = M = 32; X$_i$ = Y$_i$ = 0.11 g/cm (450 Hz/cm); scans = 2; pulse width = 23 s; t_x = t_y = 32 ms.

no hardware modifications are required; the shim coils are used for the gradients and the standard NMR probe contains the sample. A drawback is that the gradients produced are insufficient to provide an adequate frequency dispersion for the broader resonances which are encountered in many "solidus" objects. We have circumvented (11) this deficiency by building a probe which incorporates its own gradient coils, which in our system give gradients of up to 10 gauss/cm when driven from separate power supplies. Those gradients give (12) excellent spatial resolution as indicated in Fig. 7. We believe that at 270 MHz we shall soon achieve resolution of better than 50 microns for samples up to 4 mm overall diameter.

It is not appropriate to give details concerning the software developed for our General Electric Nicolet computers because it is too specific to our own system. It is worth noting, however, that many high resolution spectrometers provide a control function for "homospoil" experiments, in which one of the gradients is turned on for a brief period to eliminate magnetisation from the x, y plane. The software and hardware used to control that gradient should provide a clear indication as to how the three linear gradients can be used. Even if that is too difficult, it might be feasible to perform at least a two dimensional nmr measurement using one gradient controlled by the homospoil line and the orthogonal gradient set from the manual shim coil control.

A more complicated, but powerful, approach is to use a microprocessor designed for laboratory instrumentation control to operate the gradients and to trigger it from the main pulse programmer. This is the approach adopted for many of the whole-body proton tomographs, and examples of this approach for use with smaller magnets have been described in the literature (13).

In our own laboratory the approaches summarised above have been applied to two magnets, one a 6.2 Tesla, 35 mm bore and the other a 1.9 Tesla 300 mm bore. Besides running the gradient coils from the shim power supplies, we have also used high slew rate audio amplifiers capable of producing 20 amps; units provided by Crown Amicron have excellent performance.

It is important to note that facilities are needed to compensate for the distortions introduced by the eddy currents induced in the NMR probe and walls of the magnet, so that the final shape of a switched field gradient is rectangular. A crude "profiling" can be achieved by an analog device, but the best results require use of a programmable digital system. In this same context, similar facilities for profiling the radiofrequency pulse is also required. This is necessary to ensure that when frequency selective pulses are used to define a frequency domain, as in slice selection, the appropriate radiofrequency distribution is produced. At U.B.C. we have used a simple analog modulation system based on a ring-modulator, but the best approach undoubtedly involves a digitally programmable system, such as those used in the commercial whole-body systems.

With a console plus software, capable of driving a magnet system, it then remains to have a suitable radiofrequency probe. For

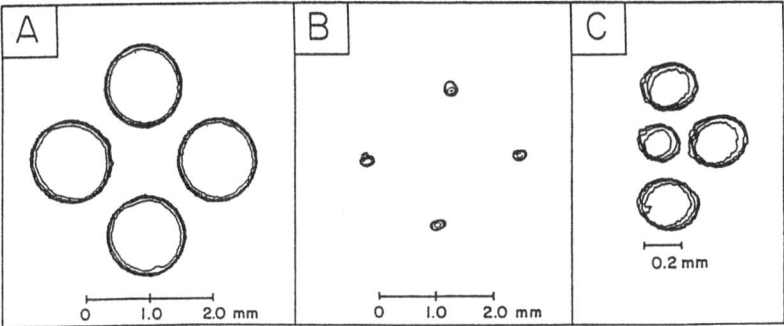

Figure 7.   Two dimensional spin-warp variant images of glass
capillary phantoms containing water enclosed in 5mm NMR tube (A) 4
capillaries (12mm ID) m; (B) 4 capillaries (250-300 m ID, 1.6 mm OD);
(C) 4 capillaries (150 m - 220 m ID); Experimental parameters (A)
sweep width = 400 Hz; Acquisition time 64.12 msec; number of scans =
4;   pulse width - 28 sec; Relaxation delay = 4 seconds; y-gradient
increment = 0.5 mTm^{-1}; maximum x-gradient = 9.3 mTm^{-1}.   (B) y-
gradient increment = 0.6 mTm^{-1}; maximum x-gradient = 11.7 mTm^{-1}.
(C) sweep width = 600 Hz; acquisition time = 42.57 msec; y-gradient
increment = 0.6 mTm^{-1}; maximum x-gradient = 38.9 mTm^{-1}.

spectrometers based on a vertical bore superconducting magnet, two
options exist. If the system is to use the magnet shim coils to
provide the imaging gradients, then the standard, high resolution
probe can be used, with the samples mounted in a conventional NMR
tube. However, if higher gradients are required, a completely new
probe will be necessary. This can be based on the existing probe,
with the purpose built gradient coils taking the place of the outer
glass dewar usually used for variable temperature studies. In either
case, the close juxtaposition between the gradient/shim coils and the
inner lining of the magnet will result in the induction of eddy
currents.

The whole concept of probe design and construction takes on new
dimensions (literally!) when magnets having a bore diameter of 30 cm,
or more, are used. Two basic factors must be remembered, regardless
of which class of probe is to be built. First, the large aperture at
each end of the solenoid provides no radiofrequency screen. Rather
than provide one for each separate probe it is advantageous to screen
the entire bore tube of the magnet inside the shim gradient coils.
This is easily achieved with a carefully grounded copper tube, and a
pair of end caps lined with copper mesh and fitted with bronze-
fingering around their circumference where they make contact with the
bore liner. The second factor is that all probes should be designed
for both spectroscopic and imaging measurements in mind. Hence non-
metallic materials should be used wherever possible to minimise the
induction of eddy currents; and when metallic devices cannot be
avoided, they should be located as far from the receiver coil as
possible, or disposed as symmetrically as possible with respect to
it.

Construction of probes which use a surface coil (13) can take
either of two forms. A solid base, capable of supporting the object,
is assembled and the surface-coil inserted into a recess on its top.
Alternatively, the coil can be mounted on the end of a flexible lead,
and then positioned in contact with the object.

Many different types and sizes of "volume" coils can be made.
For example, a plastic base can be made with a set of tuning and
matching capacitors and two mounting sockets via which various coils
can be connected. Cylindrical formers made from perspex or polyvinyl
chloride can be used to mount coils with the saddle configuration.
However, we (14) have had the most rewarding results thus far from
two types of resonator coils; both these not only make extremely
efficient use of the available radiofrequency but also give extremely
homogeneous field distribution. One version, based on the slotted
resonator principle, uses a sheet of copper foil wrapped on the
outside of a former, with the ends separated by a layer of dielectric
such as teflon; this provides the tuning capacitance, which can be
varied by controlling the pressure exerted across the copper-
dielectric-copper sandwich. A movable copper ring mounted parallel
to one end of the cylinder and connected to the spectrometer
transmitter provides tunable inductive coupling. One such coil, 7 cm
diameter and tuned to 80 MHz and coupled to a 140 watt amplifier has
a Q of 650 and provides a 90° pulse in ca 34 sec. The fact that this

coil has to be mounted transversely to the axis of the magnet is a
disadvantage for some studies; however, it is ideal for studies when
the sample must be mounted vertically, as in the column
chromatography studies reported elsewhere in this book. For samples
which require access along the axis of the magnet, we have also built
versions of the resonance coil originally designed by Alderman and
Grant (15). These have performance which rivals that of the slotted
resonator. For all imaging measurements the homogeneity of the
radiofrequency field is of crucial importance, and here too all
resonator coils we have evaluated are excellent across 60 per cent of
the diameter of the coil. We do not yet know the limits of frequency
and size which can be achieved with these designs but coils resonant
at 200 MHz of 15 cm diameter appear to be routinely feasible, and at
lower frequencies for larger diameters can be tuned.

   Although the emphasis thus far has been directed to imaging, we
also have an active interest in "point specific spectroscopy", in
which the spectrum from any selected point within an object can be
measured. We have implemented the method first suggested by Aue and
coworkers (16). We believe that this approach will ultimately
displace most of the other methods currently in use. It depends on
the fact that when a selective radiofrequency pulse is applied to a
sample which is under the influence of a linear field gradient, only
those nuclear spins which have resonance frequencies within the
transmitter bandwidth will be excited into resonance. If this
procedure is applied sequentially along all three axes, only those
spins from a defined volume will be excited.

   Thus far we have tacitly neglected the magnet which provides the
basic field. Over and above questions of field strength and magnet
bore size, the most important parameter concerns the volume of
homogeneous field. For spectroscopy the field must be homogeneous to
1 part in 10^7 and magnets of 30 cm horizontal bore now provide this
level over a ca 10 cm diameter sphere; for a 1 metre bore magnet that
volume is increased to ca 15 cm. Obviously it is possible to move
the sample with respect to this volume, but for many purposes that is
inconvenient. The homogeneity required for measurements which only
involve 1 part to 10^6 and thus the effective percentage of the magnet
bore diameter over which this is true is considerably greater than
that required for spectroscopy. In contrast, if use is made of a
vertical bore solenoiod such as that used for conventional high
resolution NMR, the diameter of sensitive volume is smaller, but the
intrinsic homogeneity over that volume is increased to 1 part in 10^8,
or better, for mobile, small molecules.

ACKNOWLEDGEMENTS
   The original experiments on our 270 MHz system were performed
whilst Subramaniam Sukumar was the recipient of a U.B.C. Killam
Postdoctoral Research Fellowship. The subsequent development of our
80 MHz system was made possible by a substantial grant jointly
provided by the Presidents of the Natural Science and Engineering
Research Council of Canada and the Medical Research Council of
Canada, to whom we are all indebted.

REFERENCES

1. L.D. Hall and S. Sukumar, J. Magn. Reson. **50** 161-164 (1982).

2. L.D. Hall, S. Sukumar and S.L. Talagala, J. Magn. Reson. **56** 275-278 (1984).

3. L.D. Hall, K. Holme and S. Sukumar, J. Magn. Reson. 61 52 (1985).

4. P.C. Lauterbur, D.M. Kramer, W.V. House Jr. and C.N. Chen, J. Am. Chem. Soc. **97** 6866 (1975).

5. (a) P. Bendel, C-M Lai and P.C. Lauterbur, J. Magn. Reson. **38** 343-356 (1980).
   (b) S.J. Cox, P. Styles, J. Magn. Reson. **40** 209-212 (1980).
   (c) A.A. Maudsley, S.K. Hilal, W.H. Perman, H.E. Simon, J. Magn. Reson. **51** 147-152 (1983).
   (d) T.R. Brown, B.M. Kincaid, K. Ugurbil, Proc. Natl. Acad. Sci. USA **79** 3523-3526 (1982).
   (e) I.L. Pykett and B.R. Rosen, Radiology **149** 197-201 (1983).

6. L.D. Hall and S. Sukumar, J. Magn. Reson. **56** 326-333 (1984).

7. L.D. Hall and S. Sukumar, J. Magn. Reson. **56** 314-317 (1984),

8. L.D. Hall, V. Rajanayagam and S. Sukumar to be published in J. Magn. Reson. **61** 188-191 (1985).

9. P. Mansfield and I.L. Pykett, J. Magn. Reson. **29** 335-373 (1978).

10. L.D. Hall and S. Sukumar, J. Magn. Reson. **56** 179-182 (1984).

11. L.D. Hall and S.L. Luck, unpublished results.

12. L.D. Hall, S.L. Luck and V. Rajanayagam, to be published.

13. J.J. Ackerman, T.H. Grove, G.C. Wong, D.G. Gadian, G.K. Radda, Nature **283** 167 (1980).

14. L.D. Hall, T. Marcus, C. Neale, B. Powell, J. Sallos and L. Talagala, J. Magn. Reson., in press.

15. D.W. Alderman and D. M. Grant, J. Magn. Reson., **36** 447 (1979); H-J. Schneider and P. Dullenkopf, Rev. Sci. Instrum., **48**, 68 (1977); **48** 832-834 (1977).

16. W.P. Aue, S. Miller, T.A. Cross and J. Seelig, J. Magn. Reson. **56** 350-354 (1984).

GATHERING METABOLIC INFORMATION USING ^{13}C AND ^{1}H HIGH RESOLUTION
SPECTRA OF LIVING SYSTEMS

J.R. Alger
Dept. of Diagnostic Radiology and
Dept. of Molecular Biophysics and Biochemistry
Yale University, P. O. Box 6666
New Haven, CT. 06511
U.S.A.

ABSTRACT. ^{13}C and ^{1}H NMR are presently being exploited for the study
of metabolism in intact living systems. This paper provides the
background which will enable the novice to understand the types of
applications which are being pursued. Some of the more recent results
are also reviewed. The discussion includes recent ^{13}C NMR experiments
which have been performed on living animals using both natural
abundance signals, and signals from metabolites which become ^{13}C
labelled as a result of the introduction of a ^{13}C enriched substrate.
New methods of obtaining ^{1}H spectra of metabolites from living systems
are also presented.

1. ^{13}C NMR IN LIVING SYSTEMS

1.1 Introduction

Metabolism has been studied in living systems by ^{13}C NMR using both the
natural abundance signals, and signals from exogeneously supplied ^{13}C
isotope for more than a decade. In this lecture the more recent of
these metabolic studies of cell suspensions, perfused organs as well as
whole animal systems will be reviewed. This lecture is biased toward
the author's own research interests which are ^{13}C studies of living
animals. However, an adequate didactic presentation requires some
discussion of a few other systems. Studies in which ^{13}C spectra of
acid extracts of cells and tissues are used to obtain metabolic
information will not be discussed because we wish to focus on in situ
spectroscopy. We do take this opportunity, however, to point out that
studies of this nature have been valuable in metabolic studies and
should not be overlooked in the design of experimental protocols.

The sensitivity is the overriding concern with in vivo ^{13}C
studies. For an equal number of spins, the ^{13}C signal is 1/4 as
intense as the ^{31}P signal, and the ^{13}C isotope is only 1.1% naturally
abundant, making the natural ^{13}C signal effectively 400 times weaker
than that of ^{31}P (1). Hence when it is desired to observe metabolites
having concentrations in the millimolar range, labelling from

231

T. Axenrod and G. Ceccarelli (eds.), NMR in Living Systems, 231–264.

exogeneously ^{13}C enriched materials is required. In such studies the ^{13}C signals tend to have a full three-fold nuclear Overhauser sensitivity enhancement, and the ^{13}C lines are often sharper than ^{31}P lines _in vivo_. These two effects improve the ^{13}C signal to the point that fully ^{13}C labelled metabolites produce signals which have intensities similar to the ^{31}P signal from an equally concentrated phosphorylated metabolite. ^{31}P NMR studies have shown that phosphorylated compounds present in cells and tissues at greater than a few millimolar provide interpretable signals in a few minutes of data acquisition (2). By these arguements, ^{13}C signals from fully labelled metabolites in the millimolar concentration range should therefore also be accessible to the NMR method, and this has been demonstrated in a number of systems (3). Thus a primary objective in the design of ^{13}C metabolic studies is the development of ways of labelling the metabolite pools with expensive ^{13}C isotope in an efficient manner. Presently, the high cost of the ^{13}C enriched substrate, and the difficulty in finding efficient labelling protocols are the most serious limitations to ^{13}C studies. When ^{13}C labelling is not used, the concentration of the metabolite to be detected must be within the range of several hundred millimolar in concentration to observe the natural abundance ^{13}C signal.

Another concern with ^{13}C NMR is the use of ^{1}H decoupling to collapse the splitting due to scalar coupling. Without this, the sensitivity arguements made above are invalid and the spectra would be difficult to interpret. The problem presented by the need for decoupling is the phenomena whereby the lossiness of the physiological sample results in significant decoupler power dissipation and therefore heating within the sample (4). The extent of heating is strongly dependent on the Larmor frequency of the ^{1}H, being disproportionately worse at high operating frequencies (5,6). It is also dependent on the shape and size of the sample and of the coil in a manner which is difficult to quantify (5,6). No studies have yet been done to determine the potential hazard that decoupling poses in human-sized subjects because it is not clear what operating frequencies will be used, and what coil designs will be employed. Presently the heating issue is being addressed by the invention of decoupling schemes which make more efficient use of ^{1}H power (7-10), and by the design of more efficient probes (5,11). At the moment, these methods are finding their way into spectrometers dedicated to in vivo studies and the verdict on how well they work with various coil designs is not yet in. A second problem associated with ^{1}H decoupling, is the need for double coil probes (12). Double coil probes most commonly have had the decoupler coil much larger than the ^{13}C coil, thus subjecting more tissue to the decoupling fields than need be. However, recently it has been shown that two coils are not always necessary, in that double-tuned circuits permit both ^{13}C detection and ^{1}H decoupling with a single rf coil (13,14).

The resolution available from the ^{13}C spectrum is greater than that available from either ^{31}P or ^{1}H, because the ^{13}C chemical shift is significantly more sensitive to molecular structure. However, the effective resolution depends not only on the chemical shift dispersion, but also on the linewidth of the resonances in the living sample. It has been commonly found that in vivo, ^{31}P linewidths are larger than ^{13}C linewidths. Generally the observed ^{13}C linewidth in vivo is not limited by the transverse relaxation time. The practical limitation to resolution has been decoupling. Incomplete decoupling causes the linewidths to be larger than they should be, thereby degrading both the resolution and the effective sensitivity. The magnetic field homogeniety in the living sample, particularly in intact animals, is the other critical factor in defining the observed in vivo linewidths. When these limitations are properly corrected, the ^{13}C lines can be quite sharp in vivo, allowing the good resolution of the ^{13}C spectra to be realized.

Why are we interested in in vivo ^{13}C spectroscopy? This question is best answered with the help of Figure 1, which shows ^{13}C spectra, from the work of Cohen et. al. (15), of a suspension of hepatocytes which had been supplied with ^{13}C labelled alanine. The large number of resonances present is a result of the superb spectral resolution of ^{13}C method and of a sensitivity about equal to ^{31}P. Most of the signals come from metabolites which became ^{13}C labelled as a result of the alanine metabolism. Each resonance line provides some information about the concentration of a metabolite. With sequentially acquired spectra of this type, it is possible to follow isotope fluxes through the pathways by observing temporal intensity changes. This type of experiment has been difficult to do with ^{31}P spectroscopy because the ^{31}P isotope is essentially 100% abundant. Thus the ^{13}C NMR methods provide a promising method for studying the metabolism of carbon skeletons in vivo in real time.

1.2 Historical Perspectives

It is not our intention to completely review the past applications of ^{13}C NMR in living systems here. We only wish to point out how a number of experiments performed over the last decade have set the stage for our present studies of metabolism in animal tissues. Originally, ^{13}C spectra were obtained from suspensions of microorganisms and red blood cells which had been fed ^{13}C labelled substrates (16-18). The general goal of these studies was not to follow the metabolism of the substrate with repetitive spectra because the sensitivity at that time was not high enough to obtain several minute time resolution. Instead, the ^{13}C spectra from the stable end products (e.g., membrane lipids and proteins) in the cells which had become labelled were obtained. Analysis of the spectra allowed some conclusions to be drawn about the structure and dynamic status of these materials in the living cells. This work, done mostly by Matwiyoff and London and their colleagues, and other very early ^{13}C metabolic work has been reviewed by Norton (19).

As NMR machines improved, it became clear that repetitive

measurements on cell suspensions or perfused tissue could be made during the metabolism of a ^{13}C enriched substrate. Thus methods were developed to perfuse organs such as livers and hearts and to maintain viable cell suspensions within NMR magnets while making ^{13}C NMR measurements (3,20–23). For the most part, studies were restricted to the fairly well-travelled metabolic pathways of glycolysis, gluconeogenesis and the Krebs cycle, and these pathways continue to be actively studied by ^{13}C NMR. While in vivo ^{13}C NMR has not resulted in the elucidation of any new pathways, it is being used to study the control of flux through these major pathways in an ever-widening range of living systems. The primary restriction of the method to the well-travelled pathways has been that the in vivo ^{13}C sensitivity is insufficient to follow pathways where the metabolite concentrations are lower. The fact that there are only a relatively small number of ^{13}C labelled substrates which are commercially available , and these only at rather large costs, has also restricted applications. Some laboratories are circumventing these limitations so as to study more exotic metabolic pathways. They synthesize their own own enriched substrates, feed the enriched substrate to a cell suspension and then extract the labelled metabolites, and analyze the extract by long term signal averaging. A recent Tetrahedron Symposia in Print review (24) provides many examples of such studies.

Actual studies directed toward obtaining in vivo metabolic rates in a number of systems have recently been reviewed by den Hollander and Shulman (25). This work which provides an excellent, yet short, overview of the metabolic work which has been done with ^{13}C NMR, dwells specifically on studies performed on yeast suspensions, hepatocyte suspensions and perfused mouse livers at 8.5 T. The authors review how repetitive spectra taken from yeast metabolizing [^{13}C-1] glucose under both anaerobic and aerobic conditions provide a determination of the glycolytic flux, and show that the yeast preferentially consume the α anomer of glucose. Additional experiments are also described in which the label distribution in carbohydrates and amino acids after feeding [^{13}C-1] glucose, [^{13}C-6] glucose or [^{13}C-2] acetate is observed in vivo or in acid extracts of the yeast. These results enabled study of the flux through various metabolic pathways. Studies done by Cohen et al (15,22) on the perfused mouse liver and hepatocyte suspensions are also reviewed there. We will discuss some of their results in detail to illustrate the capability of the ^{13}C NMR methods, and later we will contrast these results from hepatocyte studies with results from a similar study in the living rat.

Figure 1 presents spectra from their study of alanine and ethanol metabolism by hepatocyte suspensions. Gluconeogenesis from [^{13}C-3] alanine led to the formation of glucose labelled at C-1, C-2, C-5 and C-6 (Fig. 1a), consistent with the known gluconeogenic pathway (Figure 2a). The alanine metabolism also resulted in labelling of glutamate at C-2, C-3 and C-4. The label distribution in glutamate reflects the labelling of the Krebs cycle intermediate α-ketoglutarate, a metabolite of low concentration whose signals are too weak to detect. There are

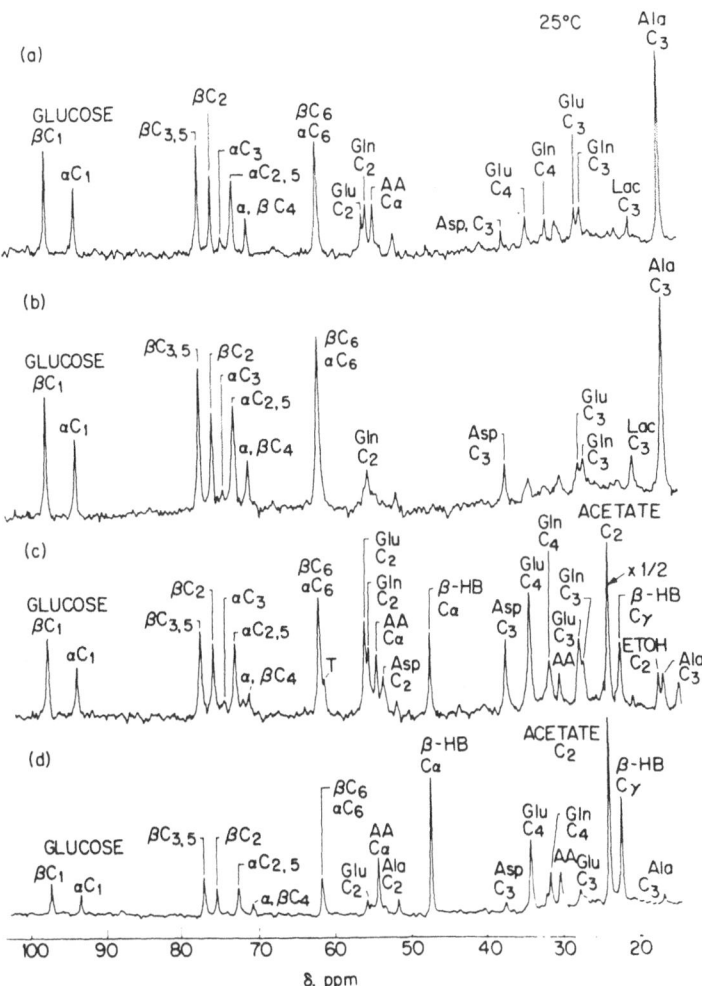

Figure 1: ^{13}C spectra of hepatocytes isolated from rats given different labelled substrates. Each spectrum was acquired during the period 145 to 175 minutes after the addition of substrate. (a) The substrate is [^{13}C-3] alanine. (b) The substrate is [^{13}C-3] alanine plus unlabelled ethanol. (c) The substrate is [^{13}C-3] alanine and [^{13}C-2] ethanol. (d) The substrate is unlabelled alanine and [^{13}C-2] ethanol. The administered alanine and ethanol concentrations were 28 mM and 20 mM respectively. The abbreviations used include: βC_1, αC_1 through βC_6, αC_6, carbons of the glucose anomers; MC_2, malate C_2; Lac C_2, lactate C_2; AA Cα, acetoacetate C_2; β-HB Cα, β-hydroxybutyrate C_2; AA Cγ, acetoacetate C_4; β-HB Cγ, β-hydroxybutyrate C_4; glu C_2 through C_4, glutamate C_2, C_3, C_4; gln C_2 through C_4, glutamine C_2, C_3, C_4; asp C_2, C_3, aspartate C_2, C_3. Taken from Cohen et. al. (15).

two routes for the [^{13}C-3] pyruvate formed from the [^{13}C-3] alanine to enter the Krebs cycle (Figure 2b). It can be carboxylated to oxaloacetate (the anaplerotic reaction) by pyruvate carboxylase, which can be shown to initially yield labelling at C-2 and C-3 (but not C-4) of glutamate. The isotope scrambling between the two positions is due to the fumarase activity. Pyruvate can also be converted to acetyl-coA by the action of pyruvate dehydrogenase and then condensed with oxaloacetate to form citrate and enter the Krebs cycle. This latter route initially produces labelling at C-4 (but not C-2 and C-3) of glutamate. When alanine alone was given to the cells (Figure 1a), glutamate C-4, C-2 and C-3 were labelled equally indicating that the fluxes through these two pathways were about equal. When unlabelled ethanol was given together with labelled alanine (Figure 1b), the glutamate C-4 signal was absent, indicating a suppression of the flow of pyruvate through the dehydrogenation pathway. Ethanol was the major source of the C-4 glutamate carbon under this condition as was shown by the experiment in which the ethanol was labelled, and the alanine was not (Fig. 1d). Figure 1c, which was obtained after giving both labelled compounds, confirms the findings discussed above. The ethanol-induced suppression of flow from alanine along the dehydrogenation pathway was interpreted as being the result of the inhibition of pyruvate dehydrogenase by the high NADH:NAD$^+$ ratio and the high acetyl-CoA:CoA ratio arising from the presence of the ethanol.

1.3 ^{13}C Labelling Studies with Living Animals

The success of the aforementioned ^{13}C studies, as well as the novel ^{31}P work being done at Oxford on living tissues encouraged us to become involved in ^{13}C studies of living animals several years ago. Additional incentives were provided by the availability of a spectrometer, the TMR-32, produced by Oxford Research Systems for whole animal studies. The magnetic field of this intrument was low (1.9 T) by high resolution spectroscopic standards, however, the bore was sufficiently large (20 cm clear diameter) for experimentation on animals as large as rabbits. Our exploratory experiment using the TMR spectrometer was to detect the ^{13}C labelling of the hepatic glycogen pool after oral administration of [^{13}C-1] glucose with a surface coil from outside the body of a rat and to observe various natural abundance ^{13}C signals from living rats and humans (26). In addition to using the TMR-32 instrument for ^{13}C metabolic studies of brain (27), heart (28) and liver (14,26,29,30) during the past two years, our group has also realized that an 8.5 T/9 cm Oxford Instrument magnet can be used quite profitably and with greater technical facility (better signal-to-noise ratio and resolution) in ^{13}C studies of cerebral metabolism in small rats (13).

The development of ^{13}C labelling methodology for living animal studies permits comparison of metabolic results obtained from intact cell or perfused organ preparations with those obtained in vivo. Recently we have performed 1.9 T studies with living rats which parallel in part the studies of alanine metabolism by hepatocytes which

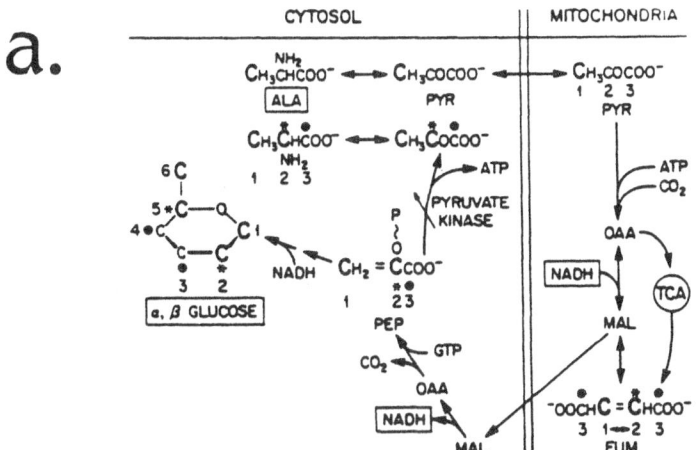

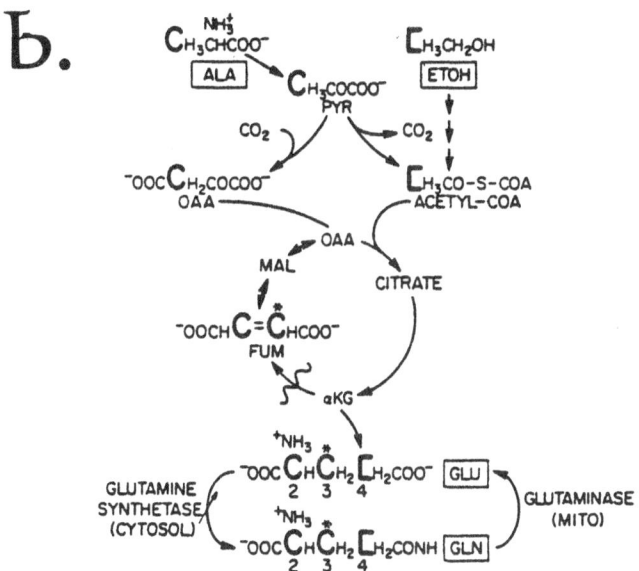

Figure 2: (a) Gluconeogenic pathway for [^{13}C-3] alanine; (b) Pathways by which alanine carbon enters the Krebs cycle, and the labelling in glutamine and glutamate which results. (Taken from Cohen and Shulman (50).)

are described above (14). Surgical procedures which place an rf coil
around two accessible lobes of the liver were developed for this study.
This approach was taken rather than the external surface coil approach
because it permits us to achieve better sensitivity and spatial
localization. [^{13}C-3] Alanine was introduced into the jugular vein of
a starved rat. Initially, a bolus dose of 120 mg was injected to bring
the plasma alanine concentration above the Michealis constant for
hepatic alanine gluconeogenesis, and then an infusion of 120 mg/hr was
performed for 1.5 hr. to maintain the plasma alanine at this elevated
level.

The in vivo ^{13}C spectrum of the liver taken during the infusion is
presented in Figure 3 together with an 8.5 T spectrum of the acid
extract of the freeze-clamped liver. Qualitatively, the spectra are
similar to those obtained when isolated hepatocytes were given ^{13}C-3
labelled alanine (Figure 1a). ^{13}C labelling at a number of positions
is detectable in vivo. These include the various positions of glucose,
glutamate/glutamine and aspartate. The absence of the C-4 signal of
glutamate in the in vivo experiment is noteworthy. In this respect,
the in vivo experiment, in which labelled alanine was given alone, is
more similar to the case of isolated hepatocytes given labelled alanine
with unlabelled ethanol (Figure 1b) than to the case of hepatocytes
given alanine alone (Figure 1a). This observation suggests that in
vivo the flow of alanine into the Krebs cycle via the pyruvate
dehydrogenase reaction is negligible. In the animal preparation, it is
likely that fatty acid oxidation is providing the acetyl-coA which
eventually becomes glutamate C-4 as ethanol did in the hepatocyte
study. However, this hypothesis is not easily confirmed without
additional labelling studies. As ^{13}C labelling methods become more
feasible for animal studies, more comparisons of the type described
here will be made in order to judge how closely the classical prefused
organ and isolated cell preparations mimic the living animal.

A second interesting point arises when the ^{1}H spectrum of the
extract shown in Figure 4 is considered. We wish to focus attention
only on the lines from the methyl group of the alanine. In the ^{13}C
labelled material, the 129 Hz ^{1}H-^{13}C J coupling splits the signal as
shown, whereas the ^{12}C labelled material is unsplit. Thus the
satellite peaks at 1.66 ppm and 1.30 ppm report the concentration of
alanine which is ^{13}C labelled at the C-3 position, and the resonance at
1.48 ppm reports that which is ^{12}C labelled. The interesting finding
is that the liver alanine is only 63% ^{13}C labelled despite the fact
that 99% labelled material was infused at a concentration 60 times the
expected physiological alanine. This label dilution is not apparent
from the ^{13}C spectra, and this simple example shows how ^{1}H NMR data can
supplement ^{13}C NMR results, with regard to determining what fraction of
the total metabolite pool is ^{13}C labelled. ^{1}H NMR will be discussed in
more detail later.

1.4 Natural Abundance ^{13}C NMR Studies of Animals

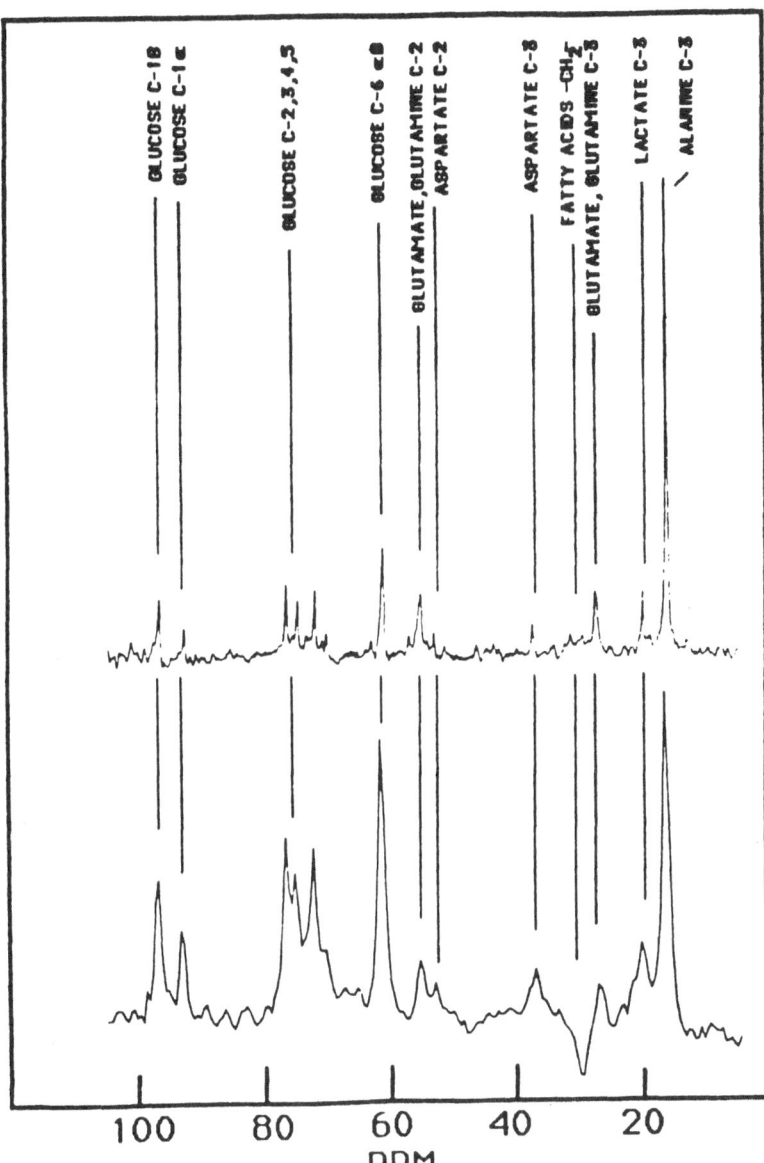

Figure 3: Lower spectrum: 1.9 T ¹³C spectra of rat liver *in vivo*. A 6% solution of [¹³C-3] alanine was infused for 90 minutes, during which the spectrum was acquired. Upper spectrum: 8.5 T ¹³C spectrum of perchloric acid extract of the liver used to generate spectrum a. This spectrum is the sum of 2048 acquisitions using 90° pulses and a recycle time of 5 seconds. Peaks are assigned as indicated. To be published (14).

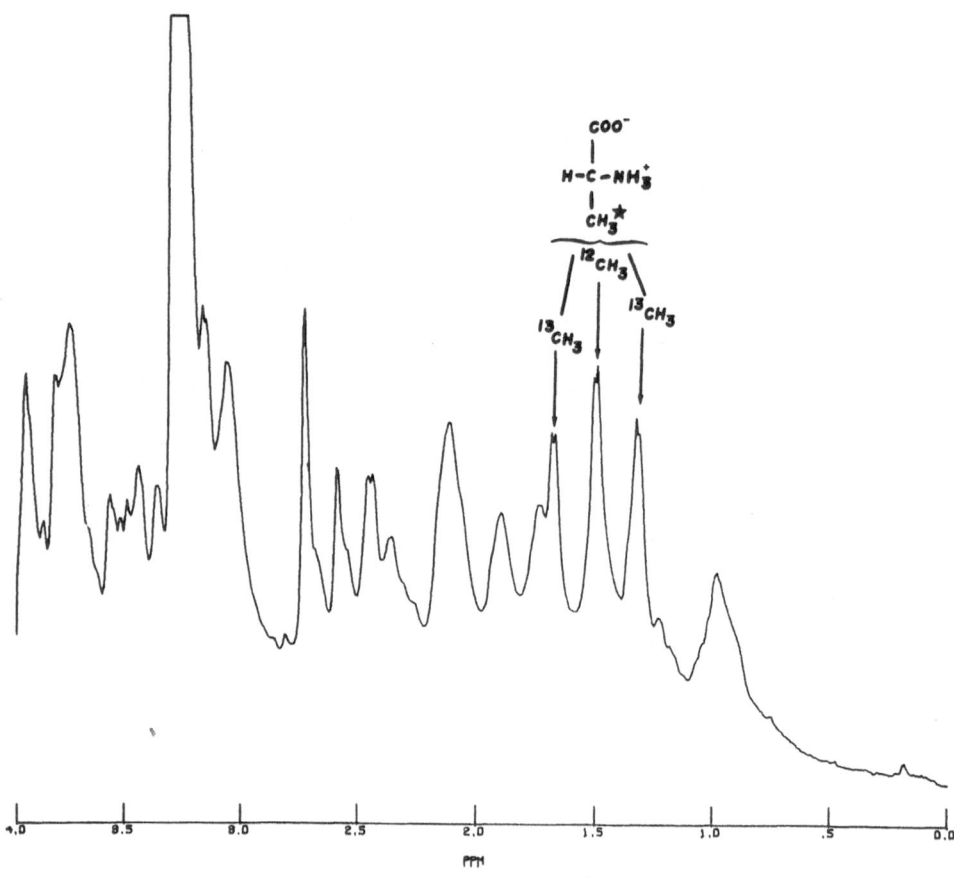

Figure 4:   8.5 T ^{1}H spectrum of the extract presented in Figure 3.   The extract   was   lyophilized and taken up in D_2O.   The spectrum is the sum of 16 acquisitions using 90° pulses with a 10 second recycle time.   The doublets indicated arise from the C-3 protons of alanine.   The peaks at 1.67 and 1.31 ppm correspond to ^{13}C labelled alanine, while the doublet at 1.49 ppm ārises from ^{12}C alanine.   (To be published (14).)

In parallel with our ^{13}C labelling studies, attention has been focussed on the ^{13}C natural abundance signals from several tissues in the living animal (26). As discussed above, the 1% natural labelling restricts the number of compounds which can be detected in this way. It is necessary for a material to be present at a level of approximately a few hundred millimolar to enable ^{13}C detection from naturally occurring ^{13}C without long acquisition times. For this reason, we have obtained spectra only from lipids and glycogen at natural abundance.

In Figure 5 we present 1.9 T spectra of two of the tissues which are of interest, liver and adipose. The resonances of the adipose tissue spectrum (Figure 5a) have all been assigned to triglyceride in the past (26,29). The terminal methyl groups yield peak 1; saturated carbons of the fatty acid chains yield peaks 2-8; the glycerol moiety's carbons give peaks 9 and 10; polyunsaturated carbon of the fatty acyl chains give peaks 11 and 12; and peak 13 comes from the carboxyl carbons at the ester linkages. Data of this type are suggestive of much quantitative information which has not yet been exploited in detail. The summed intensity in peaks 1-8 compared with the summed intensity of peaks 11 and 12 provides a measure of the saturated to unsaturated fat. Similarly, the ratio of the intensity of peak 1 to the sum of peaks 1-8 and 11-13, is the average fatty acyl chain length. The peaks 11 and 12 provide further information when they can be resolved. Peak 12 is generated by the monounsaturated olefinic carbons and the two carbons which terminate the conjugated series of olefinic bonds in the polyunsaturated fatty acids. Peak 11 is generated by the remaining olefinic carbons of the polyunsaturated acids. Thus peak 11 comes only from polyunsaturated fats, and peak 12 has contribution from both mono- and polyunsaturated fats. Hence the ratio of peak 11's intensity to that of the sum of peaks 11 and 12 yields a measure of the fraction of the total unsaturated carbons which are on polyunsaturated chains. It should be noted, however, that there is not sufficient information to calculate the relative amounts of the various polyunsaturated fatty acids (linoleic, linolenic and arachidonate). The size of the polyunsaturated pool is interesting because mammalian tissues do not synthesize these compounds. They are obtained only from the diet. Recently we have performed an experiment which showed that this part of the ^{13}C spectrum of adipose tissue in living rats was sensitive to long term modification of the dietary intake of polyunsaturated fatty acids (29).

The liver spectrum (Figure 5b) also has signals from lipids which appear to be similar to the signals from the adipose tissue. In adipose tissue, the triglyceride concentration is so high that there is little question but that the natural abundance ^{13}C signals are entirely triglyceride. However, in the liver, there are pools of phospholipids which are similar in magnitude to the triglycerides pools. The presence of signals from choline and ethanolamine (peaks 14 and 15) which are probably constituents of phospholipids provide evidence for this. The ^{13}C resolution is not sufficient to differentiate whether a fatty acyl chain is esterified to a phospholipid or a triglyceride.

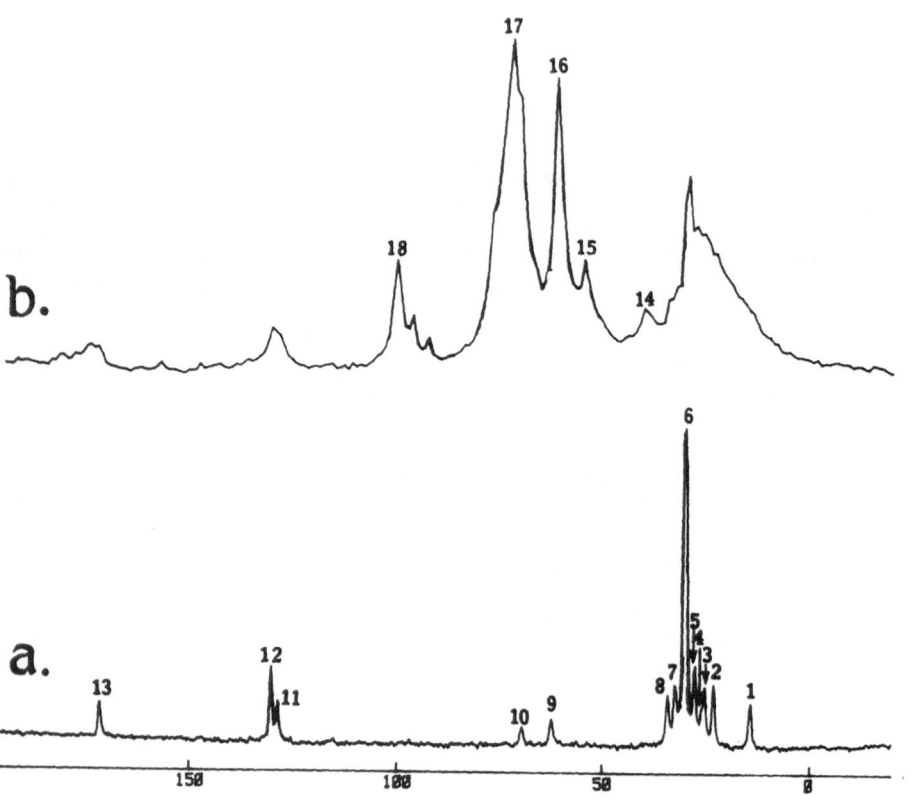

Figure 5: 1.9 T ^{13}C spectra of tissues excised from rabbit.

Thus we don't know whether the acyl carbon signals of Figure 5b are reporting the concentration of triglyceride or phospholipid. If phospholipid signals are present, we don't know whether these arise from phospholipids of the structural membranes or from various lipoproteins which are present in the tissue.

In addition to the lipid signals, the liver spectrum shows signals from glycogen. Signals from glucose monomers are also present as a result of the glycogen hydrolysis which occurs during liver excision. Peak 16 is the signal from the C-6 carbon of the glucose moiety of glycogen. Similarly, peak 18 is the C-1 signal, and peak 17 is the sum of the signals from C-2, C-3, C-4, and C-5. The presence of these signals has been shown to depend on whether the liver was taken from a fed or a fasted animal (P. Canioni, unpublished observations). The glycogen signals are absent when the animal was fasted prior to liver excision consistent with the well-known mobilization of this material during fasting. The presence of a glycogen signal is interesting because ^{13}C signals are often not obtained from macromolecules having the molecular weight of the average glycogen particle (10^8 daltons). Studies done at 8.5 T (31) and 4.2 T (32) have lead to the unexpected finding that 100% of the ^{13}C in glycogen contributes to the ^{13}C signals. Relaxation time measurements on isolate glycogen particles are consistent with intramolecular motion having a correlation time of about 10^{-8} sec.

We have demonstrated that it is possible to detect the natural abundance ^{13}C signals from hepatic glycogen from outside the body in the living rabbit using a surface coil (30). Stevens et al (32) have also reported detecting the naturally occurring signals from hepatic glycogen but they used a surgical preparation and were able to detect the signal only in a phosphorylase kinase deficient rat. Our results are presented in Figure 6. The signal-to-noise ratio for the glycogen peaks is good despite the low field. This supports the possibility that glycogen will be observable in the human liver as magnets of a similar field strength are now available for human studies. The resolution at 1.9 T is sufficient to distinguish the C-1 peak perfectly and it is likely that C-6 can be resolved from the broad line having contributions from C-2, C-3, C-4 and C-5 and the lipid peaks by resolution enhancement or line fitting techniques. There appear to be two potential experiments which arise from this preliminary finding (33). First, it should be possible to study the changes in the total glycogen pool resulting from physiological interventions by following changes in the natural abundance signals. Secondly, it should be possible to follow specific isotopic flows into C-1 or C-6 or the group C-2, C-3, C-4, C-5.

1.5 Techniques on the Horizon

The primary limitation of ^{13}C NMR is the inherent sensitivity. It is expected that much future effort will be directed to overcoming this limitation . The probable availability of higher field horizontal-bore

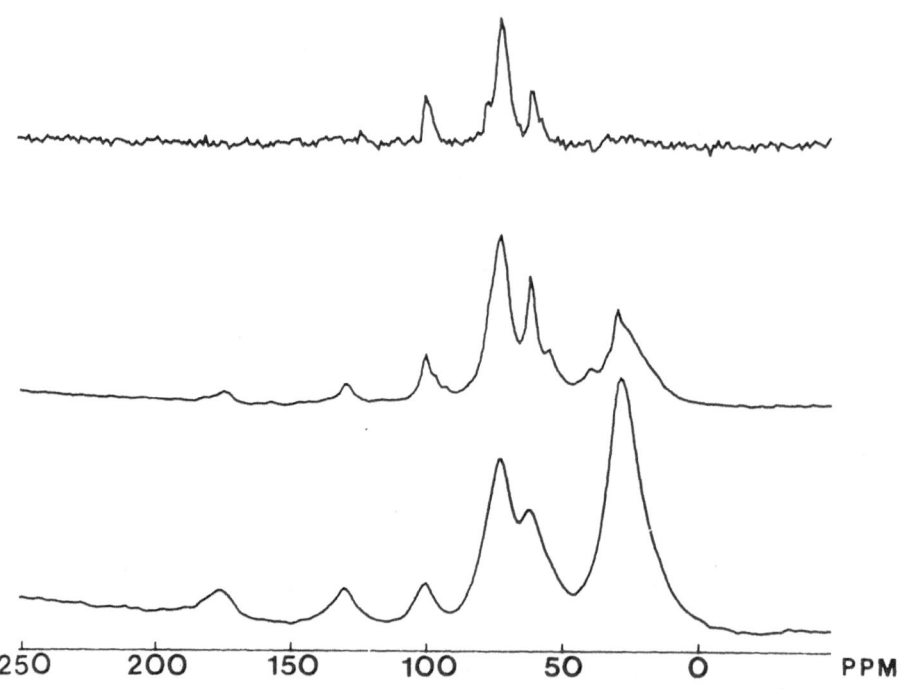

Figure 6: ^{13}C natural-abundance NMR spectra taken at 1.9 T. Lower
spectrum: Rabbit liver in vivo using a surface coil placed outside of
the body adjacent to the liver. Total accumulation time of 10 min; 60
Hz line broadening filter used in processing. Middle
spectrum: Excised liver from the rabbit used for the spectrum below.
Observed with a five-turn, 3 cm diameter solenoid with a perpendicular
Helmholtz coil decoupler; 66° pulse repeated every 0.1 sec; spectral
width, 10kHz; 1024 time-domain data points; 6000 accumulations, total
accumulation time of 10 min; 30 Hz line broadening filter used in
processing. Upper spectrum: Glycogen extracted from the liver of the
rabbit used for the spectra below. Accumulation parameters as
described for the excised liver; 10 Hz line broadening filter used in
processing. Assignments: 170-180 ppm, carboxyl carbons of fatty
acids; 125-135 ppm, unsaturated carbon of fatty acids; 95-105 ppm,
glycogen C_1 carbon; 65-80 ppm, glycogen C_{2-5} and glycerol C_2; 60-65
ppm, glycogen C_6 and glycerol $C_{1,3}$; 55.5 ppm, methyl group of choline;
40.0 ppm, methylene groups of choline and ethanolamine; 10-40 ppm,
saturated carbons of fatty acids. (Taken from Alger et. al. (30).)

magnets gives reason to expect some future sensitivity enhancement. However, additional methods of improving the sensitivity will probably be desired. Research being done at Yale suggests that indirect detection of ^{13}C magnetization via the ^1H signal by proton observe carbon decouple methods is likely to be used for sensitivity improvements, because the proton signal is much stronger. However as will be discussed below, the proton spectral resolution is poor, so methods are needed which have both the good sensitivity of the proton detection, and the good resolution of the ^{13}C detection. We will describe here these methods and present proton spectra illustrating their use without discussing the problems of proton observation in vivo which are to be discussed in the next section.

Our original approach was to give ^{13}C labelled precursors to a cell suspension and then to obtain a normal ^1H spectrum and one in which the $^{13}C - ^1H$ interaction was decoupled (34). A difference spectrum of these two spectra was then produced. The subtraction cancelled all signals which were not ^{13}C coupled, removing endogeneous background signals from various protons. However, ^{13}C-coupled protons produced a characteristic pattern having negative intensity for ^{13}C coupled protons and positive intensity for ^{13}C-decoupled protons. Decoupling could be broad banded so that all the ^{13}C coupled proton signals were present, or single frequency decoupling could be used to select a single ^{13}C coupled proton signal.

While producing the desired selectivity for ^{13}C coupled proton signals, the up-down patterns produced by our original proton observe carbon decouple method were sometimes difficult to interpret. Bendall (personal communication) has suggested that the pulse sequence shown in Figure 7 will alleviate this problem so as to produce spectra having only positive signals (35). In this method two spin echo spectra are obtained by alternately gating the ^{13}C decoupling on or off during the first τ delay. The spectrum acquired when the ^{13}C decoupling is on throughout the sequence gives the total intensity ($^{13}C+^{12}C$) of the ^1H signal (Figure 7A). However, in the other spectrum (Figure 7B), the phase modulation due to J coupling causes the ^{13}C bonded protons to give a negative signal intensity, yielding a ^{13}C decoupled signal proportional to the difference between the ^{12}C-bonded proton signal and the ^{13}C-bonded proton signal ($^{12}C-^{13}C$). Subtraction of the two subspectra results in summation of the ^{13}C bonded proton signals, with cancellation of all ^{12}C bonded signals. Broad band ^{13}C decoupling produces a spectrum of all protons coupled to ^{13}C. If this spectral presentation proves too complex, further selection of specific resonances can be achieved by decoupling a single carbon resonance so as to produce a ^1H spectrum only of the protons bound to that particular carbon.

In Figure 8, an example of the use of this method is presented (35). ^{13}C labelled glucose was infused into the venous system of a rat while 8.5T surface coil ^1H spectra of the brain were collected. The brain glutamate was labelled as a result of catabolism of the labelled

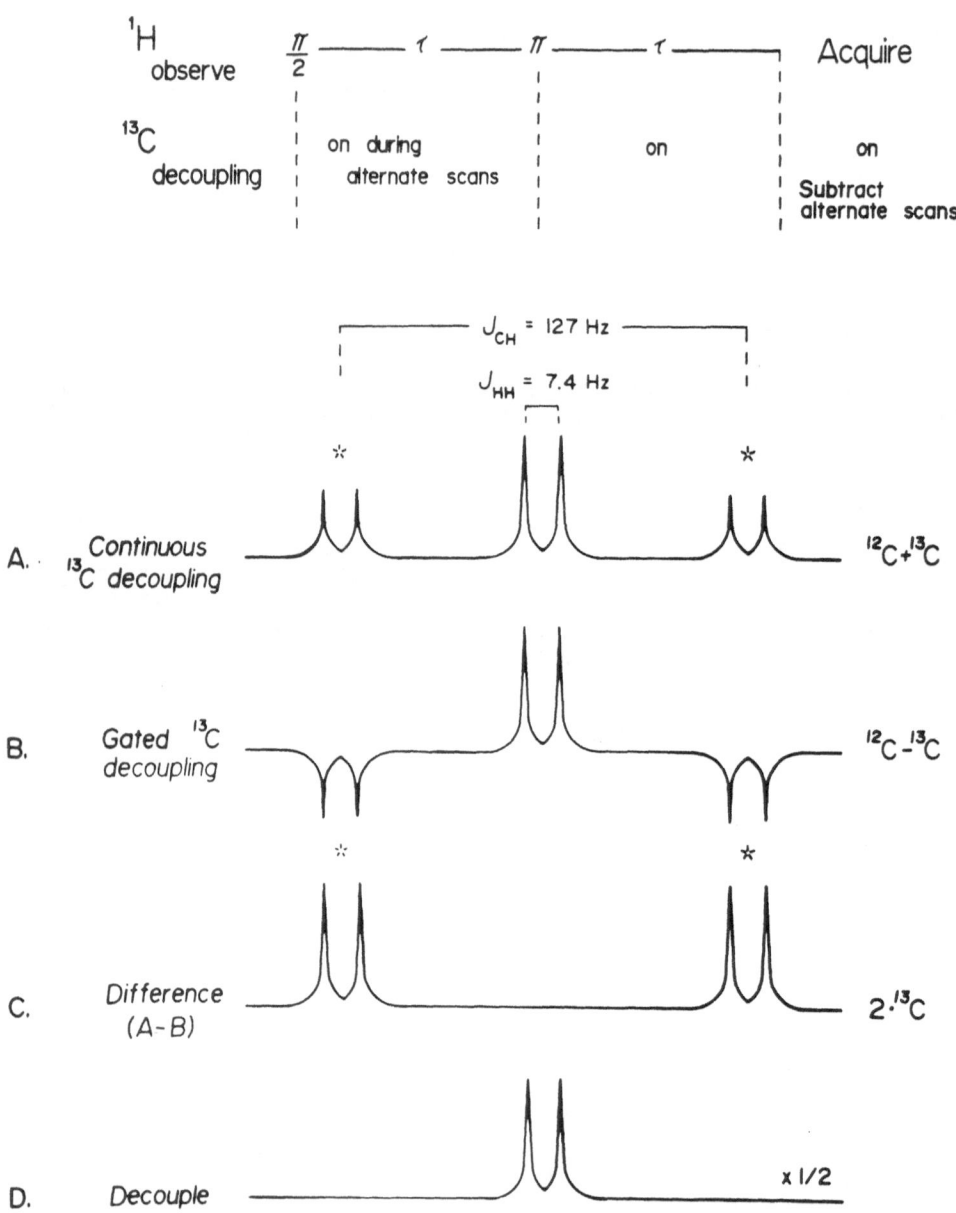

Figure 7: A proton observe ^{13}C decouple editing scheme. The spectra
in A, B, and C are presented so as to show only the effects of the ^{13}C
decoupling during the τ delay. They are presented as they would be
observed without ^{13}C decoupling during the acquisition time. Spectrum
D shows the result of decoupling during the acquisition time. (To be
published (35).)

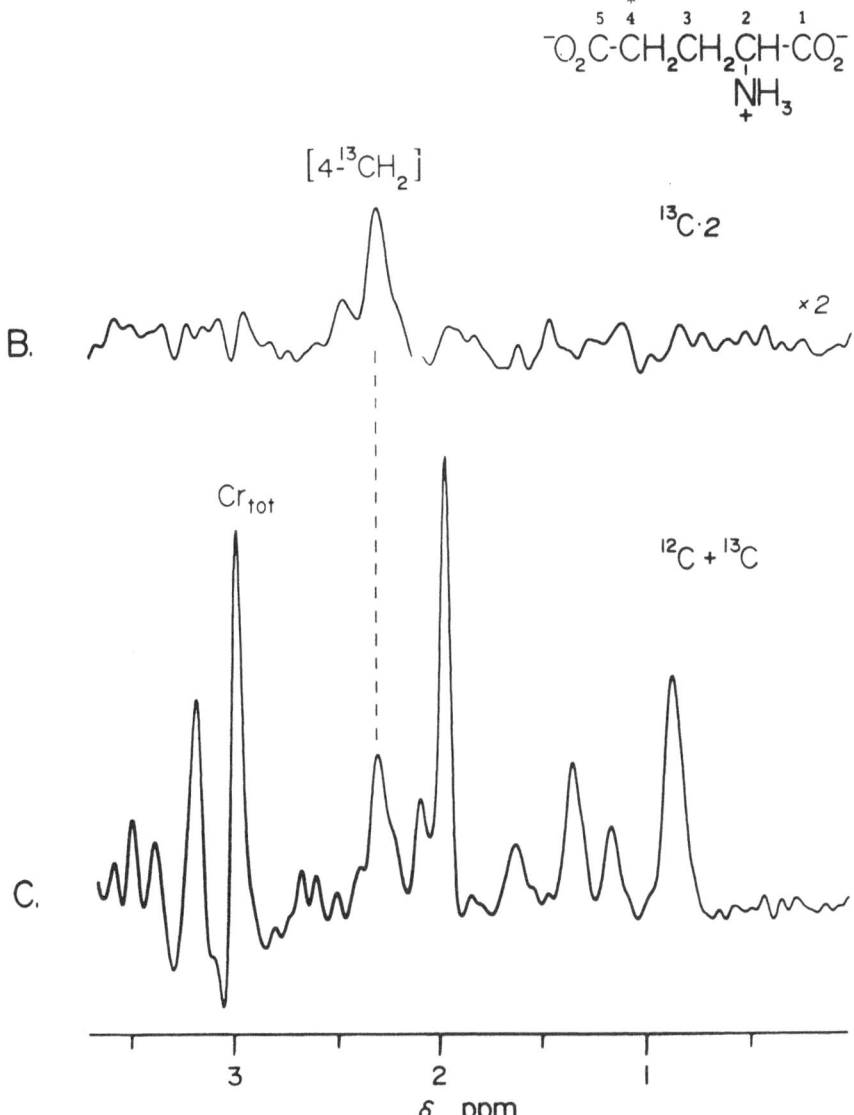

Figure 8: 8.5 T proton spectra from the rat brain after infusion of [¹³C-1] glucose obtained using the scheme shown in Figure 7. Lower spectrum: Total proton signal obtained with continuous ¹³C decoupling at the ¹³C-4 glutamate chemical shift. Upper spectrum: Difference spectrum showing selection of the ¹³CH₂ resonance of glutamate. This was obtained by subtracting the lower spectrum from a spectrum obtained with the ¹³C decoupling gated off during the first τ delay as shown in Figure 7. (To be published (35).)

glucose. The figure shows selection of the glutamate $^{13}CH_2$-4 signal by
single frequency decoupling of the ^{13}C-4 signal with elimination of all
other proton signals. While this is only a preliminary description
intended mostly to illustrate the procedure, hopefully it is clear that
a large number of ^{13}C labelled intracellular metabolites might be
studied in this way in the future.

1.6 Summary

With this lecture we have presented a review of what ^{13}C NMR technology
is providing for _in vivo_ study of metabolism. As yet many of the
studies are still at the stage of in which technical feasiability is
being developed, particularly in the cases of those studies involving
living animals. However, more detailed quantitative biochemical and
physiological information is now being obtained from various organ
preparations. The recent ^{13}C perfused liver studies by Cohen (36) are
perhaps the best example of this point. The desire to perform
metabolic studies with ^{13}C NMR is great but applications are being
restricted by the relatively low sensitivity and the need for large
amounts of expensive ^{13}C labelled compounds. We have suggested that
the stronger magnets now becoming available will improve the
sensitivity and that indirect detection via ^1H will improve it further
still. It can be shown that the high cost of most ^{13}C labelled
materials is a consequence of the cost of small scale chemical
synthesis of these compounds. We hope the future will bring a cost
reduction by the development of synthetic processes based on economies
of scale and possibly technical improvements in the synthetic
processes. With these advancements, it is likely that ^{13}C NMR will
result in a broadening of our basic understanding of metabolism, and
will also help in the understanding of a number of medically relevant
disorders.

2. ^1H NMR IN LIVING SYSTEMS

2.1 Introduction

In this lecture, new methods which are presently being explored for
obtaining ^1H spectra from small metabolites in living animals, perfused
organs or cell suspensions will be discussed. Why is it desirable to
use ^1H spectroscopy for this purpose? The primary reason is that the
sensitivity of proton detection is much higher than that of ^{13}C or ^{31}P.
The ^1H signal for an equal number of spins is 60 times stronger than
the ^{13}C signal from a ^{13}C labelled metabolite. This factor is 20 times
if the ^{13}C has a nuclear Overhauser enhancement. Thus ^1H methods show
promise of allowing the detection of lower metabolite concentrations or
of improving time resolution due to the higher signal-to-noise ratio
compared with ^{13}C detection. Furthermore, no labelling is required,
enabling the potential study of a larger number of metabolites at a
lower cost. A related point is that the ^1H signal is proportional to
the total metabolite concentration, whereas with ^{13}C NMR, the signal is
proportional to the part of the total concentration which is ^{13}C

labelled. Thus ^{1}H spectroscopy provides an easier method for following changes in the total concentration of a metabolite as opposed to ^{13}C. However, if it is desired to follow isotopic flows with ^{1}H NMR, it is possible to merge ^{1}H detection methods with ^{2}H labelling methods as Campbell and his colleagues have shown (37,38), or with ^{13}C labelling as we have discussed.

Given these advantages, why hasn't ^{1}H already been used extensively? There are two reasons: interference from the large and obligitory water signal and the poor spectral resolution characteristics of in vivo ^{1}H signals. By water signal interference we mean that the large signal from tissue water make signals from low concentration metabolites difficult to observe. By poor spectral resolution, we mean that even after the tissue water signal has been suppressed, there is usually a severe overlap of the desired metabolite signals with signals arising from fats, proteins and undesired metabolites. In the following sections, the experimental approaches to these problems will be discussed. Saturation of the water signal, spin echos and selective pulses are all being used for the suppression of the water peak. The resolution problem is being approached by spectral editing methods which are designed to detect only a single resonance among a group of overlapping ones.

2.2 Suppression of the Water Signal

The desired ^{1}H metabolite signals are about 10^6 times smaller than the water signal. The ^{1}H sensitivity leads one to expect to observe a signal from a metabolite present at the level of about 100 μm with ^{1}H NMR, because detection of 2mM ^{13}C signals from labelled metabolites is feasible and the ^{1}H signal should be on the order of 20 times stronger than the ^{13}C signal. Cooper has discussed this problem of detecting small signals in the presence of large ones when using Fourier transform methods (39). Although a number of factors come into play, the most significant in this context is the digitizer resolution. The 12 bit digitizer, which is commonly used in NMR, is capable of producing a maximum dynamic range on the order of 4×10^3. Thus when this digitizer is used, a method of reducing the water signal intensity by a factor of 250 is needed to allow detection of the small metabolite signals. A significant advancement in recent years is the appearance of 16 bit digitizers, which provide for a dynamic range of approximately 6×10^4, so that the water suppression need not be as perfect. Many methods for suppressing the water signal have been proposed. We do not intend to review them all here, but only to describe the ones that are working in our laboratory for in vivo studies with surface coils.

The first method which was used was one in which the water signal was saturated with a selective pulse prior to the acquisition of each free induction decay. A paper by Behar et. al.(40) provides an example of the use of this method at 8.5 T for obtaining ^{1}H signals from rat brain metabolites using a surface coil. The data is shown in Figure 9.

Comparison of the normal and the selectively saturated spectra (Figures 9a and 9b) show an apparent water signal suppression of several hundred fold. Further resolution enhancement by use of Gaussian filtering allows interpretation of the small metabolite signals on the high field side of the water peak as shown (Figure 9c).

A second form of water suppression which has been quite useful is to obtain spectra from spin echos. This approach accomplishes a small amount of water suppression because the water resonance _in vivo_ seems to have a significantly shorter T_2 than do several intracellular metabolites which are of interest. The short _in vivo_ T_2 of the water resonance is surprising in view of the low molecular weight of water, and this has become a point of study and discussion within the NMR imaging community. No complete explanation for the shortness of tissue water T_2 has yet arisen. However, as described by Mansfield and Morris (41), it does seem to be consistent with an exchange between free water and water bound to macromolecules. Whatever the reason, the difference between the water T_2 and the metabolite T_2 provides an effective means of selective suppression of water. Using an echo delay of 136 ms, so that the lactate methyl proton signal is refocussed in the positive direction, results in an apparent water suppresion of about 10-fold (K.L. Behar and D.L. Rothman, unpublished data) although some lactate signal intensity is lost due to its own transverse relaxation. This suppression can be supplimented by the use of pre-saturation techniques. Spin echo methods have an additional advantage in that the broad signals in the baseline from macromolecules are also reduced. These signals in many cases strongly overlap the ones of interest so that their suppression improves the apparent resolution in the spectrum.

Spin echo sequences are compatible with the use of surface coils as is discussed by Bendall and Gordon (42). Their approach is to cycle the phases of the θ and the 2θ pulses in such a way that signals from regions where $\theta = 90°$ are suppressed from the spectrum. Furthermore Rothman et. al. (43) have pointed out that this phase cycling is not needed when the echo delay 2τ is significantly longer than T_2. If the surface coil is used to deliver a spin echo sequence, care should be exercised in comparing the signal intensities with those acquired from the routine single pulse-acquire method. There are two reasons why intensity decays are observed in spectra of this type. First, the signal decays as a function of τ in the expected manner. A second more subtle reason is that the spin echo method is volume selective in that signals from volumes within the sample where θ is not approximately 90° are not present. In the extreme case where the rf field is very inhomogeneous as is the case with a surface coil, only a small fraction of the total sample may have $\theta = 90°$, and therefore a pulse-acquire method will produce a substantially larger signal than will a spin echo method, even if the delay is kept small. As a result of this effect, the amount of water suppression achieved by a spin echo should not be measured by comparing the spin echo spectrum with a pulse-acquire spectrum because the major cause of the signal loss may be due to

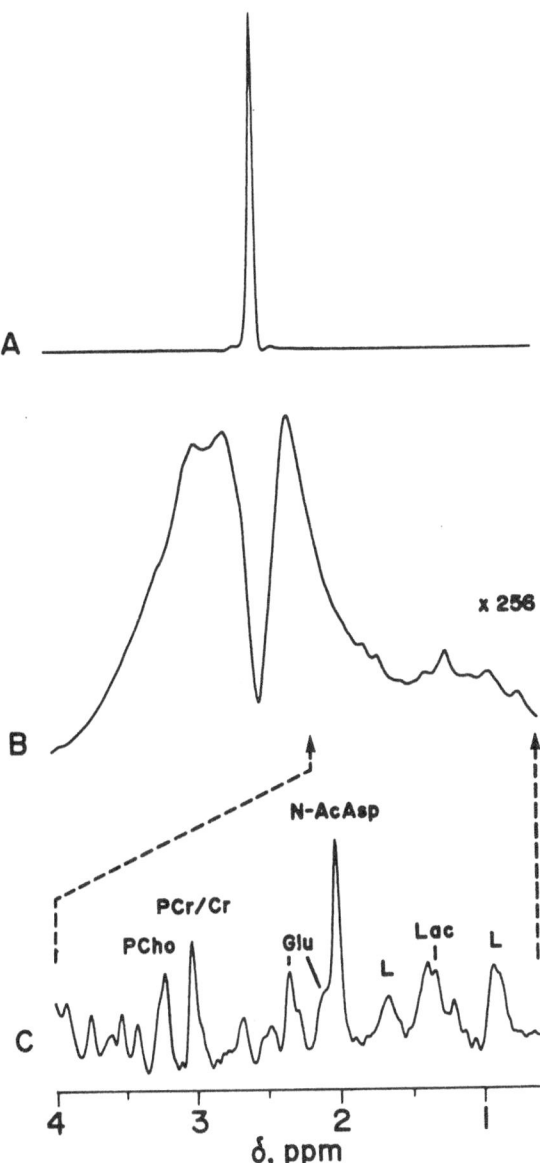

Figure 9: 8.5 T ¹H spectra of rat brain *in vivo*. A) Normal spectrum
showing   the   entire   water   peak.   B) The result of selectively
presaturating the water signal. C) Expansion of the high field part of
the spectrum B after resolution enhancement by Gaussian filtering.
Abbreviations: L, lipid; Lac, lactate;   N–AcAsp, N–acetylaspartate;
Glu, glutamate;   PCr/Cr, the sum of phosphocreatine and creatine;
Pcho, phosphorylcholine. (Data provided by K.L. Behar.)

volume selection.

Recently the spin echo and the pre-saturation method have been used together in a 1.9 T study designed to detect lactate formation in the hypoxic rabbit brain (D.L. Rothman and O.A.C. Petroff, unpublished data) following an earlier study (44). A spectrum is shown in Figure 10. By using the N-acetylaspartate signal as an approximate concentration standard, it is possible to estimate the size of the residual water signal. Such an analysis suggests that the combination of the pre-saturation, and the spin echo detection has suppressed the water signal by about 100-fold. The suppression is somewhat poorer than in the earlier high field study (Figure 9) because of less than optimum hardware characteristics of our low field instrument. Clearly, however, lactate and n-acetylaspartate can be detected in the living brain at this low field strength. The ability to detect lactate at this field has clinical significance. NMR machines which operate at this field strength for study of the human head are now available, and this result is suggestive that lactate signals will soon be sought in the human head.

Another method which is useful for water suppression is the 1331 method which was invented by Hore (45). The 1331 pulse sequence is the tailored pulse sequence

$$\theta-\tau-3\{\theta\}-\tau-3\theta-\tau-\{\theta\}-\text{Acquire}$$

where θ denotes an arbitrary nutation; $\{\theta\}$ denotes a θ nutation with a π phase shift; and 3θ denotes a nutation three times as large as θ. This sequence produces a nutation of 8θ upon a resonance located $1/2\tau$ Hertz from the carrier, and no nutation upon a resonance located at the carrier. The signal excitation envelope from this pulse sequence is approximated by the function $\sin^3(\pi f \tau)$. Water can thus be suppressed if the signal of interest is well removed on the chemical shift axis from the water signal. Furthermore, it is possible to create a Hahn spin echo sequence by doubling the "1331" to a "2662" to obtain the refocussing pulse. The reasons for wanting to do this will become apparent shortly. An example of the use of the 1331-2662 sequence from the work of Hetherington et.al. (46) is shown in Figure 11A. A surface coil placed adjacent to the brain of a sacrificed rat was used to obtain these 8.5 T spectra. Rough calibration of the water peak against the lactate peak (45-60 mM in ^{1}H) indicates this sequence has suppressed water by 2000-fold. In more recent experiments, water signal reductions of 80,000-fold fold have been observed.

The 1331 scheme has a number of advantages for water suppression. It is composed only of hard pulses from a single transmitter. Thus it is easily implemented on modern spectrometers, leaving the decoupler channel free for additional functions to be described below. Furthermore, it can be used in a straightforward manner with a surface coil. The use of the single 1331 pulse sequence with a surface coil does not result in volume selection, the sequence merely neglects to

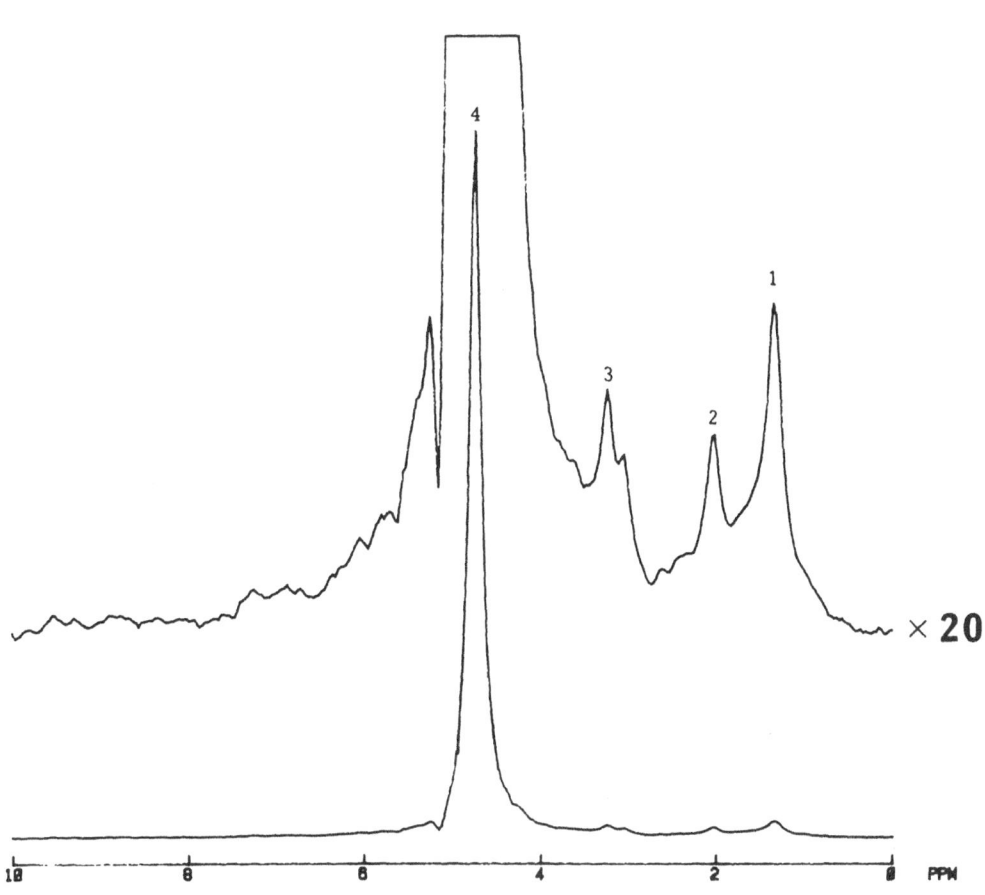

Figure 10: 1.9 T surface coil ¹H spectrum of rabbit brain _in vivo_. The skull and scalp were removed from the anesthetized rabbit so that the 1.7 cm surface coil could be placed directly against the cerebral tissue. Assignments: 1: lactate methyl protons; 2: methyl group of N-acetylaspartate; 3: sum of phosphocreatine, creatine and phosphoryl choline; 4: water.

excite resonances in certain parts of the frequency spectrum. However, if volume selection is desired, phase cycling of the type described by Bendall and Gordon (42) can be used.

2.3 Resolution Enhancement

Having suppressed the water signal by one of the above methods, it often additionally necessary to resolve a single resonance or a group of resonances from overlapping lipid peaks and the resonances of undesired metabolites. A process called "spectral editing" is used for this purpose. The general strategy is to use nuclear resonance parameters in addition to the simple chemical shift to resolve the resonance of interest. In the procedures which we will discuss, these additional parameters are the multiplicity, the coupling constant to a second spin, and the chemical shift of the second spin. The editing procedure provides a high degree of selectivity because of the unlikelihood that any other resonance would have all four parameters (chemical shift, multiplicity, J coupling constant and chemical shift of the J-coupled spin) identical to those of the resonance of interest.

We have already discussed the proton observe carbon decouple method which is a member of this class of experiments. A homonuclear variant of this experiment was recently discussed by Rothman et. al (47,48). The method edits on the basis of homonuclear coupling and the chemical shift of the coupled multiplet of ^1H resonances. The pulse sequence used is shown in Figure 12. Consider the case of an AX spin system, where it is desired to resolve the X signal from some undesired signal such as the proton signal of triglyceride. In this spin echo sequence, the two X signals will phase modulate with a period of J^{-1} during the period τ in the sequence. One spectrum is collected with the decoupling off and $\tau = (2J)^{-1}$ so that the X doublet is antiphase (negative) at the time of acquisition. Another spectrum is collected with the decoupler placed at the chemical shift so as to decouple the AX interaction and inhibit the phase modulation so that the phase of X remains unchanged (positive) during the sequence. Subtraction of the two spectra then produces a spectrum of X with cancellation of other resonances. Extention of the method to observe triplets and quartets is described in the work by Rothman et. al. (48).

The invention of this method has great relevance to ^1H studies on living animals or humans where surface coils are to be used without recourse to surgical intervention. In most animal studies there is a layer of subcutaneous fatty tissue which produces ^1H signals which tend to be strong (sometimes as large as 50% of the water intensity) because this tissue is close to the coil. Furthermore, the T_2's for this adipose tissue signal are often longer than that of the water, so they can't be removed by the spin echo sequence alone. In addition to this subcutaneous fat, many tissues have proton signals from endogeneous fatty materials which can be as large as 10% of the water signal intensity, so that even when surgical exposure is employed, one is forced to deal with very large interferences from lipid signals.

Figure 13 provides an example from the work of Rothman et. al. (48) of the use of the homonuclear editing technique to resolve the lactate ^{1}H signal from subcutaneous fat signals in the head of a sacrificed rat using a surface coil without surgery. Figure 13C shows the signal obtained with a simple pulse-acquire experiment. Some resonances are discernable, notably creatine and n-acetyl aspartate. A τ = 34 spin echo sequence (Figure 13B) shows that some of the lipid signals are reduced either by the T_2 relaxation or by the volume selectivity of the echo method, yet the lactate signal is still not resolved. As is shown by Figure 13A, single frequency decoupling of the CH proton of lactate at 4.1 ppm and subtraction from spectrum B, produces a clear signal from the lactate methyl resonance at 1.33 ppm, enabling quatitative study of this metabolite. In addition to detecting tissue lactate, Rothman et. al. (48) have shown that this method can be used to resolve a number of other endogeneous brain metabolite signals in the ^{1}H spectrum using a surface coil. These include glutamate, γ-aminobutyric acid , taurine and alanine.

Hetherington et. al. (46) have suggested an alternate editing method which provides greater spectral selectivity. The pulse sequence is shown in Figure 14. This method utilizes the 1331 sequence for the "θ" pulse and a 2662 pulse for the "2θ" pulse as described above for water suppression. Successful applications depend on tailoring the excitation spectrum of the 1331 pulses, so that the X spins receive significantly different nutations compared with the A spins. Observation of complete phase modulation of the X spins in a AX system due to J coupling with A requires that both A and X receive π pulses during the second pulse of the spin echo sequence. If A receives no nutation when X receives a π nutation, as would be the case if the 1331 pulse was very selective, X will not phase modulate at all. Thus, Hetherington et. al. has suggested that a selective DANTE pulse (49) sequence, positioned at the A resonance, should be used simultaneously with the 2662 so as to compensate for the incomplete inversion of A and thereby produce the required phase modulation in X. The DANTE excitation spectrum can be made extremely selective so that other spin systems in the vicinity of X are unlikely to receive the full π nutation.

The use of this method is illustrated by Figure 11. The experiment was performed on a sacrificed rat with a surface coil placed adjacent to the brain. The spin echo τ delay was 68 ms. At this delay, the lactate methyl protons would be antiphased if the CH proton receives a π pulse. Spectrum A shows the spin echo spectrum taken with the DANTE excitation placed on the low field side of the water signal. The excitation spectrum of the 1331 sequence is such that the CH proton receives only a very small nutation during the refocussing pulse and as a result the lactate methyl is upright. When the DANTE is moved to the position of the CH signal and adjusted so as to invert it selectively (spectrum B), phase inversion of the lactate methyl is observed. The difference between the two spectra yields a spectrum showing only the methyl protons (bottom spectrum).

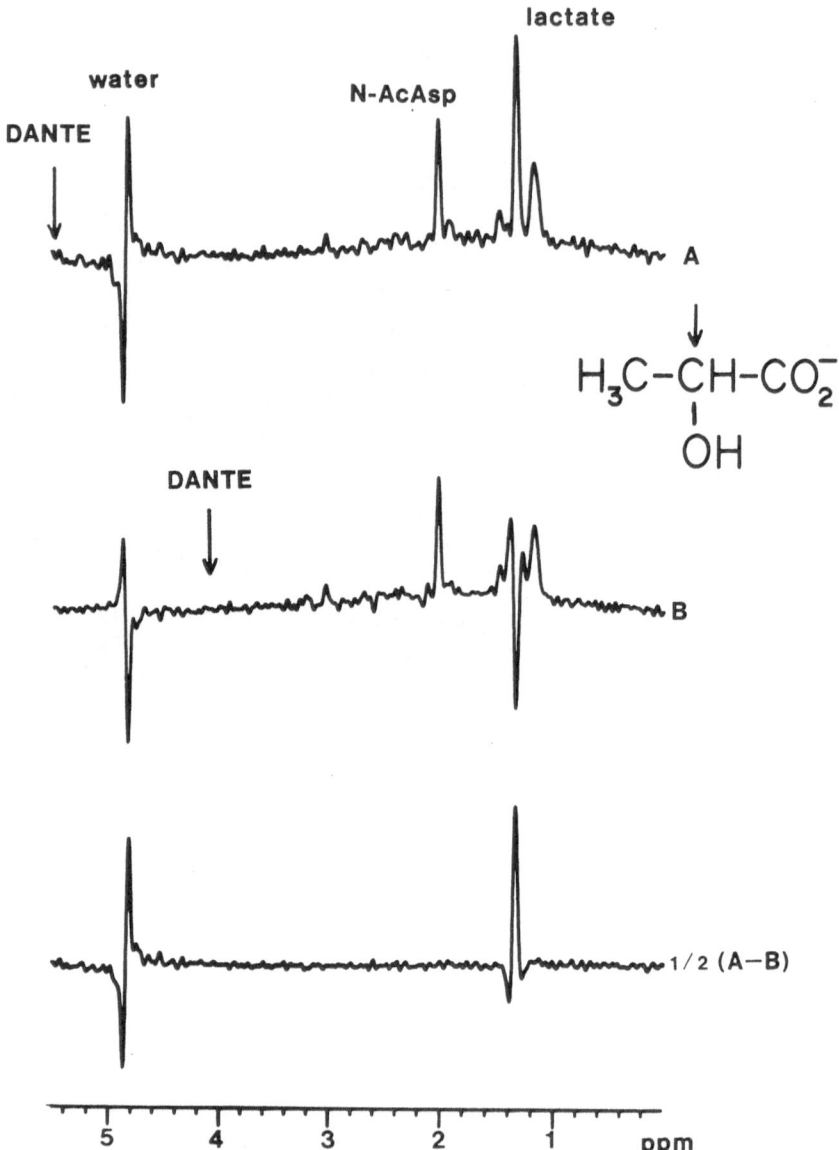

Figure 11: 1331 ^{1}H spin echo spectra of in situ rat brain of a sacrificed animal. The pulse sequence used is shown in Figure 14. Spectra taken at 8.5 T. A) Spectrum acquired with DANTE frequency placed on low field side of water so that the lactate CH resonance does not receive a refocussing pulse. B) DANTE placed at the position of the lactate CH signal so that it receives a refocussing pulse, which causes the lactate CH_3 signal to phase invert. C) Difference between A and B. (Taken from Hetherington et. al. (46).)

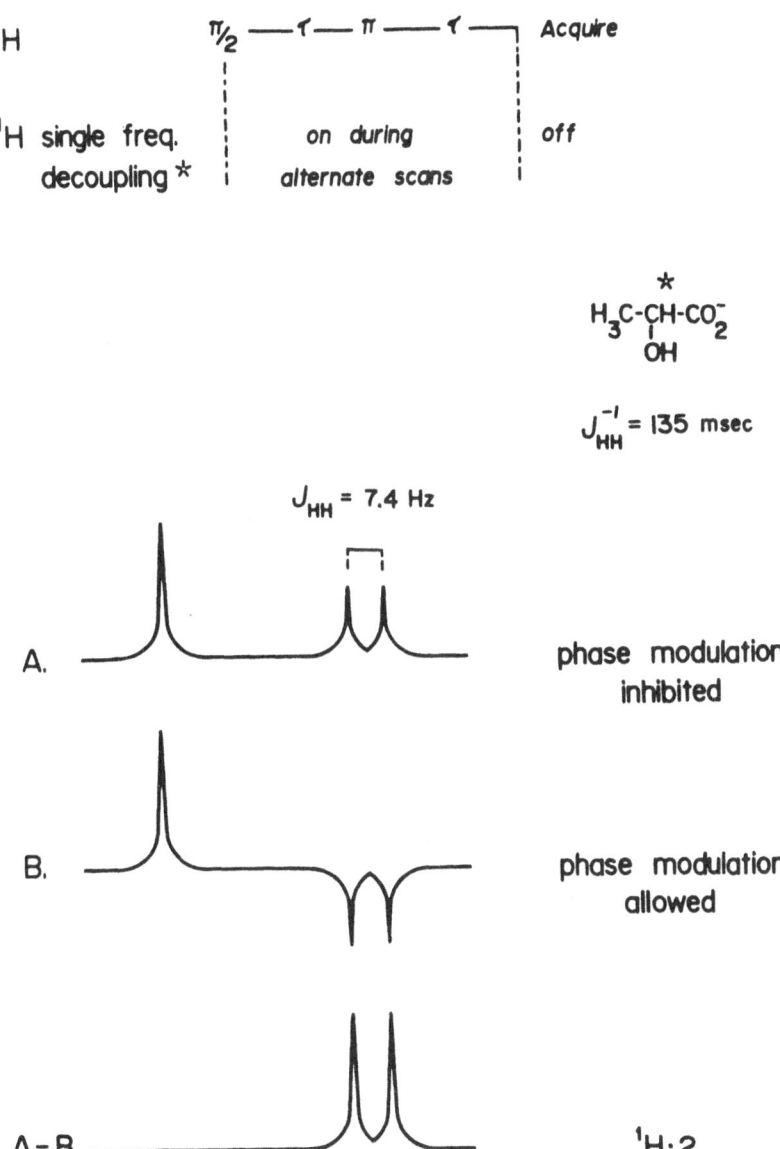

Figure 12: ¹H homonuclear editing sequence as suggested by Rothman et. al. (47,48) for selecting the lactate methyl signal out of a complex spectrum. Single frequency decoupling at the position of the CH resonance is used. A) Spectrum as would be obtained with decoupler on. B) Spectrum as would be obtained with decoupler off showing phase inversion of the methyl signal.

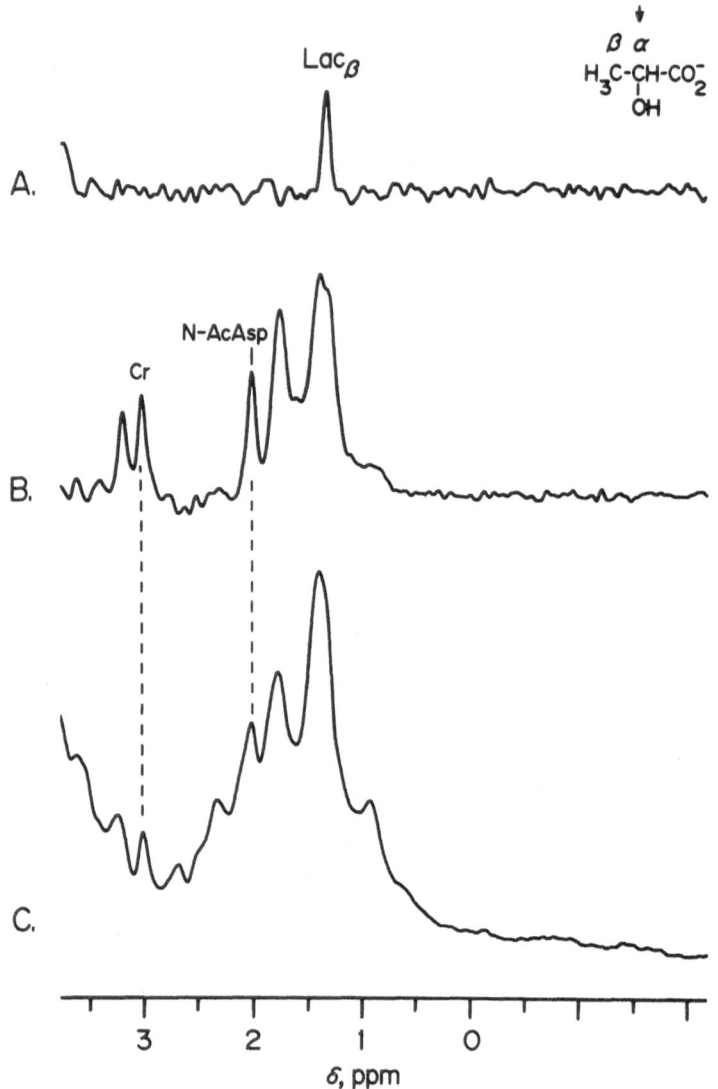

Figure 13: 8.5 T ¹H NMR spectra of the head of a rat (postmortem) with its scalp left intact. (A) The double resonance difference spectrum obtained with irradiation at 4.10 ppm to decouple the lactate α–CH proton resonance. The large signal at 1.33 ppm is the β–CH$_3$ resonance of lactate (Lacβ). (B) The τ–34 msec spin echo spectrum which is the non-irradiated component of spectrum A. Spectrum A and B are on the same intensity scale. (C) A conventional acquisition (pulse–acquire–delay) spectrum using the same π/2 pulse duration as spectrum A and B. All three spectra were processed identically. (Taken from Rothman et. al. (48).)

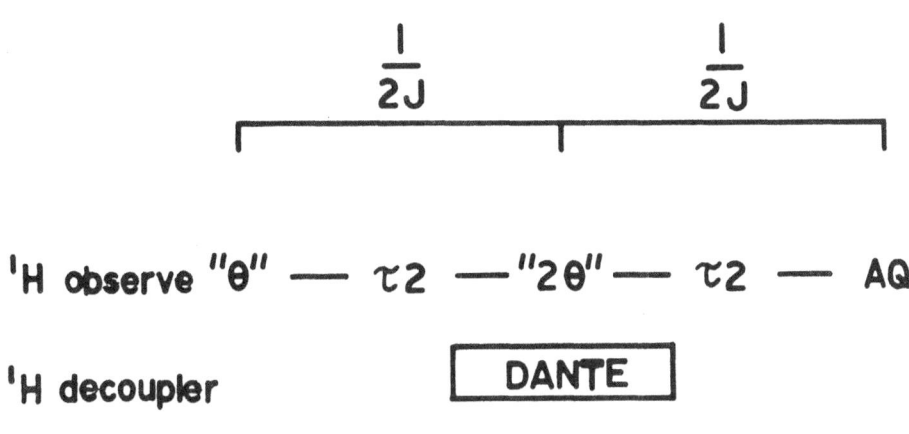

$\dfrac{1}{2J}$ $\qquad$ $\dfrac{1}{2J}$

'H observe "θ" — τ2 — "2θ" — τ2 — AQ

'H decoupler $\boxed{\text{DANTE}}$

DANTE on X resonance during alternate scans

"θ" 1-$\bar{3}$-3-$\bar{1}$

"2θ" 2-$\bar{6}$-6-$\bar{2}$

Figure 14: 1331-spin echo pulse sequence with DANTE editing for use with a surface coil as taken from Hetherington et. al. (46).

2.4 Physiological Studies

The primary purpose of this part of the lecture is to describe the ^{1}H technical methods which are now becoming available for studies of living systems. The techniques, which are at various stages of development, are being used to study a number of physiological and biochemical problems in a number of organ systems. At present, most studies have been on the brain because its proton spectrum is well-resolved and has relatively small lipid interference and so the requirements for editing are not as strict. Lactate is the metabolite which has been studied most often at both 8.5 and 1.9 T. However, resonances from glutamate, glutamine, and γ aminobutyric acid are also being exploited. With the invention of the techniques we have discussed, we seem to have just scratched the surface of the many interesting and medically relevant physiological studies.

ACKNOWLEGMENT. The author wishes to express his gratitude to R.G. Shulman, H.P. Hetherington, M.J. Avison, D.L. Rothman and K.L. Behar, who provided preprints of articles and figures prior to publication as well as many enlightening discussions. This work was supported by NIH grant GM-30278.

REFERENCES

1) D.G. Gadian, "NMR and Its Applications to Living Systems",
    Clarendon Press, Oxford.   (1982) p 8.

2) ibid. p 10.

3) R.G. Shulman, T.R. Brown, K. Ugurbil, S. Ogawa, S.M. Cohen and
    J.A. den Hollander, Science 205,160 (1979).

4) J.J. Led and S.B. Petersen, J. Magn. Reson. 32, 1 (1978).

5) D.G. Gadian and F.N.H. Robinson, J. Magn. Reson. 34, 449 (1979)

6) D.I. Hoult and P.C. Lauterbur, J. Magn. Reson. 34, 425 (1979).

7) J.S. Waugh, J. Magn. Reson. 50, 30 (1982).

8) A.J. Shaka, J. Keeler, T. Frankiel and R. Freeman, J. Magn.
    Reson. 52, 335 (1983).

9) M.H. Levitt, R. Freeman and T. Frenkiel, J. Magn. Reson. 50, 157 (1982).

10) M.H. Levitt and R. Freeman, J. Magn. Reson. 43, 502 (1981).

11) D.W. Alderman and D.M. Grant, J. Magn. Reson. 36, 447 (1979).

12) N.V. Reo, C.S. Ewy, B.A. Siegfried and J.J. H. Ackerman, J. Magn. Reson. 58,76 (1984).

13) J.A. den Hollander, K.L. Behar and R.G. Shulman, J. Magn. Reson. 57, 311 (1984).

14) M.E. Stromski, F. Arias–Mendoza, J.R. Alger and R.G. Shulman, (manuscript in preparation).

15) S.M. Cohen, P. Glynn and R.G. Shulman, Proc. Natl. Acad. Sci. USA 78, 60 (1981).

16) N.A. Matwiyoff and T.E. Needham, Biochem. Biophys. Res. Comm. 49, 1158 (1972).

17) R.T. Eakin, L.O. Morgam, C.T. Gregg and N.A. Matwiyoff, FEBS Lett 28, 259 (1972).

18) N.A. Matwiyoff and D.G. Ott, Science 181, 1125 (1973).

19) R.S. Norton, Bull. Magn. Reson 3, 29 (1982).

20) K. Ugurbil, T.R. Brown, J.A. den Hollander, P. Glynn and R.G. Shulman, Proc. Natl. Acad. Sci. USA 75, 3746 (1978).

21) S.M. Cohen, S. Ogawa and R.G. Shulman. Proc. Natl. Acad. Sci. USA 76, 1603 (1979).

22) S.M. Cohen, R.G. Shulman and A. McLaughlin, Proc. Natl. Acad. Sci. USA 76, 4808 (1979).

23) I.A. Bailey, D.G. Gadian, P.M. Matthews, G.K. Radda and
    P.J. Seeley, FEBS Lett. 123, 315 (1981).

24) A.I. Scott (editor) Tetrahedron 39, 3441 (1983).

25) J.A. den Hollander and R.G. Shulman, Tetrahedron 39, 3529 (1983).

26) J.R. Alger, L.O. Sillerud, K.L. Behar, R.J. Gillies, R.G. Shulman,
    R.E. Gordon, D. Shaw and P.E. Hanley, Science 214, 660 (1981).

27) K.L. Behar, O.A.C. Petroff, J.W. Prichard, J.R. Alger and
    R.G. Shulman (manuscript in preparation).

28) K.J. Neurohr, E.J. Barrett and R.G. Shulman, Proc. Natl. Acad.
    Sci. USA 80, 1603 (1983).

29) P. Canioni, J.R. Alger and R.G. Shulman, Biochemistry 22, 4974
    (1983).

30) J.R. Alger, K.L. Behar, D.L. Rothman and R.G. Shulman, J. Magn.
    Reson. 56, 334 (1984).

31) L.O. Sillerud and R.G. Shulman, Biochemistry 22, 1087 (1983).

32) A.N. Stevens, R.A. Iles, P.G. Morris and J.R. Griffiths, FEBS Lett
    150, 489 (1982).

33) J.R. Alger and R.G. Shulman, Brit. Med. Bull. 40, 21 (1984).

34) L.O. Sillerud, J.R. Alger and R.G. Shulman, J. Magn. Reson. 45,
    142 (1982).

35) D.L. Rothman, K.L. Behar, H.P. Hetherington, J.A. den Hollander,
    M.R. Bendall, O.A.C. Petroff and R.G. Shulman (manuscript in
    preparation).

36) S.M. Cohen, J. Biol. Chem. 258, 14294 (1983).

37) F.F. Brown and I.D. Campbell, Phil. Trans. R. Soc. Lond. B 289, 395 (1980).

38) K.M. Brindle, F.F. Brown, I.D. Campbell, D.L. Foxall and R.J. Simpson, Biochem. Soc. Trans. 8, 646 (1980).

39) J.W. Cooper in "Topics in ^{13}C NMR," (G.C. Levy, ed.) Academic Press, New York, Chapter 7 (1981).

40) K.L. Behar, J.A. den Hollander, M.E. Stromski, T. Ogino, R.G. Shulman, O.A.C. Petroff and J.W. Prichard, Proc. Natl. Acad. Sci. USA 80, 4945 (1983).

41) P. Mansfield and P.G. Morris, "NMR Imaging in Biomedicine," Academic Press, New York (1982).

42) M.R. Bendall and R.E. Gordon, J. Magn. Reson. 53, 365 (1983).

43) D.L. Rothman, K.L. Behar, J.A. den Hollander and R.G. Shulman, J. Magn. Reson. 59, 157 (1984).

44) K.L. Behar, D.L. Rothman, R.G. Shulman, O.A.C. Petroff and J.W. Prichard, Proc. Natl. Acad. Sci USA 81, 2517 (1984).

45) P.J. Hore, J. Magn. Reson. 54, 539 (1983).

46) H.P. Hetherington, M.J. Avison and R.G. Shulman, J. Magn. Reson. submitted.

47) D.L. Rothman, F. Arias-Mendoza, G.I. Shulman and R.G. Shulman, J. Magn. Reson. submitted.

48) D.L. Rothman, K.L. Behar, H.P. Hetherington and R.G. Shulman, J. Magn. Reson. submitted.

49) G.A. Morris and R. Freeman, J. Magn. Reson. 29, 433 (1982).

50) S.M. Cohen and R.G. Shulman in "Noninvasive Probes of Tissue

Metabolism" (J.S. Cohen, ed.), John Wiley and Sons, pp.   119
(1982).

NON–INVASIVE LOCALIZED VOLUME SPECTROSCOPY OF ANIMALS: PROSPECTS FROM THE VIEWPOINT OF THE HIGH RESOLUTION SPECTROSCOPIST

J. R. Alger
Dept. of Diagnostic Radiology
Dept. of Molecular Biophysics and Biochemistry
Yale University, P. O. Box 6666
New Haven, CT. 06511
U.S.A.

ABSTRACT. The successful application of high resolution NMR methodology to human metabolism studies, whether for research or clinical–diagnostic purposes, requires the development and refinement of methods for obtaining spectra from local regions within the subject. As yet no quantitatively perfect localization method has been found, although a several somewhat imperfect methods, such as surface coil and topical magnetic resonance techniques have been used, and a number of new methods based on proton imaging technologies have been suggested. This discussion critically reviews the surface coil and topical magnetic resonance methods which have been employed for high resolution spectroscopy of animal tissues. It goes on to stress that high resolution spectroscopy of small metabolites has special limitations which will be important in defining the effectiveness of those methods which have been suggested, but not yet applied in living animal experimentation.

1. INTRODUCTION

Future high resolution NMR studies directed toward clinical goals will require significant improvements in methodologies for obtaining spectral information from metabolites in specific volumes of tissue within the human body. Most of the research now being done in this area is being performed in laboratories where ^1H imaging methods were developed. Spectroscopic studies of tissue biochemistry have proceeded independently in other laboratories using imperfect localization methods such as surface coils. At this time, it seems appropriate for spectroscopists who have practical experience regarding tissue metabolite resonances to contribute to the development of the various spatial localization methods, since spectroscopic feasibility is an important part of any prospective method. Hence one function of this lecture is to discuss localization methods from the viewpoint of the body of high resolution spectroscopy knowledge which now exists. A second related function is to summarize and review the localization methods which have been attempted for metabolic studies of living animals by spectroscopists. Throughout the lecture we will be

265

T. Axenrod and G. Ceccarelli (eds.), NMR in Living Systems, 265–278.

discussing how to obtain information regarding the spatial distribution in the body of low concentration metabolites such as phosphocreatine, lactate, glutamate, inorganic phosphate, ATP and so on. We will not discuss the mapping of the heavily concentrated compounds fat and water, because this topic is covered elsewhere in the volume.

2. LOCALIZATION METHODS PRESENTLY USED IN SPECTROSCOPIC STUDIES

2.1 Surgical Methods

In own our NMR studies of tissue biochemistry, spatial localization has been achieved by using surgical procedures which expose the tissue of interest and by the design of an rf coil which optimally detects NMR signals from the exposed tissue. Using this approach, we now have methods for obtaining spectra from brain, liver, kidney and heart. For brain studies, superficial tissue on the rabbit head is retracted, so as to expose the skull and a surface coil is placed against the bone (1-4). In some cases, the skull has also been removed so that the coil can be placed directly against the cerebral tissue (O. A. C. Petroff, unpublished data). The liver of the rat is studied by placing it within a Helmholtz coil after an abdominal incision (5). Heart spectra are obtained from the guinea pig with a solenoidal coil placed around the heart after opening the chest (6-8). The rat kidney is being studied by surgically isolating the kidney in a micropunture cup containing a Helmholtz coil (9). Several other laboratories are using similar surgical approaches (10-14). In addition to providing the best possible localization now available, these surgical methods produce spectra with optimal signal-to-noise ratios because the signal is detected with the coil placed in close proximity to tissue of interest, thus maximizing the filling factor, and because high sensitivity coils, such as solenoids can be used. For these reasons the surgical approach to NMR signal localization will probably continue to be useful for studies with animals for some time to come.

2.2 Topical Magnetic Resonance

Topical Magnetic Resonance (TMR) is another method which has been used with rather limited success in spectroscopic studies. The method, as suggested by Gordon et. al. (15), produces a volume of high static field homogeneity at a specific region within an animal, with the immediately-surrounding regions experiencing steep static field gradients. Sharp NMR lines thus arise only from the volume of high homogeneity, with the unwanted regions yielding broad signals, which can be removed by FID processing. Oxford Research Systems incorporated this idea into their TMR-32 instrument. This system had a pair of opposing second and fourth order z-gradient coils which were designed to create a "sphere of homogeneity" at the center of the magnet with steep gradients surrounding the sphere. The nominal volume of the sphere could be varied by adjusting the current flowing through the profiling coils, however the design did not permit the sphere to be moved away from the center of the magnet. In addition to the original paper which described the use of the TMR method to obtain spectra of the rat liver non-invasively, we are aware of only two other reports of its use (16,17). All further development of spatial signal localization by use of static field profiling appears to have stopped.

The TMR method presently has several deficiencies which make it difficult to use routinely. The most significant of these is that there is not a practical and rapid way to ensure that the animal is positioned within the magnet in a manner that places the tissue of interest at the center of the magnet. Furthermore, there is no method for determining how large the sensitive volume actually is, or what its shape is. The question of the shape of the homogeneous volume became particularly significant with the appearence of published plots of the TMR field contours which show that the homogeneous volume created with profiling coils is not a perfect sphere (18). Another problem is that the smallest dimension of the homogeneous region is about 2 cm in diameter. This is impractical for the study of small animals because most organs of interest are not even approximately spherical and usually have at least one linear dimension smaller than 2 cm. As a result, part of the homogeneous volume is usually outside of the organ to be studied and, therefore, signals from extraneous tissues are present.

The TMR technique does have some advantages to its favor, and we feel that the basic TMR concept is promising and deserving of more research than it has received over the last few years. One advantage is that the gradients are static, so one needs not be concerned with the possibility that a pulsed field gradient has not completely relaxed at the time of signal acquisition. Similarly, the TMR method does not use complicated pulse sequences, which place stringent demands on hardware, or that restrict detection to resonances having particular relaxation times. Furthermore, the TMR method does not reduce the signal from the desired region, it simply removes signals from undesired regions, and so has the potential for producing spectra with optimal signal-to-noise ratios. As is discussed above, the problems are mostly associated with how easily the method can be routinely used. The practical implementation problems might be overcome by combining TMR field profiling with imaging methods, which map the spatial variation of the static field intensity (19), so as to define more exactly the size and shape of the homogeneous volume in each particular study. Clearly some revitalization of this type is needed if TMR is ever to become practically useful.

2.3 Surface Coil Methods

A significant contribution to living animal NMR was the invention of the surface coil by Ackerman et. al. (20). The surface coil method is the most extensively used method of achieving spatial localization of NMR signals in animals and humans. Spatial localization is achieved because this device produces an rf field intensity that varies with spatial co-ordinate. The original paper describes the sensitive region

from a circular surface coil as a disk shaped region having a diameter
equal to the coil's diameter, and a thickness equal to the coil radius.
The basic conclusion was that when a surface coil was placed against
the body and a pulse-acquire sequence used, a spectrum of the tissue in
this disk shaped region would be obtained. Later the "surface nulling
pulse" was proposed as a method of obtaining improved localization
around deeper volume elements (16). Here the excitation pulse length
is adjusted to give a π nutation, and thus minimal excitation, at the
surface, and a $\pi/2$ nutation and maximal excitation at a region located
deeper within the sample. The paper which suggests this method
supports this protocol with a plot of the excitation as a function of
position along the axis of the coil. However, the off-axis behavior of
the excitation is not presented. Since that time, a number of groups
have produced calculations of the off-axis behavior so as to better
understand the properties of the surface coil (21,22). In Figure 1 we
present a similar contour plot showing the "sensitive volume" in cross
section which is produced by a surface coil when a "surface nulling
pulse" is used. The plot shows that the volume giving strong positive
signal (the region between 60° and 120° contours) curves inward,
touching the surface at a point located 1.3 radii from the coil center.
Thus a certain amount of surface tissue is excited even if the "surface
nulling pulse" is used. Furthermore there are regions close to the
coil (inside of the 180° contour) which can produce negative signals
which cancel those from deeper regions. The behavior of the excitation
in the cross section perpendicular to the one shown in Figure 1 is even
more complicated (data not shown). This because the cylindrical
symmetry of the problem is broken by the fact that the excitation is
proportional to the projection of the rf field vector in the plane
perpendicular to the static field axis.

The spatial localization of the surface coil was further improved
by the invention of the "depth pulse" by Bendall and Gordon (23-25).
In this method a pulse sequence composed of pulses of specific lengths
and phases is delivered with the surface coil. The pulse phases are
cycled between successive FID's in such a way that signals from volumes
which experience near 90° pulses average coherently, whereas signals
from other regions, where the effective pulse length is different from
90°, average destructively. Furthermore, it is possible to adjust the
volume of the coherently averaging region, and methods of reducing the
large signals from regions close to the coil have been established
(22). Recently, Rothman et. al. (26) have pointed out that similar
effects are produced even without phase cycling if the delays between
subsequent pulses are long compared with the T_2^*. The depth pulse
method has only recently been proven to work in phantom samples, and
has yet to be used extensively in studies of living animals (24,25).
Referring to Figure 1, it can be seen that the depth pulse does not
produce perfect localization. The sensitive volume produced by the
depth pulse is depicted as the region between a pair of contour lines
(e.g., the region between the 80° and 100° contours). Clearly these
volumes are not regular geometric shapes, but are complicated curved
surfaces of varying thickness. Despite the irregular shape of the

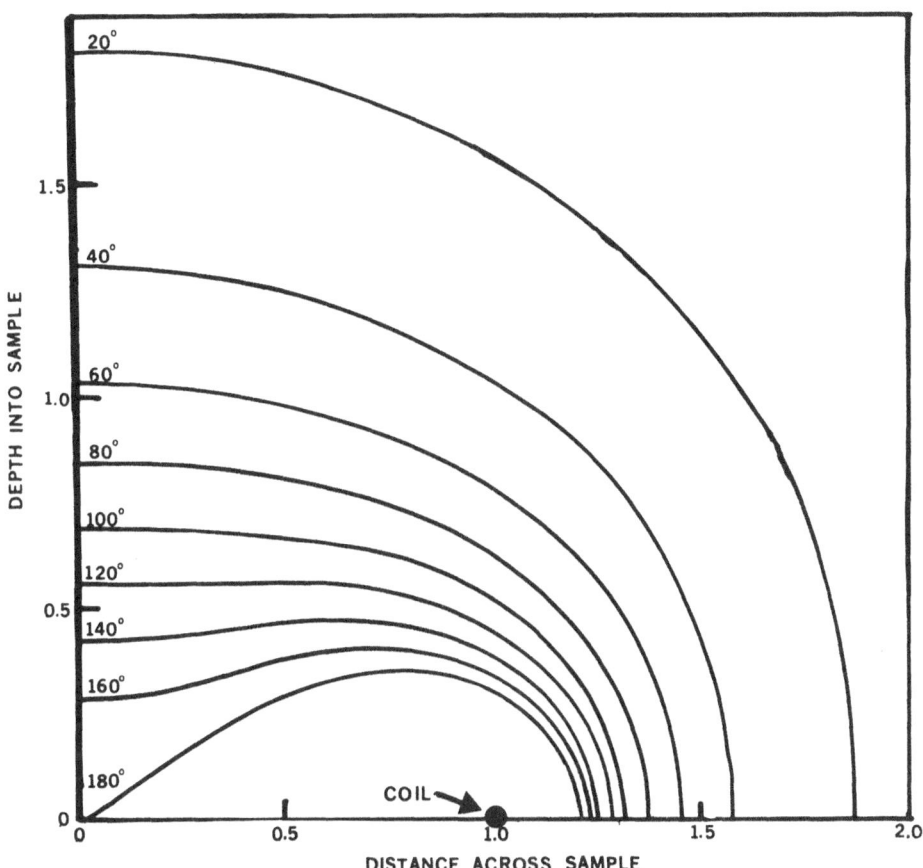

Figure 1. Contour plot of the spatial dependence of the nuclear excitation from a surface coil. The coil is circular with a radius of 1 unit, and a rotation axis congruent with the ordinate of the plot. Thus the coil can be envisioned as curving out of the page toward the reader. Only one quadrant is plotted because the contours are symmetrical about the ordinate. The section shown passes through the coil's center and is perpendicular to the axis of the static magnetic field. The contour lines depict the nutation angles resulting from a single pulse which produces a 180° nutation at the center of the coil. The contours were calculated by using a computer program to numerically integrate Ampere's law in a "brute force" fashion.

localized region, the depth pulse method shows great promise because
the method conserves all the signal from the localized region, and
because it obviates the need for pulsed field gradients.

A further refinement of surface coil localization has recently
been proposed by Haase et. al. (27). In their method, FIDs are
obtained as the exciting pulse length in a pulse-acquire sequence is
varied, and then a 2-dimensional Fourier transform is performed to
produce a plot of intensity against both chemical shift and 90° pulse
width. This provides the ability to determine the location of the
metabolite within the sample because the 90° pulse width is dependent
upon the rf field intensity. Note should be taken of the fact that
this "surface coil imaging" method is very similar to the concept of
Rotating Frame Zeugmatography as proposed by Hoult (28). This method
has not yet been used in a living animal system.

3. TENABLE LOCALIZATION METHODS AND SPECTROSCOPIC LIMITATIONS

Many ways have now been proposed for achieving spatial localization of
NMR signals. The methods which have been proposed to date fall into
two broad categories. Multiple volume methods collect signals
simultaneously from all volumes within the sample (27-33). Gradients
in the static field are commonly used in these methods to spatially
encoded the NMR signals (29-33). Gradients in the rf field have also
been shown to be suitable for this purpose (27,28). Sensitive volume
methods, on the other hand, collect data from a single volume element
at a time (15,20,34-36). Here spatial information is encoded by use of
selective rf pulses and gradients in the static field (34), by use of
shaped static field gradients (15), by use of oscillating gradients in
the static field (35,36), or by use of rf field gradients (23).
Clearly, most of the methods of both types rely on the use of gradients
in the static field. We note that these gradients can not be present
during signal acquisition, as this would prohibit obtaining high
resolution data. Usually there is a preparation period where the
signals are spatially encoded with the help of a gradient, and then the
gradient is turned off to permit acquisition of high resolution data.

Each proposed method has potential advantages as well as
disadvantages and these will ultimately define what methods will be
used for "metabolite imaging." At this time, much of the research
needed to ascertain how well various methods will work in living
systems to detect metabolites present at physiological concentration
has yet to be performed. Some of these techniques have been
successfully used only in phantom systems, and some have been used to
obtain maps of only the very strong ^1H signals from water and fatty
material in living tissues. Others which we have already discussed,
actually have been used in studies of tissue metabolism. As a result
of this paucity of data, the most that can be said is that it seems
unlikely that any single method will be universally useful because of
the differences in spectral width, sensitivity, and relaxation behavior
of the various metabolite signals which have been identified in ^{13}C,

[1]H, or ^{31}P spectra of living tissues. Therefore we will not criticize each prospective method specifically, but instead we will present some criteria based on our _in vivo_ spectroscopic experience which should be considered in the evaluation of prospective methods.

3.1 Spectral resolution and gradients in the static field

In Figure 2 we present a ^{1}H spectrum of rabbit brain taken at 1.9 T, which has the methyl lactate signal elevated as a result of hypoxia (D.L. Rothman and O.A.C. Petroff, unpublished data). This spectrum was obtained using only surface coil localization, after careful shimming of the static field. The linewidths of the water, N-acetylaspartate and lactate signals are all on the order of 7 Hz (prior to exponential processing), yet our spin echo studies show that the natural linewidth is on the order of 2 Hz (K.L. Behar and D.L. Rothman, unpublished observations). Thus 70% of the observed linewidths of these signals is generated by inhomogeniety in the static field. In Figure 3 a 1.9 T ^{31}P spectrum of the rabbit brain is presented (K.L. Behar, O.A.C. Petroff, unpublished data). The phosphocreatine linewidth is 0.2 ppm (without exponential filtering), which is equal in ppm to the linewidth of the ^{1}H water signal measured from an ^{1}H spectrum (data not shown) taken immediately prior to the ^{31}P spectrum. Thus it seems likely that the phosocreatine as well as the water linewidths are mostly the result of inhomogenity in the static field. It appears that in the brain of the living rabbit, the field inhomogeniety over the region sensed by the surface coil (about 10 ml.) is on the order of 0.1-0.2 ppm. In our studies of liver in the intact rabbit, the static field inhomogeniety was about an order of magnitude larger (37). The fact that the inhomogeniety depends on what part of the animal is studied, and the fact that our magnet can be shimmed to better than 0.08 ppm over a 32 ml volume on test samples, suggest that the inhomogeniety is a consequence of the presence of the animal itself. In summary, it appears that the spectral resolution is presently limited by field inhomogeniety, and this is the case even when pulsed field gradients are not being used.

These observations have ramifications for the use of localization methods which encode spatial information with the help of pulsed gradients in the static field. When attempting any such method, it will be extremely important to guarantee that the pulsed gradient relaxes completely before signal acquisition so that the resolution is not further degraded. Further loss of resolution will be particularly difficult to deal with at the low fields likely to be used in human metabolite imaging studies. Inspection of Figure 3, for instance, shows that pH measurement would become more difficult if the resolution was very much poorer because of overlap between the inorganic phosphate signal and those of the phosphodiester and phosphomonoester. It is also worth noting that broadening of the resonances will decrease the signal-to-noise ratio. Because of this stiff requirement for good static field homogeniety, methods which employ only rf gradients seem to enjoy some advantage. Put simply, the arguement is that the

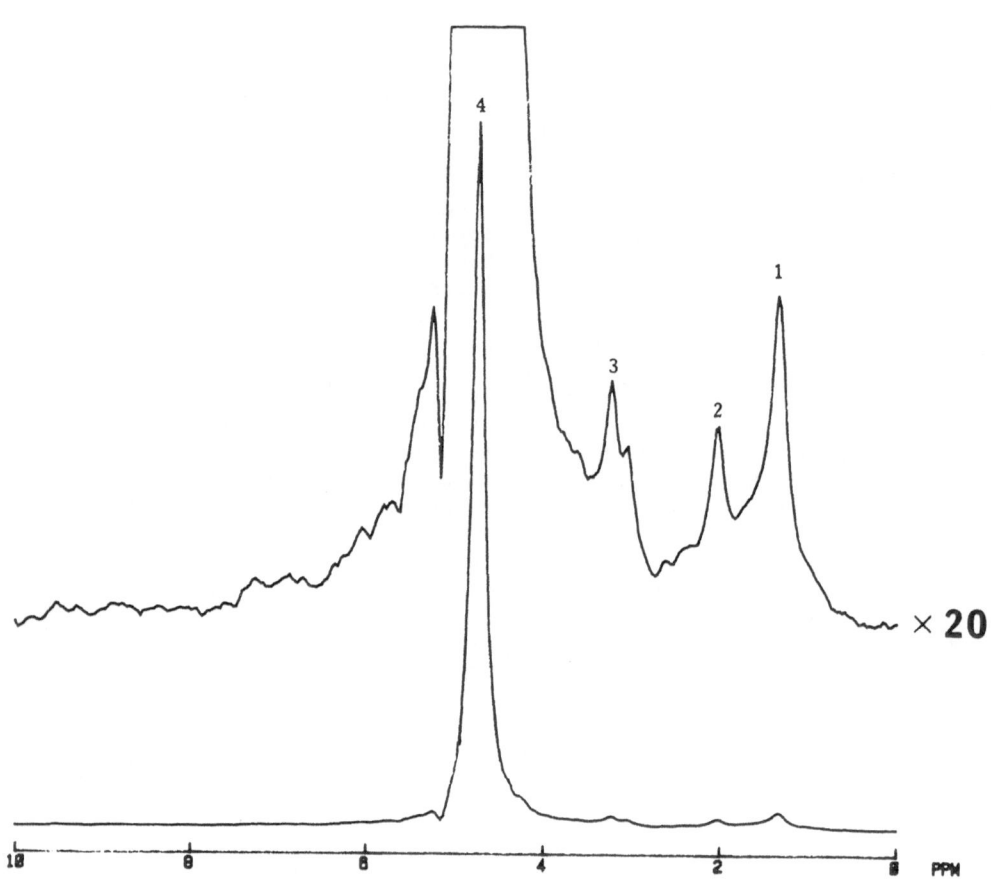

Figure 2. 1.9 T surface coil ¹H spectrum of rabbit brain in vivo. The spectrum was obtained with a 1.7 cm diameter surface coil placed against the brain after surgical removal of scalp and skull. The animal was maintained under nitrous oxide analgesia, with pancuronium bromide/tubocurarine chloride induced paralysis, and was mechanically respirated during the data collection. Assignments: 1: lactate methyl protons; 2: methyl group of N-acetylaspartate; 3: sum of phosphocreatine, creatine and phosphorylcholine; 4: water.

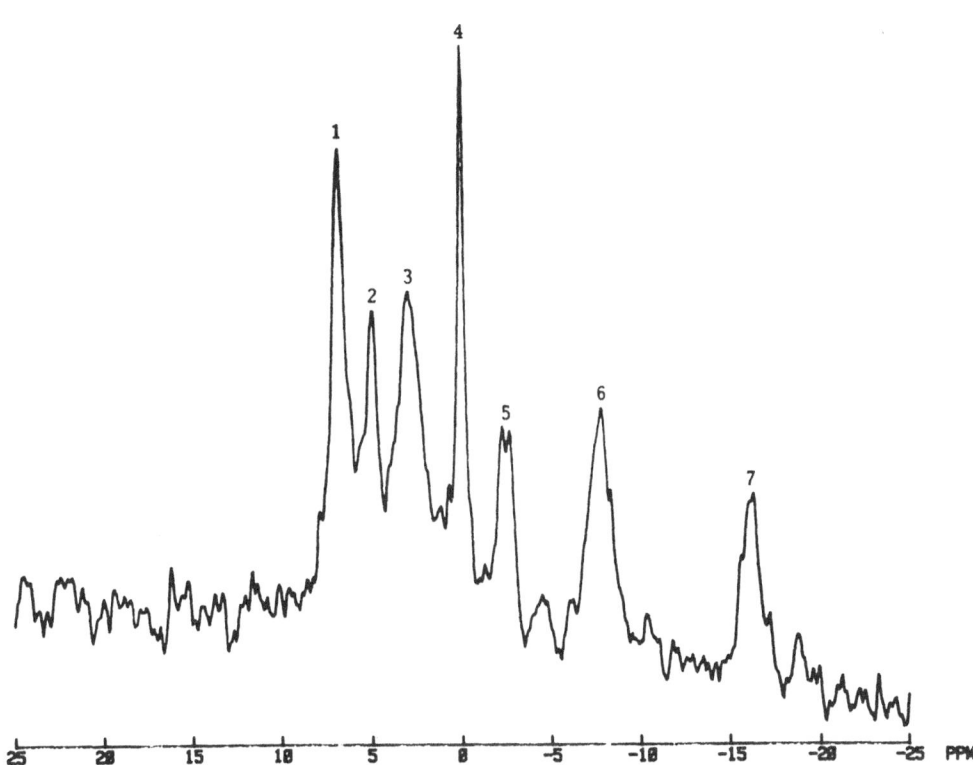

Figure 3. 1.9 T surface coil ³¹P spectrum of the rabbit brain. The animal preparation is described in Figure 2. NMR parameters are as follows: excitation pulse width, 7µs; 256 scans; interpulse delay, 25 sec; total accumulation time, 1.8 hr. Resonance assignments: 1: phosphomonoeslers; 2: inorganic phosphate; 3: phosphodiesters; 4: phosphocreatine; 5: γ–ATP; 6: α–ATP; 7: β–ATP.

spectroscopist devotes a great effort to making the static field homogeneous, so why spoil it?

Another concern with methods which select volumes using pulsed gradients and selective pulses is the problem of disentangling chemical shift and spatial information. Selective pulses are selective on the basis of frequency only, and so they cannot differentiate a chemically-shifted resonance from a gradient-shifted resonance. When ^{31}P and ^{13}C spectroscopy are used, larger gradients will be needed because these nuclei have larger chemical shift dispersions than does the proton. For example, if it is desired to obtain 10 mm spatial resolution, the gradient in the static field must vary over 10 mm by an amount significantly greater than the chemical shift dispersion of the nucleus being studied. For ^{31}P then, the gradient must be much greater than 30 ppm per cm, and for ^{13}C, it must be greater than 200 ppm per cm. At 2 T, these requirements dictate that a gradient much greater than 0.6 gauss per cm is needed for ^{31}P and that a gradient much larger than 4 gauss per cm is needed for ^{13}C.

3.2 The signal-to-noise ratio and spatial resolution

In this section we will discuss the signal-to-noise levels which can be expected in spectra of low concentration metabolites in living tissues, and then point out how the expected levels might affect the spatial resolution in metabolite mapping. The signal-to-noise ratio achieved for a particular resonance from a localized volume will have little dependence on the method used to localize the designated volume, because at a particular field, sensitivity is most strongly defined by the nuclear gyromagnetic ratio, the volume in the selected region, the spin concentration and the rf coil design, and not the method used to isolate the volume. We will not discuss rf coil design, but will simply assume that receiver systems at least as good as presently are used in ^{1}H imaging will be available for spectroscopic work. We wish to focus on the dependence of the signal strength on the nuclear gyromagnetic ratio, the volume of the selected region, and the spin concentration.

It seems unlikely that metabolite concentrations will be mapped with the same spatial resolution which tissue water now is, because of the dramatically lower concentrations of metabolites with respect to water. In metabolite mapping work then, it will be necessary to increase the size of the selected region to attain the same signal-to-noise ratio as is now achieved for the tissue water mapping. For instance, consider the hypothetical experiment designed to map the lactate methyl proton signal. In ischemic tissue the lactate concentration is on the order of 10 mM, so that its proton signal is about 3,000-fold smaller per unit volume than is the tissue water signal. In non-ischemic tissue the lactate level is lower and difficult to detect (2,4). Thus to obtain a lactate signal-to-noise ratio from a volume within the ischemic area similar to that currently achievable in water mapping, the voxel in the lactate mapping experiment must on the order of 3000 times larger. This corresponds to a linear spatial resolution of about 17 (the cube-root of 3000) times larger. Presently the state-of-the-art water imaging linear spatial resolution is about 1 mm, so that our hypothetical lactate mapping study is expected to have a spatial resolution not better than 17 mm. For ^{31}P mapping, the lower gyromagnetic ratio will result in an even lower sensitivity per unit volume and, therefore, an even larger spatial resolution will be required. For the most part, these estimates of spatial resolution are independent of the localization method used. While some methods may be capable of producing better spatial resolution, there will just not be enough signal in a volume smaller than we have estimated, to produce an interpretable spectrum. Although a number of important parameters have not been included, we hope we have given the reader a feeling for the importance of the lower ^{31}P gyromagnetic ratio and the low metabolite concentrations.

4. SUMMARY

While this has only been a brief discussion of a young and complex area of technical development, we hope that it has brought out a few of the aspects of high resolution spectroscopic studies of animals which have substantial importance for the design of metabolite mapping methods. We have discussed how metabolite concentrations, which are low with respect to tissue water, will lead to rather coarse spatial resolution. Consideration of the field homogeneity is also important. In view of the rather low fields that will be used in human NMR studies, excellent static field homogeneity will be required to obtain high quality spectral data, and methods using pulsed field gradients will have to have excellent recovery of the field homogeniety after the pulses.

ACKNOWLEDGEMENT. The author is grateful to M. R. Bendall, K. L. Behar and M. J. Avison for stimulating discussions regarding these subjects. Professor O. A. C. Petroff kindly provided the spectra for Figures 2 and 3. This work was supported by NIH grant GM 30287.

REFERENCES

1) J. W. Prichard, J. R. Alger, K. L. Behar, O. A. C. Petroff and R. G. Shulman, Proc. Natl. Acad. Sci. USA 80, 2748 (1983).

2) K. L. Behar, J. A. den Hollander, M. E. Stromski, T. Ogino, R. G. Shulman, O. A. C. Petroff, and J. W. Prichard, Proc. Natl. Acad. Sci. USA 80, 4945 (1983).

3) O. A. C. Petroff, J. W. Prichard, K. L. Behar, J. R. Alger and R. G. Shulman, Ann. Neurol. 16, 169 (1984).

4) K. L. Behar, D. L. Rothman, R. G. Shulman, O. A. C. Petroff and
    J. W. Prichard, Proc. Natl. Acad. Sci. USA 81, 2517 (1984).

5) M. E. Stromski, F. Arias-Mendoza, J. R. Alger and R. G. Shulman,
    (manuscript in preparation).

6) K. J. Neurohr, E. J. Barrett and R. G. Shulman, Proc. Natl. Acad.
    Sci. USA 80, 1603 (1983).

7) K. J. Neurohr, G. Gollin, E. J. Barrett and R. G. Shulman, FEBS
    Lett. 159, 207 (1983).

8) K. J. Neurohr and R. G. Shulman, to be printed in "Advances in
    Myocardiology" (R. Dhalla, ed.), Plenum Publ. Co.

9) N. J. Siegel, M. J. Avison, H. F. Reilly, J. R. Alger and R. G.
    Shulman, Am. J. Physiol. 245, F530 (1983).

10) A. N. Stevens, R. A. Iles, P. G. Morris and J. R. Griffiths, FEBS
    Lett. 150, 489 (1982).

11) N. V. Reo, C. S. Ewy, B. A. Siegfried and J. J. H. Ackerman, J.
    Magn. Reson. 58, 76 (1984).

12) H. L. Kantor, R. S. Balaban and R. W. Briggs, J. Magn. Reson. in
    Med. 1, 183 (1984).

13) A. P. Koretsky, S. Wang, J. Murphy-Boesch, M. P. Klein, T. L. James
    and M. W. Weiner, Proc. Natl. Acad. Sci. USA 80, 7491 (1983).

14) R. B. Rehr, R. M. Peshock, J. A. Jackson, L. M. Buja, J. T.
    Willerson, P. W. Parkey, J. E. Dowdey and R. L. Nunnally, J.
    Magn. Reson. in Med. 1, 235 (1984).

15) R. E. Gordon, P. E. Hanley, D. Shaw, D. G. Gadian, G. K. Radda,
    P. Styles, P. J. Bore and L. Chan, Nature 287, 367 (1980).

16) R. S. Balaban, D. G. Gadian and G. K. Radda, Kidney Int. 20, 575
    (1980).

17) P. Canioni, J. R. Alger and R. G. Shulman, Biochemistry 22, 4974 (1983).

18) R. E. Gordon, P. E. Hanley and D. Shaw, Prog. NMR Spectros. 15, 1 (1982).

19) A. A. Maudsley, S. K. Hilal, H. E. Simon and S. Wittekoek, J. Magn. Reson. in Med. 1, 202 (1984).

20) J. J. H. Ackerman, T. H. Grove, G. C. Wong, D. G. Gadian and G. K. Radda, Nature 283, 167 (1980).

21) J. L. Evelhoch, M. G. Crowley and J. J. H. Ackerman, J. Magn. Reson. 56, 110 (1984).

22) M. R. Bendall, J. Magn. Reson. 59 (in press).

23) M. R. Bendall and R. E. Gordon, J. Magn. Reson. 53, 365 (1983).

24) M. R. Bendall, Chem. Phys. Lett. 99, 310 (1983).

25) M. R. Bendall and W. P. Aue, J. Magn. Reson. 54, 149 (1983).

26) D. L. Rothman, K. L. Behar, J. A. den Hollander and R. G. Shulman, J. Magn. Reson. 59, 157 (1984).

27) A. Haase, C. Malloy and G. K. Radda, J. Magn. Reson. 55, 164 (1983).

28) D. I. Hoult, J. Magn. Reson. 33, 183 (1979).

29) T. R. Brown, B. M. Kincaid and K. Ugurbil, Proc. Natl. Acad. Sci. USA 79, 3523 (1982).

30) A. A. Maudsley, S. K. Hilal, W. H. Perman and H. E. Simon, J. Magn. Reson. 51, 147 (1983).

31) L. D. Hall and S. Sukumar, J. Magn. Reson. 50, 162 (1983).

32) P. Bendel, C-M. Lai and P. C. Lauterbur. J. Magn. Reson. 38, 343 (1980).

33) J. C. Haselgrove, J. C. Subramanian, V. Harihara, J. S. Leigh Jr., L. Gyuli and B. Chance, Science 220, 1170 (1983).

34) W. P. Aue, S. Mueller, T. A. Cross and J. Seelig, J. Magn. Reson. 56, 330 (1984).

35) P. A. Bottomley, J. Magn. Reson. 50, 335 (1982).

36) K. N. Scott, H. R. Brooker, J. R. Fitzsimmons, H. F. Bennett and R. G. Mick, J. Magn. Reson. 50, 339 (1982).

37) J. R. Alger, K. L. Behar, D. L. Rothman and R. G. Shulman, J. Magn. Reson. 56, 334 (1984).

NMR METHODS FOR MEASURING CATION CONCENTRATIONS IN BIOLOGICAL SYSTEMS

J. Feeney
Physical Biochemistry Division
National Institute for Medical Research
Mill Hill, London NW7 1AA
U.K.

ABSTRACT. A brief review is presented of the various NMR methods available for measuring intracellular pH by monitoring pH-sensitive chemical shifts of nuclei in metabolites naturally occurring in cells. The use of fluorine containing chelator molecules for measuring intracellular cation concentrations is also considered with particular reference to the measurement of free intracellular $[Ca^{2+}]$.

1. INTRODUCTION

There is considerable interest in developing methods for measuring the concentrations of free intracellular cations (such as $[H^+]$ and $[Ca^{2+}]$) since such information is crucial for understanding many biological processes within cells. For example, intracellular pH is known to play an important role in the regulation of cellular metabolism and proliferation (1). Similarly intracellular free Ca^{2+} is an important regulatory ion and can act as a second messenger for external stimuli (2). The role of Ca^{2+} in mitogenic stimulation of lymphocytes is just one of several important areas of study in which specific cations have been implicated in biological processes (3).

Several non-destructive methods have been developed for making such measurements and these include (i) introducing pH- or metal ion-sensitive microelectrodes into cells and making direct measurements (ii) studying the distribution of weak acids or bases (iii) introducing various probe molecules (dyes, proteins, chelators) into cells and using colorimetric or fluorometric techniques to monitor changes in absorption, luminescence or fluorescence which accompany cation binding (2,4). However, none of these methods can claim to be truly non-invasive. It was therefore not surprising that a great deal of excitement was generated when the early NMR experiments of Moon and Richards (5) and the subsequent detailed investigations of other workers (Radda ; Hoult (27); Gadian; Wilkie; Shulman, Navone) showed that ^{31}P chemical shift measurements on endogenous metabolites in cells could provide a reliable basis for such non-invasive measurements. More recently, additional NMR methods have been developed which are based on introducing suitable

279

T. Axenrod and G. Ceccarelli (eds.), NMR in Living Systems, 279–289.
© *1986 by D. Reidel Publishing Company.*

chelating probe molecules into cells (6,7,8) and then measuring changes
in their chemical shifts when they bind to metal ions: these promise
to have enormous potential for the measurement of selective cation concentrations. Although the latter methods offer considerable improvements in selectivity over other techniques they do share the problems
associated with probe molecules (such as the need to investigate
potential perturbations caused by the probe and the need to establish
the distribution of the probe molecules in the cells and tissues
examined).

2. INTRACELLULAR pH MEASUREMENTS

2.1 Use of Phosphate ^{31}P Chemical Shifts

The ^{31}P assignments for the metabolites detected in studies of cells
and tissues have been well-documented (see Gadian (9)) and these are
given on the ^{31}P spectrum from a beating ferret heart shown in Figure
1 (10).

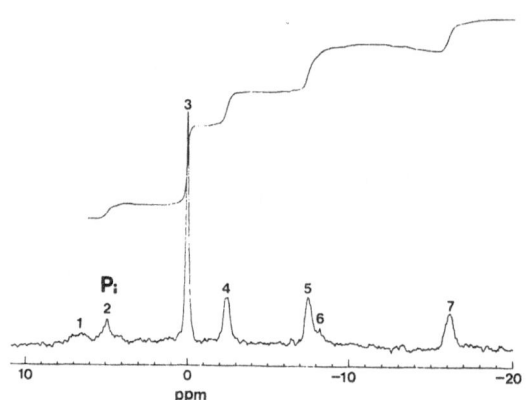

Figure 1. The ^{31}P NMR spectrum (80 MHz) of a beating ferret heart.
Assignments: 1. Sugar phosphate; 2. Inorganic phosphate, P_i;
3. Phosphocreatine; 4,5,7. γ-, α- and β- phosphates of ATP respectively; 6. NAD pyrophosphate. (P.G. Morris, private communication).

    The chemical shift of the inorganic phosphate (P_i) signal is
sensitive to pH in the physiological pH range and thus provides an
internal pH meter within the cell. The equilibrium responsible for
this variation in ^{31}P chemical shift is

$$H_2PO_4^- \; \rightleftharpoons \; H^+ + HPO_4^{2-} \quad (pK \sim 7)$$

These two phosphate anions have different ^{31}P chemical shifts (separated by ~ 2.4 ppm) and they are in fast exchange on the NMR time scale.

This results in a single ^{31}P signal being observed for the two exchanging species and its chemical shift is an average of the shifts in the two forms weighted according to their fractional populations (x and (1 - x))

$$\text{Observed shift} = \Delta = x\delta_{H_2PO_4^-} + (1 - x)\delta_{HPO_4^{2-}}$$

Thus a plot of the ^{31}P chemical shift as a function of pH gives the titration curve shown in Figure 2. Such a curve can be used to obtain the pH within a cell if the ^{31}P chemical shift of its P_i signal can be measured. Various factors influence the accuracy of such measurements and these have been discussed by Gadian (9).

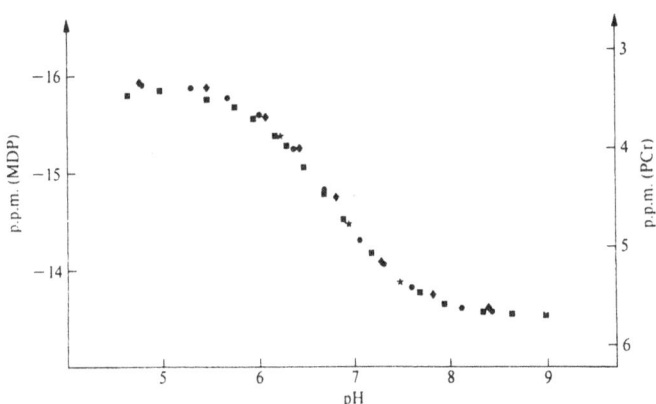

Figure 2. The titration curve of the ^{31}P chemical shift of inorganic phosphate (10 mM) as a function of pH at various ionic strengths. Chemical shifts referred to methylene diphosphonate (MDP) or phosphocreatine. PCr. key: ◆ 120 mM KCl, ■ 160 mM KCl, ● 200 mM KCl, ✱ 160 mM NaCl (As adapted by Gadian (9) from data of Garlick, Radda and Seeley (11)).

(i) *Measurement of chemical shifts*
The positions of the ^{31}P signals can usually be measured to better than ± 0.02 ppm and such errors would contribute negligible errors to the pH measurements (± 0.01 pH unit). However the actual chemical shifts measured from a reference compound can have substantial errors if the referencing is not done carefully. The best reference to use is an internal one such as the phosphocreatine ^{31}P signal or the ^{1}H signal from water or from a suitable proton containing metabolite. It is also important to use the same reference procedure in the pH determination as was used in obtaining the pH calibration curves. Errors from these

sources can be large if care is not taken.

(ii) *Effects of ionic strength and temperature*
The pH titration curves depend on the ionic strength and temperature of the solution and it is important to measure the calibration curve under ionic strength conditions similar to those found in cells and at the same temperature. Although it is difficult to match the ionic strength conditions perfectly the work of Garlick and co-workers (11) indicates that uncertainties about the exact ionic strength are probably not important (see titration curves in Figure 2).

(iii) *Effects of chemical shift contributions from bound phosphate*
One cannot eliminate the possibility that some of the ^{31}P chemical shift contribution arises from inorganic phosphate bound to molecules in the cell in fast exchange with free phosphate ions. It is difficult to estimate directly the errors in pH measurement from these effects. However in cases where the pH has been measured independently on the same system using NMR and other methods or where two different NMR pH probes have been used simultaneously there is good agreement between the pH values. For example Nicolay and co-workers (12) found quantitative agreement between transmembrane ΔpH values in *Rhodopseudomonas sphaeroides* measured using ^{31}P NMR and a flow dialysis 'distribution' method, Gillies and co-workers found identical agreement between intracellular pH values in Ehrlich ascites tumour cells measured using either inorganic phosphate or intracellular 2-deoxyglucose-6-phosphate (introduced into the cells by suspending them in 2-deoxyglucose which is taken up and phosphorylated by a cellular hexokinase (13)). The results of Hollis (14) who found similar pH titration curves for phosphate examined in aqueous solutions and in homogenised dog heart preparations are also encouraging in this regard. Because of the problems mentioned above there will be appreciable errors in the absolute accuracy of the pH measurements. These are difficult to estimate but they are probably about ± 0.1 pH unit if the calibration curve and the chemical shift measurements are made carefully, while the measurement of changes in pH can probably be made to ± 0.05 pH units (see Gadian (9)).

There are some advantages of an analytical method which depends on measuring chemical shifts under fast exchange conditions rather than signal intensities of species in slow exchange. Chemical shift changes can usually be measured more accurately than intensity changes and do not require spectra with high signal to noise ratios, a factor which contributes to the time resolution of the method. The fast exchange situation also allows us to study compartmentation since the ^{31}P signals from phosphate in two different non-exchanging compartments will have different chemical shifts reflecting the different pH values in the two compartments. Two ^{31}P signals are often seen for intra- and extracellular phosphate and an example is shown in the ^{31}P spectrum of succinate-grown *E. coli* cells (15). In favourable cases phosphate signals from different intracellular compartments such as mitochondria and cytoplasm have been observed (16). Such compartmentation measurements could not be made directly if the two ionised forms ($H_2PO_4^-$ and

HPO_4^{2-}) were in slow exchange since the different compartments would give signals of different intensities for these forms but located at the same frequencies.

2.2 Other Metabolites used for Measuring Intracellular pH

The NMR spectra of several other endogenous metabolites have been used to measure intracellular pH. Brown and co-workers [17] have measured the proton chemical shifts of the histidine imidazole C2 protons of haemoglobin in red blood cells for this purpose. Anserine [18] and carnosine [19] are histidyl containing metabolites whose imidazole ring protons can be detected in the ^{1}H spectra of tissues and these can similarly be used for intracellular pH measurements. Anserine was found in chicken pectoralis muscle [18] and carnosine was found in brain slices [19]. Legerton and co-workers [20] have introduced various ^{15}N labelled amino acids into *Neurospora* where they accumulate as pools of free amino acids in the cells. The distribution of the amino acids in the various pools is known (alanine, for example, is mainly in the cytoplasm while arginine locates in the vacuole) and thus they were able to measure cytoplasmic and vacuolar pH by monitoring the ^{15}N shifts of alanine, arginine, histidine and proline in the cells.

Several methods of measuring intracellular pH based on incorporating probe molecules into cells have been proposed. The most elegant are those which use the Tsien method [21] of loading polar molecules into cells (see next section). For example intracellular pH in human peripheral blood lymphocytes has been measured by Deutsch and co-workers [16] by monitoring the ^{19}F chemical shift of D,L-2-amino-3-3-difluoro-2 -methylpropanoic acid trapped within the cells and the accuracy of this approach has been checked using equilibrium distribution methods involving 5,5-dimethyloxazolidine-2,4-dione. Metcalfe and co-workers [8] have also loaded cells with ^{19}F containing chelators in order to measure intracellular cation concentrations such as $[H^+]$, $[Ca^{2+}]$ and $[Zn^{2+}]$ and these experiments are described in the following section.

3. DETERMINATION OF INTRACELLULAR FREE METAL ION CONCENTRATIONS

The ^{31}P chemical shifts of ATP [22,23] and phosphocreatine [24] are dependent on the extent of metal ion binding. Only Mg^{2+} ions are at sufficiently high concentrations to give these effects and the bound and free species are in fast exchange on the NMR time scale. Because of uncertainties in the ^{31}P chemical shift contributions arising from other interactions involving these molecules it is difficult to quantitate the data. The measurements indicate that more than 90% of the ATP is usually bound to Mg^{2+}: Gupta and Moore [23] estimated that 93% of muscle ATP is complexed to Mg^{2+} which corresponds to an intracellular $[Mg^{2+}]$ of 0.6 mM.

There is a good deal of interest in developing methods which can measure cation concentrations more selectively and which can be used for cations at fairly low intracellular concentrations (such as Ca^{2+} and

Zn2+). Metcalfe and co-workers (8) have devised such a method which involves the use of fluorine containing molecules related to analogues of 1,1-bis(o-aminophenoxy)ethane-N,N,N',N'-tetraacetic acid (BAPTA) (see Scheme I). This chelator, which binds much more tightly to Ca^{2+}

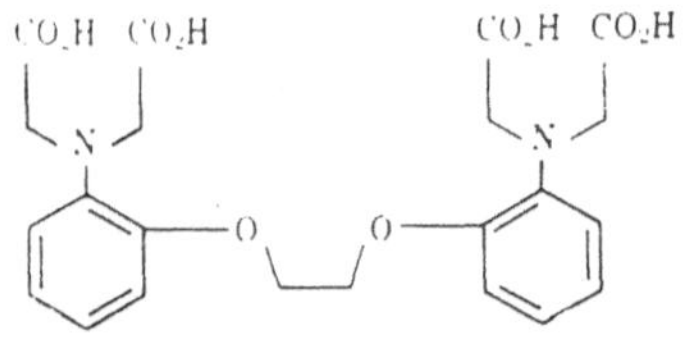

BAPTA

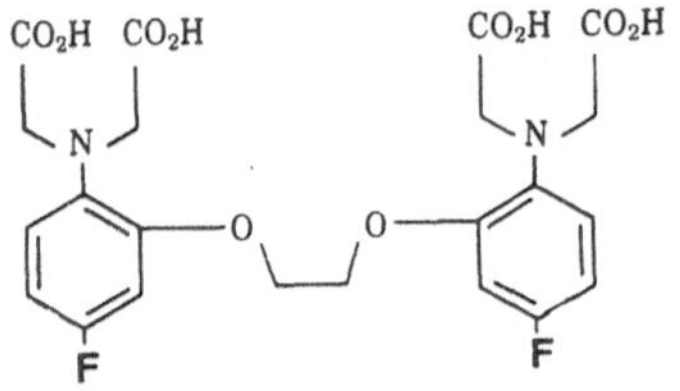

5F BAPTA

Scheme I

than to Mg^{2+} and H^+, had been designed by Tsien (21) as a fluorescence indicator for measuring intracellular calcium concentrations.

3.1 Tsien's Method for Measuring Intracellular Ca^{2+} Concentrations
Tsien and his co-workers have written an elegant series of papers (21, 25,26) describing how to load BAPTA and related indicators into various cells and explaining how to obtain intracellular Ca^{2+} concentrations from the fluorescence measurements. The indicators were loaded by incubating cells in the presence of the tetraacetoxymethyl ester of BAPTA. The ester on entering the cells is hydrolysed to the acid by endogenous esterases in the cell and the released BAPTA, being polar, is then trapped within the cell. Using this method it was possible to load BAPTA to concentrations in excess of 1 mM in the cells. Tsien and co-workers have shown (25) that the BAPTA enters the cytoplasm and that the BAPTA does not change the concentration of intracellular free Ca^{2+} cations. The Ca^{2+} ions which bind to the BAPTA enter the cell from the outside medium. The binding constant of BAPTA to Ca^{2+} is

known and thus if we have a spectroscopic method of determining the
intracellular concentrations of BAPTA and its Ca^{2+} bound form then we
can obtain the free intracellular Ca^{2+} concentration. Tsien and co-
workers have applied this fluorescence technique to a series of systems.
More recently other workers (3) have pointed out some of the practical
limitations of this approach. One of the problems is that the method
is non-selective and this can have serious consequences when operating
at low BAPTA concentrations (< 0.5 mM) where binding of the small
amounts of tightly binding cations such as Mn^{2+} can interfere with the
intracellular Ca^{2+} measurement. The NMR method using fluorine
labelled BAPTA analogues can overcome this particular problem (7,8).

3.2 NMR Method for Measuring Intracellular Free $[Ca^{2+}]$ using Fluoro
BAPTA Analogues

Metcalfe and co-workers (7,8) have examined the ^{19}F NMR spectra of
various fluoro analogues of BAPTA in the presence of a wide range of
cations. The 5F-analogue (see Scheme I) proved to have ideal properties
for use as an NMR probe in the measurement of intracellular cation
concentrations.

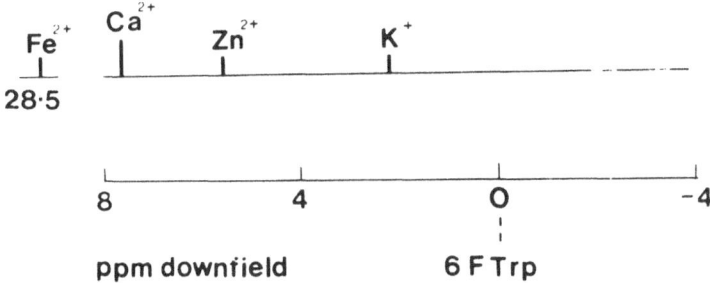

Figure 3. The ^{19}F chemical shifts of 5F-BAPTA saturated with Ca^{2+},
Zn^{2+} and Fe^{2+} measured relative to 6-fluorotryptophan external reference (Smith, Hesketh, Metcalfe, Feeney and Morris (8)).

Figure 3 summarises the ^{19}F chemical shifts of 5F-BAPTA (relative to
6-fluorotryptophan) for the complexes with the high affinity cations
Ca^{2+}, Zn^{2+} and Fe^{2+} obtained by using saturating concentrations of the
cations. Large characteristic ^{19}F chemical shifts are observed for
each of the complexes and because the signals are in slow exchange
(between the BAPTA M^{2+} complex and that in the KCl/Hepes buffer) they
provide direct information about the ionic species chelated and form
the basis of a method for selective detection of different cations
within the cell (see Figure 4). An advantage of using a ^{19}F probe is
that there are no problems relating to background signals.
      These chelators have now been used successfully in several systems
to estimate free intracellular $[Ca^{2+}]$. Figure 5 shows the ^{19}F spectrum
of 5F-BAPTA (1 mM) loaded into mouse thymocytes (10^8 cells ml^{-1}): the
signals for Ca^{2+} bound 5F-BAPTA can be resolved clearly and their
relative intensities give the ratio of bound to free species directly.

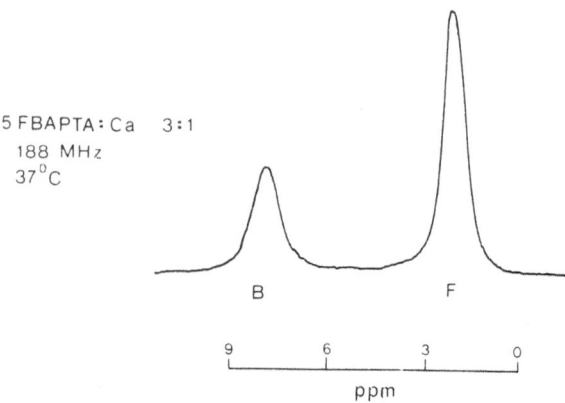

Figure 4. The ^{19}F signals at 188 MHz from 5F-BAPTA in its free and Ca^{2+} complexed forms (Smith, Hesketh, Metcalfe, Feeney and Morris (8))

Since the binding constant for Ca^{2+} is known

$$K_{Ca} = \frac{[Ca\ 5F\text{-}BAPTA]}{[Ca^{2+}][5F\text{-}BAPTA]} = 10^{6.15}$$

then [Ca^{2+}] can be estimated once the ratio of bound to free 5F-BAPTA has been measured from the NMR spectrum. The intracellular free [Ca^{2+}] in the thymocytes was 250 nM (previously estimated at 150 nM using the fluorescence technique) and this value was increased to 350 nM by the addition of mitogenic concentrations of succinylated concanavalin A. When the Ca^{2+} ionophore A23187 was added the chelator was saturated with Ca^{2+} from the external medium. The intracellular free [Ca^{2+}] measurements are unaffected by free [Mg^{2+}] < 10 mM, by pH 6-8 and by contaminating divalent ions of high affinity (Zn^{2+}, Fe^{2+}, Mn^{2+}).

An improved probe and sample cell has been designed to increase sensitivity and allow long term experiments (over several hours if necessary). The increased sensitivity results from using a horizontal solenoid for the receiver coil (in a superconducting magnet with B$_0$ in the vertical direction) and the cells are maintained in a viable state for long periods by continuously supplying dialysate via hollow fibres immersed in the agitated cell suspension. This flow technique will also remove any free 5F-BAPTA which leaks from the cells (8). Using this method we can obtain ^{19}F spectra with adequate signal to noise ratio in about 2 mins (1 mM BAPTA in 10^8 cells ml^{-1} suspensions) and there is scope for increasing the sensitivity even further which would lead to an improvement in the time resolution of the method.

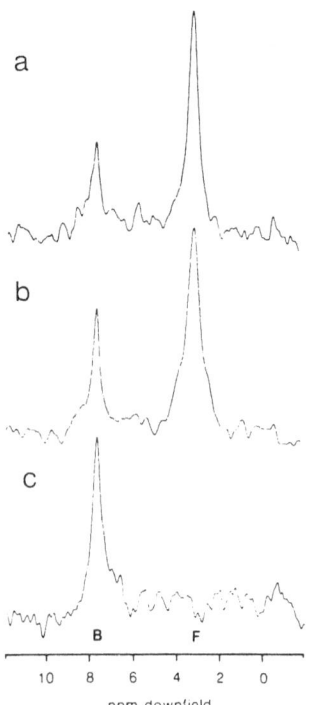

Figure 5. The ^{19}F spectra at 188 MHz of 5F-BAPTA (a) Incorporated into mouse thymocytes (b) After addition of mitogenic concentrations (100 μm/ml of succinylated concanavalin A (c) After addition of A23187, a Ca^{2+} ionophore. (Smith, Hesketh, Metcalfe, Feeney and Morris (8)).

Using this probe Metcalfe and co-workers (8) have examined rat basophil leukaemic cells (2H3 cells) primed with IgE and measured the changes in intracellular free $[Ca^{2+}]$ which result from challenging the cells with ovalbumin: in this system the changes take place over periods of a few minutes and can easily be measured.
    No doubt these chelators have considerable Ca^{2+} buffering capacity and this could impede their usefulness for measuring very rapid changes in $[Ca^{2+}]$ in other systems: the potential of these indicators for measuring Ca^{2+} fluxes is currently being explored.
    Preliminary measurements have indicated the feasibility of extending these measurements to other cations (such as Zn^{2+}) and to other cells and tissues including whole organs (8). Suitable chelators

for binding selectively to H^+ have also been prepared , and efforts to produce selective chelators for Mg^{2+} and Na^{2+} are under way (8). It should be mentioned that as with any other probe technique it is important to carry out experiments at different concentrations of the chelators to ensure that they are not perturbing the system (for example BAPTA does have some mitogenic effects on lymphocytes).

In summary the NMR method can give a selective determination of free intracellular cation concentrations with direct identification of the ionic species chelated. It has the further advantage over the fluorescence method that (i) the estimate of the free/bound BAPTA ratio can be made without requiring lysis of the cells (ii) contaminating ions such as Mn^{2+} are non-interfering (iii) the method has potential application in opaque cell suspensions (8).

REFERENCES

1. R.J. Gillies, 'Intracellular pH and growth control in eukaryotic cells in the transformed cell'. Academic Press, N.Y. (1981) 347. Editors: I.L. Cameron and T.B. Pool
2. C.C. Ashley and A.K. Campbell, Editors. 'Detection and measurement of free calcium ions in cells' (1979). Elsevier, Amsterdam
3(a) J.C. Metcalfe, T. Pozzan, G.A. Smith and T.R. Hesketh. (1980) Biochem. Soc. Symposium 45, 1.
  (b) T.R. Hesketh, G.A. Smith, J.P. Moore, M.V. Taylor and J.C. Metcalfe (1983) J. Biol. Chem. 258, 4876.
4. R.D. Cohen and R.A. Iles (1975) Crit. Rev. Clin. Lab. Sci. 6, 101
5. B.B. Moon and J.H. Richards (1973) J. Biol. Chem. 240, 7276.
6. C. Deutsch, J.S. Taylor and D.F. Wilson (1982) Proc. Nat. Acad. Sci. U.S.A. 79, 7944.
7. G.A. Smith, R.T. Hesketh, J.C. Metcalfe, J. Feeney and P.G. Morris (1983) Proc. Nat. Acad. Sci. U.S.A. 80, 7178.
8. J.C. Metcalfe, G.A. Smith, T.R. Hesketh, P.G. Morris and J. Feeney Unpublished results.
9. D.G. Gadian (1982) 'NMR and its Application to Living Systems' Clarendon Press, Oxford
10. P.G. Morris. Unpublished results.
11. P.B. Garlick, G.K. Radda and P.J. Seeley (1979) Biochem. J. 184, 547.
12. K. Nicolay, J. Lolkema, K.J. Hellingwerf, R. Kaptein and W.N. Konings. (1981) FEBS Letters, 123, 319.
13. R.J. Gillies, T. Ogino, R.G. Shulman and D.C. Ward (1982) J. Cell. Biol. 95, 24.
14. D.P. Hollis (1979) Bull. Mag. Reson. 1, 27.
15. K. Urgurbil, R.G. Shulman and T.R. Brown in 'Biological Applications of Magnetic Resonance' Academic Press (1979), 537. Editor R.G. Shulman.
16. P.B. Garlick. Private communication.
17. F.F. Brown, I.D. Campbell, P.W. Kuchel and D.C. Rabenstein (1977) FEBS Letters, 82, 12.

18. C. Arus, M. Barany, W.M. Westler and J.L. Markley (1984) J. Mag. Reson. 57, 519.
19. H.S. Bachelard, D.W. Cox, P.G. Morris and J. Feeney. Unpublished results.
20. T.L. Legerton, K. Kanamori, R.L. Weiss and J.D. Roberts (1983) Biochemistry, 22, 899.
21. R.Y. Tsien (1980) Biochemistry, 19, 2396.
22. M. Cohn and T.R. Hughes (1962) J. Biol. Chem. 237, 176.
23. R.J. Gupta and R.D. Moore (1980) J. Biol. Chem. 255, 3987.
24. S.M. Cohen and C.T. Burt (1977) Proc. Nat. Acad. Sci. U.S.A. 74, 4271.
25. R.Y. Tsien, T. Pozzan and T.J. Rink. (1982) J. Cell Biol. 94, 325.
26. R.Y. Tsien, T. Pozzan and T.J. Rink (1982) Nature, 295, 68.
27. D.I. Hoult, S.J.W. Busby, D.G. Gadian, G.K. Radda, R.E. Richards and P.J. Seeley (1974) Nature, 252, 285.

NMR SPECTROSCOPY OF INTRACELLULAR SODIUM IONS IN LIVING CELLS

Raj K. Gupta
Department of Physiology and Biophysics
Albert Einstein College of Medicine of Yeshiva University
New York, New York 10461
U.S.A.

ABSTRACT. Na-23 NMR, in combination with extracellularly localized paramagnetic shift reagent dysprosium bis(tripolyphosphate), has emerged as a
convenient and rapid method for studying intracellular sodium ions without
contamination from extracellular ions. The unusually large paramagneic
hyperfine shifts in the frequency of the Na-23 resonance caused by this
reagent are ascribed to its highly anionic nature as well as its ability
to bind sodium ions in close proximity of the paramagnetic dysprosium. A
sizeable pool of intracellular sodium ions may be NMR-invisible due to
broadening of its resonance via nuclear quadrupolar interactions. Such
interactions do not, in all cases, cause a 60% reduction in the intensity
of the observed Na-23 signal due to broadening only of transitions involving the outer magnetic energy levels of the sodium nucleus. NMR-visible
cell sodium responds to changes in tissue physiological state. Thus, insulin deficiency causes a decrease in the NMR-visible sodium in isolated
cardiac myocytes, and blood lymphocytes in chronic lymphocytic leukemia
contain only half the normal level of NMR-visible sodium ions. Changes in
the NMR-visible sodium concentration may sometimes occur without a corresponding change in the total cell sodium content. NMR may, therefore, be a
unique noninvasive technique in studies of the role of sodium ions in cell
regulation.

INTRODUCTION

Intracellular Na^+ ions and their electrochemical gradients across the
plasma membrane appear to play an important role in a variety of cellular
activities, such as nerve transmission and generation of action potentials.
The concentration of Na^+ ions is different in different types of tissues
and responds to changes in physiological state. Intracellular Na^+ ion
imbalance has been associated with cancer, hypertension and diabetic states
as well as with sickle cell disease (1-6). Na^+ ion concentrations appear
related to the cell proliferation state and have been implicated in the
mechanisms of mitogenic as well as oncogenic phenomena (1). The association between Na^+ ions and hypertension is well recognized and it has been
postulated that an increase in intracellular Na^+ of arteriolar smooth
muscle may be the primary cellular defect in hypertension (4). It has long

291

T. Axenrod and G. Ceccarelli (eds.), NMR in Living Systems, 291–308.

been known that, in contrast to normal erythrocytes, sickle red blood
cells gain intracellular Na^+ in the deoxygenated state (6). A recent
suggestion also implicates an alteration in intracellular Na^+ in the
diabetic state (5). Noninvasive NMR studies of intracellular Na^+ are
therefore of direct physiological significance.

The magnetic properties of the Na-23 nucleus are equally attractive,
with a natural abundance of 100% and a resonance frequency close to that
of C-13. While the sensitivity of the Na-23 nucleus in a single pulse NMR
experiment is an order of magnitude lower than that of protons, its relaxation times are about two orders of magnitude shorter than those of protons
in a similar environment. Therefore, in time-averaging experiments, the
Na-23 NMR signal acquired per unit time is comparable to that generated
from a similar population of protons.

NMR OBSERVATION OF INTRACELLULAR SODIUM IONS

Measurement of intracellular Na^+ concentration is generally hampered
by the large magnitude of the Na^+ concentration difference across the
plasma membrane. A small contamination by occluded extracellular fluid containing a high Na^+ concentration significantly distorts the measurement of
the intracellular Na^+ levels by techniques which are not specific to the
intracellular compartments, such as flame photometry and atomic absorption
spectroscopy. To avoid calculated correction factors or extensive washing
to remove extracellular Na-23 a noninvasive direct measurement of intracellular Na^+ concentration is most advantageous. NMR spectroscopy offers
such a noninvasive technique.

Early Na-23 NMR studies of intact cells and tissues were carried out
in a number of laboratories (7-12). However, two reservations precluded
the use of Na-23 signal as a quantitative measure of intracellular Na^+.
First, the exact volume of cells in the NMR-window, from which the observed
signal was originating, was difficult to estimate with reasonable accuracy.
Second, a sizeable contamination of the Na-23 signal by extracellular ions
was unavoidable. The interesting Na-23 resonance of intracellular ions was
masked by the uninteresting but much larger resonance of extracellular
ions. Until recently, this lack of spectral discrimination between intra-
and extracellular Na-23 resonances precluded the use of NMR in the study
of intracellular Na^+ ions. Our recent discovery of a highly anionic paramagnetic shift reagent dysprosium bis(tripolyphosphate) $Dy(PPP_i)_2^{7-}$
effectively circumvents this problem (13) and for the first time allows
direct observation of separate Na-23 resonances from intra and extracellular Na^+ in living cells (figure 1). This permits a study of the intracellular Na^+ without interference from the extracellular ions and paves
the way for future NMR studies of monovalent cations in cells, tissues and
organisms (14). The detection of separate resonances from intra- and
extracellular Na^+ exploits the fact that the anionic paramagnetic reagent
causes a hyperfine shift in the frequency of the resonance of Na^+ accessible to it. The reagent, because of its highly anionic character, does
not enter intact cells over the time scale of NMR measurements, and remains
localized only in the extracellular compartments so that the NMR absorption of extracellular Na^+ is shifted away from the resonance of intracellular Na^+. Because the technique is noninvasive, consecutive steps in a

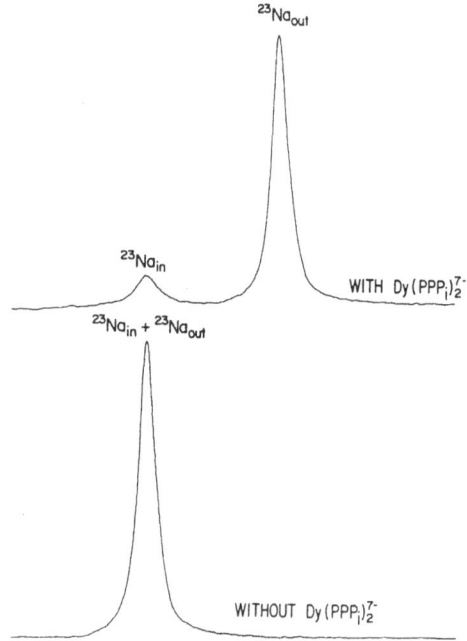

Figure 1. Na-23 NMR spectra of red cells in heparinized whole human blood with (top) and without (bottom) 3 mM Dy(PPP$_i$)$_2$ showing spectral separation of extra- and intracellular Na$^+$ ions by the paramagnetic shift reagent.

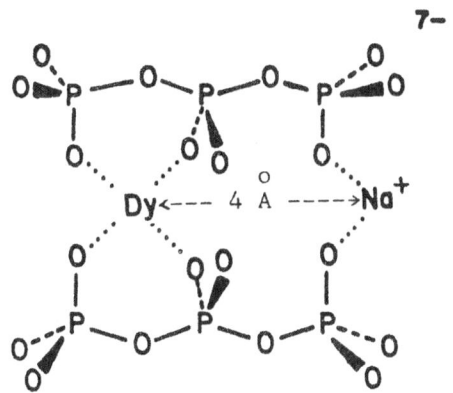

Figure 2. A possible structure of the complex of the anionic shift reagent Dy(PPP$_i$)$_2^{7-}$ with the Na$^+$ ion, consistent with the paramagnetic effects of the analogous relaxation reagent Gd(PPP$_i$)$_2^{7-}$ on the Na-23 nucleus.

protocol can be carried out on the same cell sample.

Dysprosium bis(tripolyphosphate) causes especially large hyperfine shifts in the NMR absorption of Na-23. This is ascribed to its highly anionic nature and its ability to bind Na^+ in close spatial proximity of dysprosium. In order to obtain information on the structure of the complex of Na^+ with dysprosium bis(tripolyphosphate), the paramagnetic effect of the S-state ion Gd(III) on the longitudinal nuclear relaxation rate of the Na-23 nucleus in a complex of Na^+ with gadolinium bis(tripolyphosphate) was measured. From the magnitude of the paramagnetic effect (about 10,000/ sec), using the rotational correlation time estimated from Stokes law, a Gd(III) to Na-23 distance of 4 Å has been obtained using the theory of distance-dependent paramanetic dipolar interactions (15,16). A structure of the complex consistent with this distance is shown in figure 2.

$Dy(PPP_i)_2$ causes an upfield paramagnetic shift in the frequency of the extracellular Na-23 resonance and only minimal line-broadening. A complex of the same ligand with thulium $Tm(PPP_i)_2$, however, causes a downfield paramagnetic shift presumably due to differences in orientation of the principal axes of the electronic g-tensor but thulium bis(tripoly-phosphate) is only half as effective as dysprosium bis(tripolyphosphate), as judged by the magnitude of the resulting paramagnetic shifts (14,17).

QUANTITATION OF INTRACELLULAR SODIUM IONS BY NMR

Once the separation of intra- and extracellular Na-23 resonances by the shift reagent has been achieved, a comparison of the intensity of the reso-nance from extracellular ions (A_{out}) with that of a cell-free control (A_o) containing the same concentration of Na^+ ions as present in the extracel-lular medium [Na_{out}] (figure 3) directly yields the fractional space in the NMR-window that is extracellular (S_{out}). It should be noted that the extracellular space defined in this way is the space seen by the Na-23 ions themselves and includes the space occupied by the medium as well as any interstitial spaces. The intensities of the Na-23 resonances of intra-cellular (A_{in}) and extracellular ions together with a knowledge of the fractional space that is extracellular then directly yield the concentra-tion of intracellular Na-23 ions [Na_{in}] that contribute to the observed resonance signal. The following equations provide the relationship between the observed resonance intensities and the "NMR-visible" intracellular Na-23 ion concentration (13,14):

$$S_{out} = \frac{A_{out}}{A_o} \qquad [1]$$

$$[Na_{in}] = \left[\frac{A_{in}}{A_{out}} \frac{S_{out}}{(1-S_{out})} \right] [Na_{out}] \qquad [2]$$

When [Na_{out}] is expressed in mM, the units of [Na_{in}] are mmols/l cells. A knowledge of water content of the cells enables a calculation of [Na_{in}] on the basis of kilogram cell water.

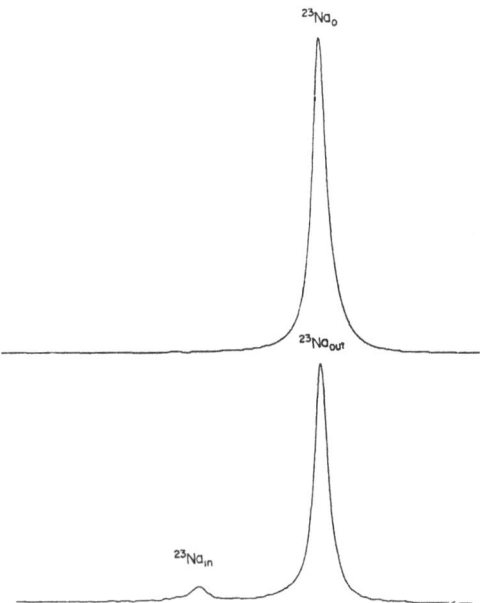

Figure 3. Comparison of Na-23 NMR spectrum of red cells suspended in serum containing 4 mM dysprosium bis(tripolyphosphate) (lower trace) with that of the suspension medium alone (upper trace). The ratio of the intensities of the Na_{out} and Na_o signals directly gives the fractional extracellular space.

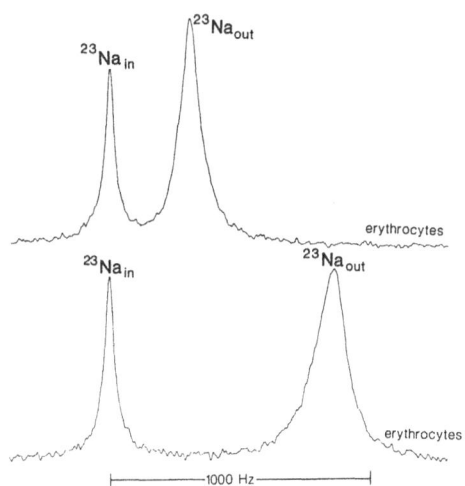

Figure 4. Na-23 NMR spectra of human erythrocytes with 2 mM (upper trace) and 5 mM (lower trace) dysprosium bis(tripolyphosphate) showing no change in the intracellular Na^+ signal with increasing reagent concentration.

SODIUM IONS IN HUMAN ERYTHROCYTES

Exposure to $Dy(PPP_i)_2$ does not affect the ATP, 2,3-DPG or free Mg^{2+} level
in the human red blood cell (14). The reagent would thus appear to be non-
toxic to cellular energy metabolism. The chemical shift and intensity of
the intracellar Na-23 resonance are also independent of the concentration
of $Dy(PPP_i)_2$ in the extracellular medium, showing that the presence of
the reagent does not perturb the concentration or environment of intracellular Na^+ ions (figure 4). The resonance at right (upfield) corresponds
to extracellular Na-23 ions, which interact with the reagent, while the
resonance at left (downfield) arises from intracellular Na-23 ions (13).
The Na-23 NMR spectrum of well-packed fresh human blood or erythrocytes
shows reduced extracellular space as expected (figure 5). From the spectrum in figure 5, an intracellular Na^+ ion concentration of 4.1 mmols/l
cells has been estimated (18). This NMR-visible Na^+ concentration in
human erythrocytes is significantly (20-30%) lower than the total concentration of the ions in the same cells estimated using atomic absorption.
The simplest explanation for the results is that the entire pool of intracellular Na-23 ions is not contributing to the observed resonance and the
cell makes a part of the intracellular Na^+ somehow invisible to the NMR
technique (14,18). The resonance of this Na-23 ion pool must be experiencing quadrupolar broadening sufficient to cause its disappearance. In order
to explain the observations (18), however, the exchange of NMR-invisible
and NMR-visible Na^+ pools must be slow on the NMR time scale; otherwise
the observed Na-23 resonance would be expected to reflect the entire concentration of intracellular Na^+ ions.

In the absence of a paramagnetic shift reagent, human red blood cells
exhibit only a single Na-23 resonance due to overlap of the signals from
intra- and extracellular ions. Hemolysis of packed, ATP-rich, human red
cells by repeated freeze-thawing caused a $17\pm 2.4\%$ increase in the overall
Na-23 NMR signal (18,19) (figure 6). This observation indicates that an
NMR-invisible pool of intracellular Na-23 ions exists in the human red
cell and that ions in this pool become observable upon cell lysis. Using
dysprosium bis(tripolyphosphate) to distinguish between intra- and extracellular ions, the contribution of extracellular Na^+ to the observed signal
from well-packed erythrocytes has been estimated to be about 24%. Since
the contribution of the extracellular Na^+ to the observed signal is expected to be invariant, the NMR-invisible pool represents 17/0.76 or about
22% of the total intracellular Na^+ concentration. Essentially all of the
Na^+ becomes observable by NMR in the lysed state. A similar (about 20%)
increase in the Na-23 NMR signal is observed when well-packed red cells
are lysed by detergent solubilization of the cellular membranes. The NMR-
invisible Na^+ is not present in ATP-depleted red cells or in ATP-containing
cells depolarized by treatment with 2.5 or 10 uM gramicidin, as indicated
by the absence of any increase in the Na^+ signal upon freeze-thawing (19).
These results indicate the existence of a compartment dependent upon the
presence of an intact membrane potential that contains NMR-invisible Na^+
experiencing a large quadrupolar interaction within the red blood cell.
The inability of this Na^+ pool to exchange rapidly with the free cytosolic Na^+ makes it NMR-invisible.

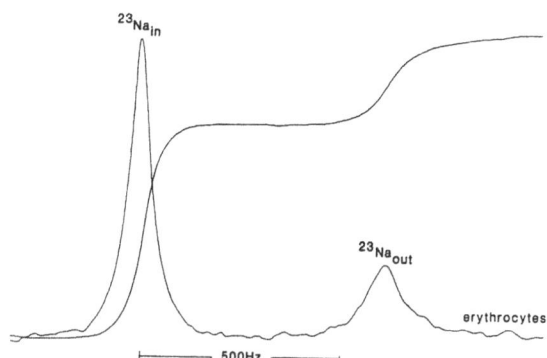

Figure 5. Na-23 NMR spectrum of well-packed human erythrocytes suspended in serum containing 4 mM dysprosium bis(tripolyphosphate) [from (18)].

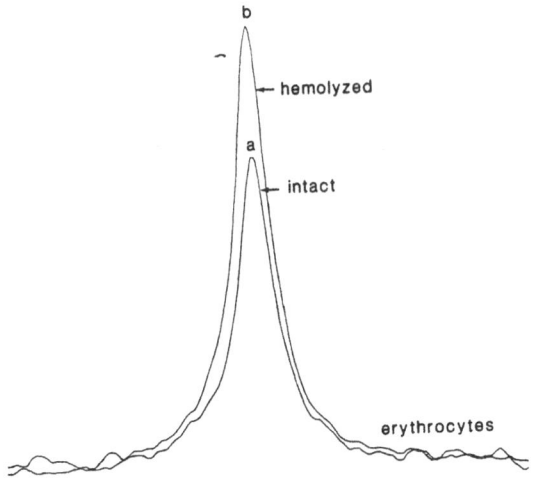

Figure 6. Na-23 NMR spectra of well-packed human erythrocytes without any reagent: a, intact cells; b, lysate after 3X freeze-thawing [from (18)].

SODIUM IONS IN HUMAN NORMAL AND LEUKEMIC LYMPHOCYTES

The Na-23 NMR technique is readily applicable to living lymphocytes and acceptable spectral signal to noise ratio is easily attainable (14,18). Several considerations have led to the hypothesis that an abnormality in the control of intracellular monovalent cations may play a role in the abnormal maturation of some leukemic cells. In order to test this hypothesis, NMR-visible Na^+ contents of human normal and leukemic lymphocytes have been measured using $Dy(PPP_i)_2$. Lymphocytes from patients with chronic lymphocytic leukemia (CLL) have been compared with normal controls (18). In this study lymphocytes were suspended in their own serum in order to reflect the in vivo situation as closely as possible Na-23 NMR spectra from normal and abnormal (CLL) samples of lymphocytes yielded significantly different NMR-visible intracellular Na^+ ion concentrations (17.5± 1.2 mmols/l cells for normal and 8.7± 0.8 mmols/l for abnormal cells (figures 7) (18). These results appear to indicate that the NMR-visible Na^+, which is presumed to be predominantly free, is only at half the normal level in leukemic lymphocytes. Accordingly, the Na^+ electrochemical gradient across the plasma membrane is two-fold larger in leukemic lymphocytes than in normal lymphocytes. It has been suggested that an increased Na^+ electrochemical gradient would enhance the entry of many nutrients into the cell and may be associated with the neoplastic process in vivo (18). The ability of the Na^+ NMR technique to non-invasively monitor the state of intracellular ions in abnormal lymphocytes may be useful as a simple in vitro assay for determining the effectiveness of action of cancer chemotherapeutic agents (18).

INTRACELLULAR SODIUM IONS IN MAMMALIAN CARDIAC MYOCYTES

The maintenance of electrochemical gradients in heart muscle is crucial to the maintenance of resting potential, the development of action potential, and initiation of contraction. The unambiguous measurement of intracellular sodium ions by the noninvasive NMR technique offers a new opportunity to monitor precisely the maintenance and fluctuations of intracellular Na^+ levels in cardiac cells. Dysprosium bis(tripolyphosphate) does not permeate heart cells when added to suspensions of intact adult rat cardiac myocytes. Using Na-23 NMR in conjunction with this shift reagent, the concentration of Na^+ in cardiac myocytes at rest, as well as the magnitude and reversibilty of changes in intracellular Na^+ level induced by insulin-deficiency and by removal of extracellular Ca^{2+} have been studied (20,21).

Figure 8a (right) illustrates the Na-23 NMR spectrum of rat cardiac myocytes in a calcium and insulin-containing medium. In the presence of 0.3-1 mM Ca^{2+} and 5-10 mU/ml insulin in the extracellular medium, the intracellular Na^+ level has been measured to be 8.8± 1.2 mmols/l cells (21). When these myocytes were transferred to a Ca^{2+}-free medium there was a marked increase in the NMR-visible Na^+ to a level of 22.8∓ 2.6 mmols/l cells as shown in figure 8b (right). This magnitude of increase was observed even when the calcium concentration in the extracellular medium was changed only from 300 uM to 10 uM. The increase in intracellular Na^+ was reversed by the addition of 0.3 to 1 mM $CaCl_2$ to the medium. The myocytes thus appeared to remain alive in a Ca^{2+}-free medium in the NMR tube (21)

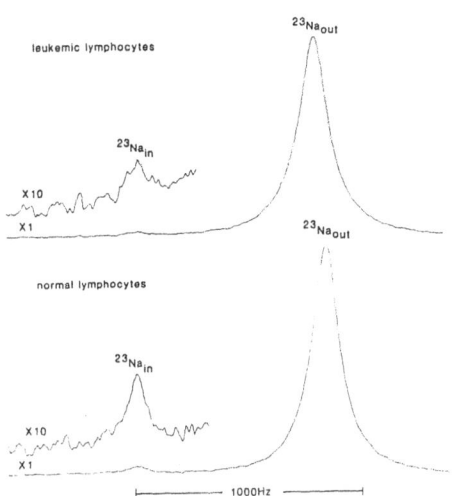

Figure 7. Na-23 NMR spectra of human normal (lower trace) and leukemic (CLL) lymphocytes (upper trace) suspended in their own serum containing 4 mM dysprosium bis(tripolyphosphate) [from (18)].

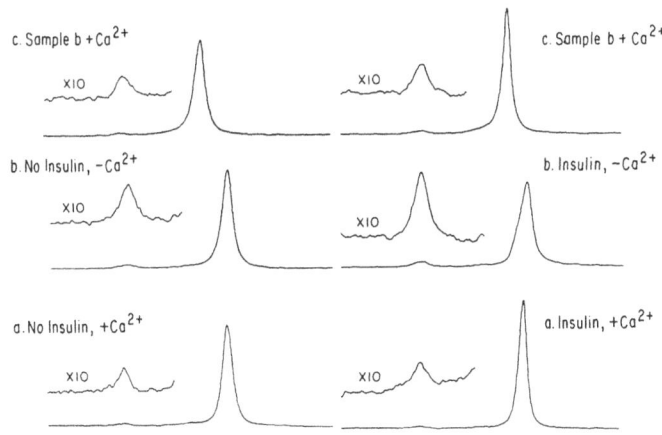

Figure 8. Na-23 NMR spectra of rat cardiac myocytes showing the effects of extracellular calcium and insulin-deficiency on intracellular Na^+ concentration. Myocytes were maintained in insulin-containing (right) or insulin-deficient medium (left) without calcium (b) or with 1 mM calcium (a) or resuspeded in calcium after initial removal of calcium (c) [from (21)].

and were able to pump their Na^+ down to the characteristic low level when
they were transferred again to a Ca^{2+}-containing medium (figure 8c, right).
Since cardiac cells have functional insulin receptors and insulin is known
to affect membrane ion-transport processes (22-25), the effect of insulin-
deficiency upon intracellular Na^+ in myocytes was studied (20,21). Insulin-
deficiency in the extracellular medium caused a detectable (21%) decrease
in the NMR-visible intracellular Na^+ to a level of 6.9 ± 0.5 mmols/l cells
in a normal Ca^{2+}-containing physiological medium (figure 8a, left). In a
Ca^{2+}-free, insulin-deficient, medium, the NMR-visible Na^+ was again increased but to a level (14.6 ± 2.0 mmols/l cells) markedly (64%) lower than
that found in insulin-containing cells (22.8 ∓ 0.6 mmols/l cells) under
similar conditions (figure 8b, left & right). Thus in a Ca^{2+}-free medium,
the insulin induced a substantial increase in the NMR-visible cell Na^+.
A large increase in intracellular Na^+ was observed even when Ca^{2+} in
the extracellular medium was changed only from 300 uM to 10 uM.

The isolated cardiac myocytes used in this study were functionally
intact rectangular cells which contracted repeatedly, synchronously and
specifically in response to electrical stimulation in 1 mM calcium and
possessed nearly normal high energy phosphate content. During the NMR
mesurements, which routinely took about 10 minutes, the cells might have
become hypoxic but remained well supplied with glucose substrate. After
NMR measurements, the cells had somewhat reduced high energy phosphate
stores but a majority of them retained normal morphology in those experiments in which changes in internal sodium levels were reversible. The fact
that cells left in the NMR tube retained low Na^+ for at least 0.5 h indicated that these levels of high energy phosphates are sufficient to sustain
the energy flux required to maintain Na^+ gradient across the plasma membrane at least in calcium-containing medium. Cell viability under the conditions used to record the NMR spectra was indicated by a comparison of
two successive NMR measurements on the same sample over an interval of 20
mins which yielded essentially identical values for the level of internal
Na^+ (21).

The NMR-measured value of $[Na_{in}]$ in cardiac myocytes, 8.8 ∓ 1.2 mmols/l
cells, is comparable to a recent measurement of total sodium of about 8.1
mmols Na per kilogram rat myocytes by flame photometry carried out after
washing the cells in LiCl to remove extracellular sodium. These results
suggest that nuclear quadrupolar interactions did not reduce the NMR signal
of the entire pool of intracellular Na-23 ions by 60% in heart cells. A
major fraction of the intra- cellular Na^+ in cardiac myocytes therefore
appears to be NMR-visible (21).

NMR readily measured sodium loading of isolated adult cardiac myocytes
when extracellular calcium was removed and demonstrated sodium extrusion
when extracellular calcium was restored. Extrusion of intracellular Na^+
was accompanied by uptake of Ca^{2+} from the extracellular medium and might
occur, in part, via the sodium/calcium exchange system in the sarcolemma.
While these effects can be measured by chemical techniques the NMR method
has the advantage that sequential Na^+ loading and unloading may be demonstrated in the same sample of cells without interference from extracellular sodium.

Cardiac cells in 0.3 mM external calcium, despite their ability to
maintain normal internal sodium, ATP and creatine phosphate levels, do not
contract in response to electrical stimulation. They do, however, contract

spontaneously in 10 uM norepinephrine. Cells in 0.3 mM Ca^{2+} do exhibit a high input resistance, maintain a normal resting potential, and display normal action potentials. Excitation and contraction pathways are therefore separately functional at 0.3 mM external Ca^{2+}. Cells suspended in 1 mM external calcium also have normal internal sodium levels, exhibit normal resting and action potentials, but do contract in response to electrical stimulation. It is considered that Ca^{2+}, bound to the sarcolemma, is required for excitation-contraction coupling and that external Ca^{2+} has two distinct functions. At 300 uM external Ca^{2+}, intracellular Na^+ is maintained at its normal level, contraction is possible, and resting and action potentials are normal. However only at 1 mM external Ca^{2+} is excitation coupled to contraction (21).

Insulin-deficiency caused only a small decrease (21%) in intracellular Na^+ in Ca^{2+}-containing medium but a marked decrease (36%) in Ca^{2+}-free medium. These results are consistent with insulin stimulation of Na^+ influx in mammalian cardiac myocytes. In the presence of calcium, the level of intracellular Na^+ is low and the Na^+-pump may not be saturated with this cation. If so, any increase in internal Na^+ by insulin-stimulation of Na^+ influx would shift the operating point resulting in enhanced activity of the Na^+-pump which together with 3 Na^+/1 Ca^{2+} exchange would tend to reduce the steady state intracellular Na^+ level towards the value measured in the absence of insulin. In a Ca^{2+}-free medium, however, 3 Na^+/1 Ca^{2+} exchange cannot extrude Na^+ and the increased $[Na_{in}]$ may saturate the Na^+ site of the Na^+-pump so that it is operating close to V_{max}. Therefore, an increased Na^+ influx causes a more marked increase in the steady state level of this cation. It is interesting to note that increased stimulation of Na^+/K^+ exchange across cell membranes due to increased internal Na^+ would cause depletion of extracellular K^+ and may explain the well known hypokalemic effect of insulin in man (22).

SODIUM IONS IN AMPHIBIAN OOCYTES, OVULATED EGGS AND EARLY EMBRYOS

Sodium ions appear to play an important role in the regulation of early embryonic development. Rana oocytes constitute a particularly favorable cell system for Na-23 NMR study in part because of their high intracellular Na^+ content (74-88 mM) relative to amphibian plasma (110 mM). A Rana female contains up to 2-3 thousand large (1.8 mm diameter) oocytes arrested in first meiotic prophase. They can be readily superfused in the NMR tube and induced to undergo nearly synchronous meiotic and mitotic divisions by introduction of hormones. While, in the amphibian oocyte, progesterone provides the primary physiological stimulus, it is interesting that insulin can also act to release the block at prophase arrest and reinitiate the meiotic divisions. Insulin action on the plasma membrane causes a rapid change in its ion-permeability and electrical properties and the possibilty that it affects intracellular Na^+ has been investigated (24,25).

Dysprosium bis(tripolyphosphate) has been used to separate and study the resonances of intra- and extracellular Na^+ ions in Rana oocytes, ovulated eggs and early embryos (24-27). Since the technique enables a noninvasive analysis of intracellular Na^+ in-situ and allows detection of small changes in cell Na^+, an accurate analysis of Na^+ levels in the amphibian egg in meiotic prophase arrest, second meiotic metaphase arrest and during early cleavage was possible.

Figure 9 illustrates the Na-23 NMR spectra of gently packed suspension of isolated Rana ovarian follicles (spectrum a) and "denuded" oocytes (spectrum b) in a Ringer's solution containing 4.0 mM shift reagent at pH 7.4 (The denuded oocytes were obtained by removing surrounding epithelial cell layers). Two well-resolved Na-23 resonances are directly observable in each spectrum showing the spectral separation of intra- and extracellular Na^+ in the intact follicle and the denuded oocyte suspensions by the shift reagent. Spectrum c shows the Na-23 NMR signal from denuded oocytes in Na^+-free Ringer's solution without shift reagent. As can be seen from a comparison of spectra b and c, the intensity of the intracellular resonance is not altered by the presence of the paramagnetic shift reagent. Further, 4 mM dysprosium bis(tripolyphosphate) had no effect on oocyte membrane potential or conductance, or on the phosphocreatine level as observed by P-31 NMR for periods of at least 2 h (24,25). The reagent also did not inhibit insulin or progesterone-induced nuclear breakdown. Thus, the shift reagent appears to be non-toxic to Rana oocytes.

NMR data indicated that only 14-17% of the total slowly exchanging Na^+ in the follicle-enclosed, prophase-arrested oocyte is detectable by NMR (24-27). In contrast to intact follicles, about 39-47% of the total Na^+ of denuded oocytes was calculated to be NMR-visible. The increase in total Na^+ in the denuded oocyte compared to the follicle (16-17 mmols/kg cells) is in good agreement with the increase in NMR-visible Na^+ (17-20 mmols/kg cells) and suggests that the Na^+ taken up by the oocyte during removal of the follicle cells is largely "free". Following hormonal release of the prophase block there is an initial further decrease in NMR-visible Na^+ prior to nuclear breakdown followed by a four-fold increase in NMR-visible Na^+ during nuclear breakdown. These changes in NMR-visible Na^+ occur without a change in total oocyte Na^+. By in-vivo ovulation (second metaphase arrest), total intracellular Na-23 increases and NMR-visible Na^+ now accounts for 31% of the total Na^+. The increase in NMR-visible Na^+ is largely accounted for by a net increase in Na^+ uptake by the egg during ovulation. During early cleavage there was a small decrease in total Na^+ but NMR-visible Na^+ rose to account for about 70% of the total. NMR-visible Na^+ thus increases markedly during early development.

To study the role of Na^+ ions in insulin action in re-initiation of meiotic divisions, NMR-observable and total intracellular Na^+ levels in untreated and insulin-treated follicles and denuded oocytes were compared. Treatment of denuded oocytes with 10 uM insulin for 1 h increased NMR-visible Na^+ by about 9 mmols/l cell water. An analysis of total Na^+ by atomic absorption indicated that there was a net increase in oocyte Na^+ from 100.4 ± 0.4 to 109 ± 0.4 mmols/l oocyte water under the conditions. When follicles were allowed to accumulate Na^+ in a Ca,Mg-free medium, by 2 h the NMR-visible Na^+ level increased from 11.7 to 66.6 mmols/l cell water. The follicles lost preloaded Na^+ when transferred back to Ca,Mg-containing medium but the decrease in Na^+ occurred much more slowly in the presence of 10 uM insulin (figure 10). Thus, 3 h after transfer to Ca,Mg-containing medium, insulin-deficient oocytes retained only 37.4 mmols Na^+/l cell water, while in insulin-containing oocytes the intracellular Na^+ was at a markedly higher level of 51.8 mmols/l cell water (24,25).

About 1.8% of the total oocyte fluid volume (1.4 ul/oocyte) exchanges per hour via endocytosis. The fluid uptake has been estimated to be $25\overline{+}1.6$

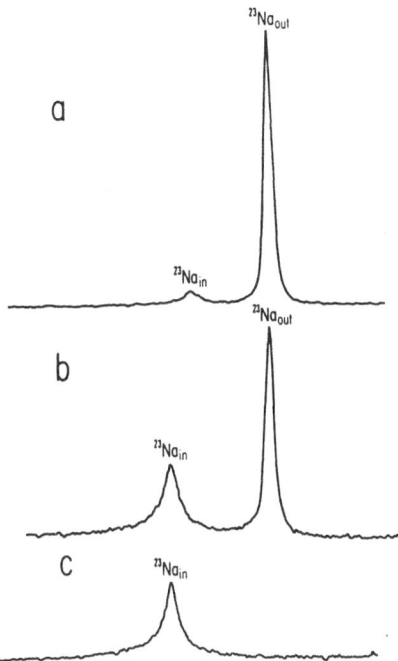

Figure 9. Na-23 NMR spectra (53 MHz, 21°C) of gently packed prophase-arrested Rana oocytes in three physiological states (pH 7.4): a, follicle-enclosed oocyte or b, denuded oocytes in a Na^{+}-containing medium with 4 mM shift reagent; and c, denuded oocytes in a Na^{+}-free medium without shift reagent. To obtain each spectrum, 1,000 pulses of NMR signal with a recycle time of 0.2 s were accumulated and an exponential filter of 5 Hz was used.

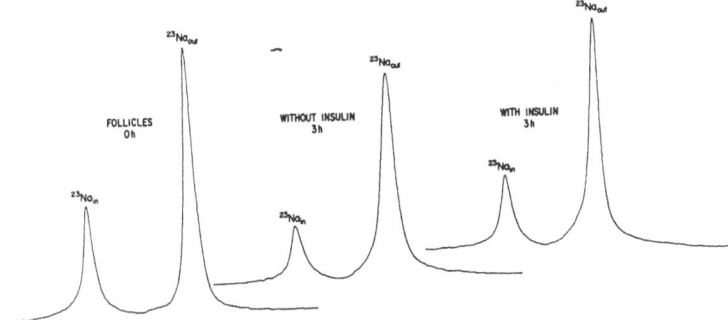

Figure 10. Na-23 NMR spectra (53 MHz, 21°C) showing the effect of insulin (10 uM) on follicle-enclosed Rana oocytes. Follicles were loaded with Na^{+} by 3 h preincubation in a Ca,Mg-free medium without insulin and subsequently transferred to the Ca,Mg-containing medium for 3 h with or without insulin. At the end of the incubations, the intracellular Na-23 resonance was significantly larger in oocytes from insulin-containing medium.

nl/oocyte/h (24). Since the medium contains about 110 mM Na^+, fluid uptake
via endocytosis could account for about 2 mmols Na^+ uptake/kg/h in the
prophase-arrested oocyte. Thus about one-third of the Na^+ uptake by the
prophase oocyte may be via endocytotic vesicles. Insulin is known to increase fluid uptake and turnover by stimulating endocytotic pathway 2 to
3-fold over the first h after treatment. Enhanced endocytosis could be
contributing significantly to the insulin-induced increase in NMR-visible
Na^+. About half of the increase in both total and NMR-visible Na^+ levels
in response to insulin (about 4.5 mmoles/kg/h) may be due to enhanced Na^+
uptake (2.3 mmols/kg/h) during increased endocytosis. Insulin, however,
also causes an increase in intracellular pH (28). In Rana oocytes insulin-
induced elevation of pH_i was Na^+ dependent indicating that intracellular
pH may be regulated by Na^+:H^+ exchange and that, as proposed for muscle
(22), insulin may act at least in part by stimulating the Na^+:H^+ exchange
system in the oocyte plasma membrane. Thus, the increase in NMR-visible
Na^+ may be due in part to increased Na^+ uptake in exchange for H^+ as well
as increased fluid phase turnover. Insulin stimulation of Na^+:H^+ exchange
in the oocyte plasma membrane may occur via a decrease in the activation
energy of this system which would allow Na^+ moving down its free energy
gradient into the cell to provide energy to move protons outward, against
their free energy gradient, with a resulting increase in intracellular
pH. Since the buffering capacity of the oocyte is relatively large, the
increase in pH_i from 7.4 to 7.6 (24) can be accompanied by a significant
Na^+ uptake.

It is clear that in amphibian oocytes, NMR-visible Na^+ concentration
is significantly lower than the total concentration estimated by atomic
absorption. This suggests either that all of the intracellular Na^+ is
not contributing to the observed resonance, or that the observed resonance
does not represent full absorption associated with all of the magnetic
transitions of the Na-23 nucleus due to broadening beyond detection of
some of the transitions by nuclear quadrupolar interactions. Theoretical
considerations indicate that the loss of signal intensity due to broadening of only two outer nuclear transitions by first order nuclear quadrupolar interactions involving the entire pool of cell Na^+ is expected to
be either 60% or none (10,12). The observation of an intensity loss of
only 30% or as much as 85%, depending upon the physiological state, in
comparison to the expected full signal, must be interpreted in terms of
compartmentation and quadrupolar broadening of the NMR-invisible Na-23.
Quadrupolar interactions could cause sufficient broadening of all nuclear
transitions resulting in total disappearance of the Na-23 resonance of a
given compartment. The quadrupolar broadening effect may be enhanced by
asymmetric electric field gradients and/or immobilization of Na-23 ions.
In order to explain our results, however, the compartmentalized Na^+ pool
undergoing quadrupolar broadening must exchange slowly with the NMR-visible
Na^+ on the NMR time scale; otherwise the observed Na-23 resonance would
be expected to reflect the entire concentration of intracellular Na^+ ions.

The possibility that a change in the quality factor Q of the NMR
receiver coil arising from the presence of oocytes in the sample tube could
affect the measurements was also considered. In order to check this possibility, the intracellular Na-23 signal as well as the Na-23 signal from a
cell-free sample were measured as a function of radio-frequency pulse
width over a wide range of values (corresponding to pulse nutation angles

of $30°$ to $360°$). Cellular as well as noncellular samples of similar ionic composition yielded identical pulse widths for the same nutation angle showing that the coupling of radio-frequency power to the NMR coil is not affected by the presence of oocytes in the sample tube. Since the NMR spectrometer had a single coil probe, one would expect that the sensitivity of the detection channel would also be unaffected by the cellular nature of the sample. Thus, the determinations of extracellular space and intracellular Na^+ concentrations would appear not to be affected by the heterogeneous nature of the cellular sample. This was supported by the good agreement between the fractional extracellular space values obtained from NMR and from dilution of radioactive inulin.

The identity of intracellular organelles responsible for compartmentation of ions within mature oocytes is unknown. The yolk platelets occupying a large part of the oocyte are a likely site of compartmentalization although the nucleus may also play a role. Atomic absorption techniques showed that about 35% of the total oocyte Na^+ was contained in the yolk platelet fraction when isolated by differential centrifugation at room temperature in Na^+-free isotonic sucrose. NMR analysis did not yield a detectable Na-23 signal from these intact platelets. Treatment of platelets with fuming nitric acid did, however, render most of the platelet Na^+ NMR-visible as indicated by the appearance of a sizeable Na-23 signal. These studies indicated that, while yolk platelets are rich in Na^+, this Na^+ does not contribute to the oocyte Na-23 NMR signal (27). It may be that the Na^+ associated with yolk platelets in prophase-arrested oocytes is released in part into the cytosol by ovulation or during early development. Such a release would be consistent with the increased NMR-visibilty of intracellular Na^+ in these physiological states. It should be noted that, unlike NMR, microelectrodes can sense the properties of only a small volume of intracellular fluid and the composition of this fluid may not be representative of the total intracellular fluid since subcellular compartmentalization is present. The finding that NMR-visible Na^+ increases during the first meiotic division and this increase coincides with the disappearance of the Na/K-ATPase suggests an inverse relationship between the level of NMR-visible Na^+ and active Na^+ transport.

Partially relaxed Na-23 FT NMR spectra were recorded to determine if they would reveal the existence of intracellular compartments with different magnetic environments and relaxation behaviour within an intact oocyte. Such studies detected at least two distinct compartments in denuded oocytes containing most of the NMR-visible Na^+ (27). Since platelet Na^+ appears to be NMR-invisible, as indicated by experiments with isolated platelets, one of the two observed compartments might be the nucleus, an interpretation that remains to be confirmed by examination of enucleated eggs. If so then NMR may offer at least in priciple the possibility of studying subcellular compartmentation of Na^+ noninvasively.

INTRACELLULAR SODIUM IONS IN MAMMALIAN RENAL CELLS

The distal nephron in the human kidney is responsible for the fine control of the total body fluid volume and electrolyte balance, a function regulated partly by adrenal steroids. In defining the regulatory mechanisms operative in the distal tubule, the measurement of the intracellular Na^+

level is of paramount importance, since this level regulates Na/K-ATPase activity, the final determinant of the amount of Na^+ reabsorbed by the kidney.

Measurements of intracellular Na^+ levels in suspensions of separated tubules from the outer medullary segment of the thick ascending limb of the loop of Henle of the rat kidney have been carried out using dysprosium bis(tripolyphosphate) to distinguish between intra- and extracellular ions (29-31). The intracellular Na^+ level was 42 ± 1 mmol/l cell water at $22°C$. There was a significant decrease in the intracellular Na^+ level measured after 30 min equilibration of the tubular preparation at $37°C$. The level measured was 26 ± 1 mmol/l cell water at $37°C$, consistent with a sizeable increase in Na/K-ATPase activity with an increase in temperature from $22°C$ to $37°C$, with a concommitant a decrease in intracellular Na^+ level (29).

The intracellular Na^+ measured at $22°C$ in the suspension of outer medullary kidney tubules was responsive to defined physiological stimuli. Furosemide (10 uM), an inhibitor of the $Na^+/K^+/Cl^-$ co-transport system, the major Na^+ transporting system in the thick ascending limb, reduced the intracellular Na^+ level from a control value of 41 ∓ 1 to one of 27 ± 6 mmol/l cell water. In addition, amiloride (1 mM), an inhibitor of the Na^+ channels at low concentrations and also an inhibitor of the $Na^+:H^+$ exchange process at the concentrations used, reduced the intracellular level of Na^+ from 40 ∓ 1 to 25 ± 4 mmol/l cell water. Thus the $Na^+:H^+$ exchange mechanism may be an important regulator of intracellular Na^+ levels in the thick ascending limb of the loop of Henle. In contrast, 1 mM ouabain, a specific Na/K-ATPase inhibitor, caused a marked rise in the measured intracellular Na^+ to 64 ± 3 from a basal level of 41 ± 1 mmol/l cell water.

In validation of the measurement of the intracellular Na^+ levels, the accessibility of the entire extracellular space to the shift reagent was tested by comparing the extracellular space containing Cl-35 ions with the extracellular space defined by the shift reagent. The measurement of extracellular space using Cl-35 NMR was based on the expectation that the resonance of intracellular Cl-35 ions may be too broad to observe due to its interactions with intracellular proteins and other components which would cause a large quadrupolar broadening. Indeed when the extracellular Cl-35 signal was broadened beyond detection by adding the $ZnHbO_2$ complex, there was no detectable Cl-35 NMR signal in the tubular suspension. These results indicated that the intracellular Cl-35 signal was broadened beyond detection. The invisibility of intracellular Cl^- meant that the Cl-35 NMR signal provided a measure of the extracellular space available to this ion. The extracellular space containing Cl^- ions was very similar to that defined by $Dy(PPP_1)_2^{7-}$ (29-31).

Incubation of outer medullary kidney tubules at room temperature in a medium containing 1 mM ouabain plus 10 uM amphotericin B, which would tend to equilibrate cytosolic free Na^+ concentration with that in the extracellular medium raised the NMR-visible intracellular Na^+ to 118 ∓ 10 mmol/l cell water (figure 11), a level equal to $87 \pm 7\%$ of that in the incubation medium (135 mM). These observations exclude the possibility that nuclear quadrupolar interactions reduce the NMR signal of the free intracellular Na^+ pool by 60%. The observed somewhat lower estimate of intracellular Na^+ in comparison to the extracelluar Na^+ under conditions which would tend to equilibrate Na^+ across the plasma membrane, could arise from incomplete equilibration of ions among intracellular compartments.

Packed Tubules (~50% Cells)

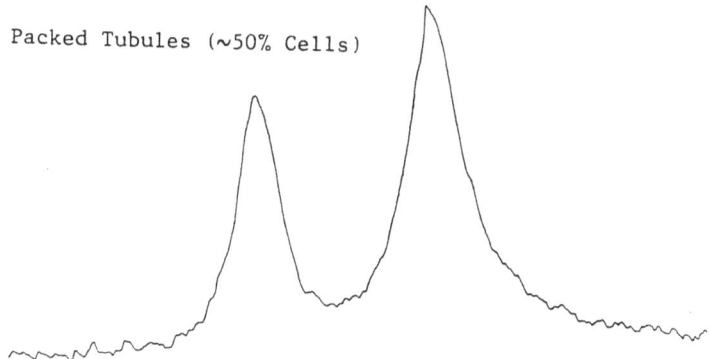

<u>Figure 11.</u> Na-23 NMR spectrum showing resonances of intra- (left peak) and extracellular (right peak) Na$^+$ in suspensions of rat outer medullary kidney tubules incubated in medium containing 1 mM ouabain for 1 h and subsequently in medium containing 1 mM ouabain plus 10 uM amphotericin B for 3 h.

The chronic increase in intracellular Na$^+$ levels elicited by superfusion of rat kidney tubules in medium containing 100 uM ouabain has previously been demonstrated to increase the apparent number of Na/K-ATPase enzyme sites by 75%, over an interval of 18 h at 37°C. The intracellular Na$^+$ levels in the same suspensions of tubules under parallel superfusion conditions have been measured using the Na-23 NMR technique. Over superfusion intervals of 2-4 h, at 37°C, the intracellular was markedly raised from a control value of 26 $\overline{+}$3 to one of 52 $\pm$3 mmol/l cell water. However, over intervals of 18-20 h, the incubation period required for the Na/K-ATPase response, the intracellular Na$^+$ level decreased to a level of 25 $\overline{+}$ 1 mmol/l cell water, a level not significantly different from the control value of 26 $\pm$2 mmol/l cell water. These data are consistent with the notion that an initial increase in intracellular Na$^+$ level induces an increase in the apparent number of Na/K-ATPase sites of sufficient magnitude to reduce the intracellular Na$^+$ level close to the control value (31).

Na-23 NMR has also been used to show that dexamethasone, a glucocorticoid, raises intracellular Na$^+$ significantly. In a suspension of outer medullary tubules, in paired experimets, 50 nM dexamethasone raised intracellular Na$^+$ from a control value of 36 $\pm$1 to 47 $\pm$1 mM. This effect appeared to be glucocorticoid specific. Incubation in a medium containing 50 nM aldosterone did not change intracellular Na$^+$ (38 $\pm$1 mM). These data implicate glucocorticoids in the regulation of ion-transport in the thick ascending limb of the loop of Henle (30).

Thus, Na-23 NMR, in combination with dysprosium bis(tripolyphosphate), would appear to offer a new and useful quantitative approach to the analysis of Na$^+$ handling by renal epithelial cells.

REFERENCES

1. Boynton, A.L., McKeehan, W.L. and Whitfield, J.F., eds. 1982, "Ions, Cell Proliferation and Cancer", New York, Academic Press, 551 pp.
2. Cameron, I.L., Smith, N.K.R., Pool, T.B. and Sparks, R.L. 1980, Cancer Res. 40, pp. 1493-1503.
3. Gupta, R.K., Gupta, P. and Negendank, W. 1982, See Ref. 1, pp. 1-12.
4. Blaustein, M.P. 1977, Am. J. Physiol. 232, pp. C165-75.
5. Moore, R.D., Munford, J.W. and Pillsworth, T.J. 1983, J. Physiol. (London) 338, pp. 277-98.
6. Tosteson, D.C. 1955, J. Gen. Physiol. 39, pp. 55-65.
7. Jardetzky, O. and Wertz, J.E. 1960, J. Am. Chem. Soc. 82, pp. 318-21.
8. Cope, F.W. 1967, J. Gen. Physiol. 50, pp. 1353-75.
9. Rotunno, C.A., Kowalewski, V. and Cereijido, M. 1967, Biochim. Biophys. Acta 135, pp. 170-73.
10. Berendsen, H.J.C. and Edzes, H.T. 1973, Ann. NY Acad. Sci. 204, pp. 459-85.
11. Yeh, H.J.C., Brinley, F.J. and Becker, E.D. 1973, Biophys. J. 13, pp. 56-71.
12. Civan, M.M. and Shporer, M. 1978, Biol. Magn. Reson. 1, pp. 1-32.
13. Gupta, R.K. and Gupta, P. 1982, J. Mag. Res. 47, pp. 344-49.
14. Gupta, R.K., Gupta, P. and Moore, R.D. 1984, Ann. Rev. Biophys. Bioeng. 13, pp. 221-46.
15. Gupta, R.K. and Mildvan, A.S. 1978, Methods Enzymol. 54, pp. 151-92.
16. Mildvan, A.S. and Gupta, R.K. 1978, Methods Enzymol. 49, pp. 322-59.
17. Chu, S.C., Pike, M.M., Fossel, E.T., Smith, T.W., Balschi, J.A. and Springer, C.S. 1984, J. Mag. Res. 56, pp. 33-45.
18. Gupta, R.K., Gupta, P. and Negendank, W. 1982, in "Ions, Cell Proliferation and Cancer" (A.L. Boynton, W.L. McKeehan and J.E. Whitfield, eds.), Academic Press, NY, pp. 1-12.
19. Petrovich, D.R. and Gupta, R.K. 1985, Fed. Proc., in press. (Abstr.)
20. Gupta, R.K. and Wittenberg, B.A. 1983, Fed. Proc. 42, p. 2065. (Abstr.)
21. Wittenberg, B.A. and Gupta, R.K. 1985, J. Biol. Chem. 260, in press.
22. Moore, R.D. and Gupta, R.K. 1980, Int. J. Quant. Chem., Quant. Biol. Symp. 7, pp. 83-92.
23. Moore, R.D. 1983, Biochim. Biophys. Acta 737, pp. 1-30.
24. Morrill, G.A., Kostellow, A.B., Weinstein, S.P. and Gupta, R.K. 1983, Physiol. Chem. Phys. Med. NMR 15, pp. 357-62.
25. Morrill, G.A., Weinstein, S.P., Kostellow, A.B. and Gupta, R.K. 1985, Biochim. Biophys. Acta, in press.
26. Gupta, R.K., Kostellow, A.B. and Morrill, G.A. 1983, Biophys. J. 41, p. 128a. (Abstr.)
27. Gupta, R.K., Kostellow, A.B. and Morrill, G.A. 1985, Fed. Proc., in press. (Abstr.)
28. Morrill, G.A., Kostellow, A.B., Mahajan, S. and Gupta, R.K. 1984, Biochim. Biophys. Acta 804, pp. 107-17.
29. Rayson, B.M. and Gupta, R.K. 1984, Fed. Proc. 43, p. 301. (Abstr.)
30. Rayson, B.M. and Gupta, R.K. 1984, Kidney Int. 25, p.600. (Abstr.)
31. Rayson, B.M. and Gupta, R.K. 1985, Fed. Proc., in press. (Abstr.)

APPLICATIONS OF CARBON–13 AND SODIUM–23 NMR IN THE STUDY OF PLANTS, ANIMAL, AND HUMAN CELLS

Laurel O. Sillerud, James W. Heyser, Chung H. Han, and Mark W. Bitensky
Division of Life Sciences, Los Alamos National Laboratory, University of California, Los Alamos, New Mexico 87545

0.0   ABSTRACT

Carbon–13 and sodium–23 NMR have been applied to the study of a variety of plant, animal and human cell types. Sodium NMR, in combination with dysprosium shift reagents, has been used to monitor sodium transport kinetics in salt–adapted, and non–adapted cells of P. milliaceum and whole D. spicata plants. The sodium content of human erythrocytes and leukemic macrophages was measured. Carbon–13 NMR was used to determine the structure and metabolism of rat epididymal fat pad adipocytes in real time. Insulin and isoproterenol–stimulated triacylglycerol turnover could be monitored in fat cell suspensions. [1–^{13}C] glucose was used as a substrate to demonstrate futile metabolic cycling from glucose to glycerol during lypolysis. Cell wall polysaccharide synthesis was followed in suspensions of P. milliaceum cells using [1–^{13}C] glucose as a precursor. These results illustrate the wide range of living systems which are amenable to study with NMR.

1.0   INTRODUCTION

In light of the relatively large cost of modern high–field NMR systems, especially those suitable for use on human patients, it is important to understand the reasons why the utility of NMR justifies its expense in applications to living systems. An examination of the available methods for the investigation of the interior of the body reveals that only a handful can give structural information in a non–invasive manner: these include NMR, x–ray, computed tomography, ultrasound, and neutron scattering. Other spectroscopic methods use probes of high energy or short wavelength which cause physical or chemical changes in cells. NMR is one of the only technologies that can provide functional information without the need for radiation, cell or tissue disruption, or damage to the system. In addition, it is selective for various nuclei in different chemical or biochemical environments and gives data in real time with respect to the integrity of chemical bonds.

T. Axenrod and G. Ceccarelli (eds.), NMR in Living Systems, 309–333.

A complete picture of the applicability of NMR to living systems must also include an exposition of limitations of the technology. While all of the major bionuclei have isotopes that have non-zero spin, and hence, give rise to NMR signals, these nuclei differ greatly in terms of their sensitivity, natural abundance, and biochemical concentrations in tissues of interest. Some, such as hydrogen, and phosphorus-31 have narrow signals due to the fact that they posess a nuclear spin of 1/2, while others such as sodium-23 and oxygen-17 are quadrupolar nuclei with much broader lines. Carbon-13 is present in nature at an abundance of 1.1% of all of the carbon so that signals from this nuclide will be difficult to obtain without the use of enrichment or large samples. This general lack of sensitivity limits NMR to the detection of only the most abundant chemical species. Furthermore, the width of a nuclear magnetic resonance signal increases as the correlation time of the nucleus decreases; this leads to the conclusion that NMR observes high-resolution signals from only the most mobile components of cells and tissues. In general these components are the small molecules such as glucose, metabolic precursors or products, free ions or mobile side chains on proteins or lipids. All modern NMR studies of living systems are done with the aid of signal averaging and Fourier transformation with finite pulse repetition rates. Consequently, the nuclear magnetization virtually never returns to equilibrium after the last pulse before the next is applied, and one must know the rate of spin relaxation in order to correct the observed signal intensities to obtain accurate measurements of the tissue concentrations of metabolites. Once these factors are taken into account in the design, execution, and analysis of an NMR experiment, the full substantial potential of NMR examination of living systems can be realized.

Our investigations to date have been directed at applications of NMR to living systems that have not been examined previously. There are active plant biotechnology and diabetes groups working at Los Alamos National Laboratory so that studies in these fields were chosen as initial demonstrations of the uses of NMR in new directions. Sodium toxicity is an important issue confronting all agricultural endeavors which utilize irrigation. We applied sodium-23 NMR at natural abundance to the study of the sodium content and tissue transport of salt tolerant monocotyledonous grasses of agricultural and economic importance in the American West and Southwest. We also used sodium-23 NMR, in combination with dysprosium-based anionic shift reagents, to measure the sodium content of normal human erythrocytes and human leukemic macrophages.

Carbon-13 NMR was chosen as the method by which the metabolism of adipose tissue could be monitored in order to assess the defects responsible for, and contributing to, diabetes. In this area Los Alamos National Laboratory is in the unique position of a lead laboratory with respect to the large-scale production of carbon-13. We have been producing carbon-13 at an isotopic enrichment of greater than 99% for the last 15 years for both internal and external use. At the same time, our National Stable Isotopes Resource has promoted the incorporation of this stable, spin 1/2, magnetic isotope into biomolecules of interest to the NMR community. We have sought to use this C-13 in the study of the metabolic regulation of adipose tissue. We also have examined the biosynthesis of cellular polysaccharides in millet (Panicum miliaceum) cell suspensions using [1-^{13}C]-D-glucose as a metabolic precursor. Natural-abundance carbon-13 NMR is an alternative to the somewhat expensive enrichment that is done for metabolic studies. We illustrate an application of natural-abundance C-13 NMR to the study of hormone-stimulated lipolysis in adipocytes.

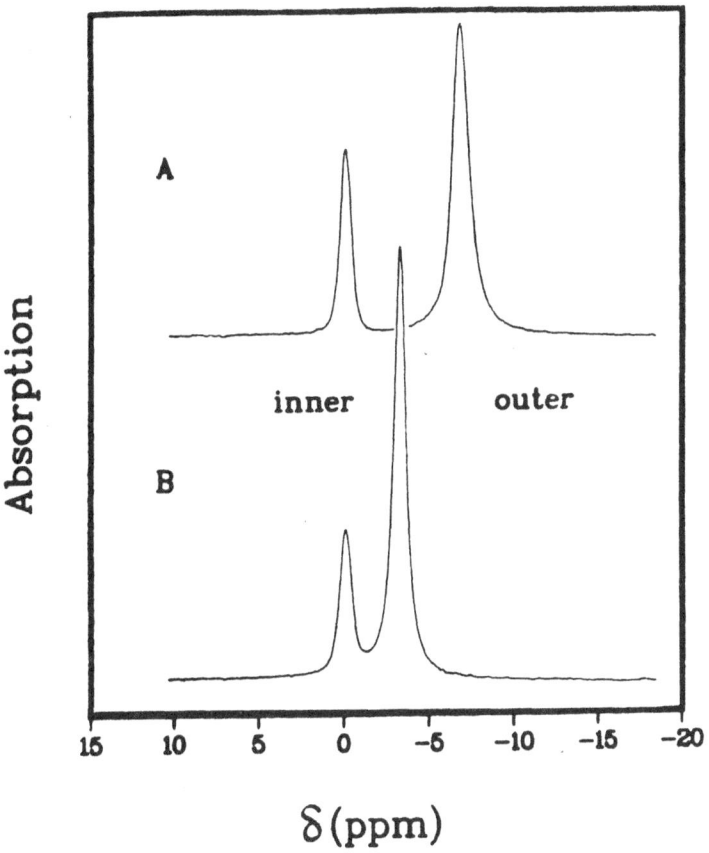

Fig. 1. Natural abundance sodium-23 NMR spectra of a suspension of millet cells, grown on 130 mM NaCl, in the presence of 5 mM DyTP at a temperature of 292K. (A) Cell spectrum taken for 3 min prior to the initiation of efflux. (B) Cell spectrum taken for 3 min commencing 90 min after the initiation of sodium efflux by means of a two-fold dilution of the exterior medium with sodium-free medium. Inner and outer here refer to the intracellular and extracellular sodium compartments, respectively.

2.0   SODIUM–23 NMR OF PLANT AND HUMAN CELLS AND WHOLE PLANTS

        The cytosolic enzymes of many plant cells are inhibited by
high intracellular concentrations of sodium. How certain plants deal
with this sodium represents a key feature in their relative ability to
grow in saline environments such as occur during the salinity increase
accompanying prolonged irrigation of the soil with water which contains
some dissolved salts. Sodium–23 NMR provides a rapid, non–invasive
method for the determination of the amount, and distribution, of sodium
ions in cells: data can be obtained with a time resolution of seconds,
in real–time, without the need for extraction or disruption of the
plant cells. Furthermore, efflux or influx time courses can be
obtained in vivo from single samples of cells. The minimum
concentration that can be measured is about 1 mM with a signal to noise
ratio of about 10:1 in 1–2 min. The interior and exterior sodium
signals from millet cells were separated with the aid of dysprosium
(III) triphosphate (DyTP) (1,2) so that the sodium concentration in
each compartment could be determined simultaneously. The DyTP was not
taken up by the cells.
        In order to follow changes in the amounts of sodium in the
millet cells, we added 5 mM DyTP to the suspension and observed the
intracellular and extracellular sodium–23 signals as a function of
time. This amount of the shift reagent split the sodium resonance into
two signals separated by about 7 ppm (Fig. 1) and about 1 ppm in width.
The alterations in the sodium signals caused by the shift reagent are
such that several factors must be determined before the areas of the
sodium resonances can be used to quantitatively follow the flux of
sodium ions. These include the time constant for spin–lattice

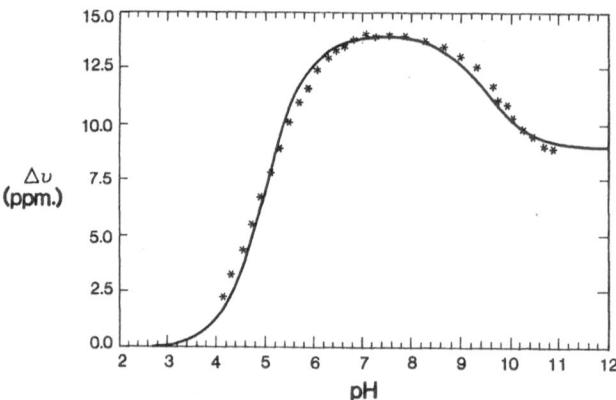

Fig. 2. Chemical shift difference between the DyTP–resolved sodium–23
NMR signals as a function of pH. The sample was a dual–compartment
(coaxial) NMR tube, with 100 mM NaCl in one compartment, and NaCl +
DyTP in the other in which the pH was varied with NaOH or HCl. The
solid line is a fitted curve corresponding to two pKs, one of 5.0 and
another of 9.5.

relaxation (T1), the extracellular pH, and the included and excluded
volumes of the cells. We determined the sodium T1 to be 42 ± 0.6 ms in
Linsameir and Skoog medium containing 195 mM sodium at a temperature of
292 K. The acquisition time for our data accumulations was 340 ms, so
that the sodium nuclear spins reached thermal equilibrium after every
pulse.

Binding of sodium to the DyTP is a complex process that is
influenced by the pH of the solution (3). For this reason, the
chemical shift difference between the two sodium resonances is a
function of pH (Fig. 2). The data can be fitted to a two-site
titration model with a span of 14.0 ppm and a pK1 of 5.0, for the first
site, and a span of –5.0 ppm with a pK2 of 9.5 for the second. In the
pH range from about 6.2 to 8.0 there is only a small change in the peak
separation with pH; fortunately, this falls nicely around the range of
biological interest. At a given pH the binding of sodium to the DyTP
shift preagent follows a Michaelis-Menton saturable binding curve; at
pH 7.8, 100 mM NaCl, the affinity was found to be 7.56 mM, with a

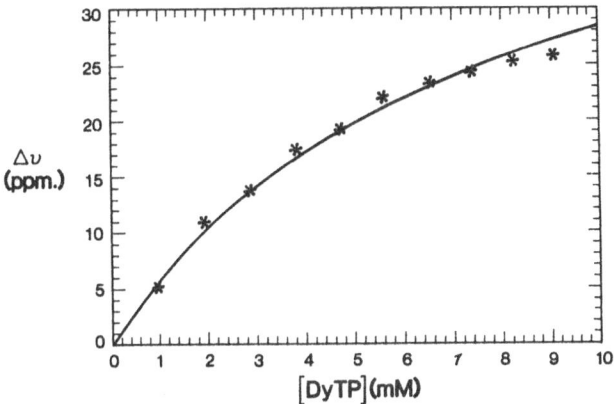

Fig. 3. Sodium binding to DyTP as measured from the chemical shift
difference between two sodium signals from a sample similar to that
described in Fig. 2, in which the DyTP concentration was varied in one
compartment. The solid line is a linear least squares fit to the data
points of a saturation-binding curve with an affinity of 7.56 mM and a
maximum splitting at infinite DyTP concentration of 50.0 ppm.

maximum splitting of 50.0 ppm (Fig. 3). Sodium is a quadrupolar
nucleus (I=3/2, Q=0.12) so that any electric field gradient across the
nucleus will distort the nuclear energy levels and cause the appearance
of additional transitions that occur at higher and lower fields than
those of the symmetric, rotationally averaged ion in solution. These
other lines are not always easily observable and can give rise to a

pH TITRATION OF SODIUM/DyTP.

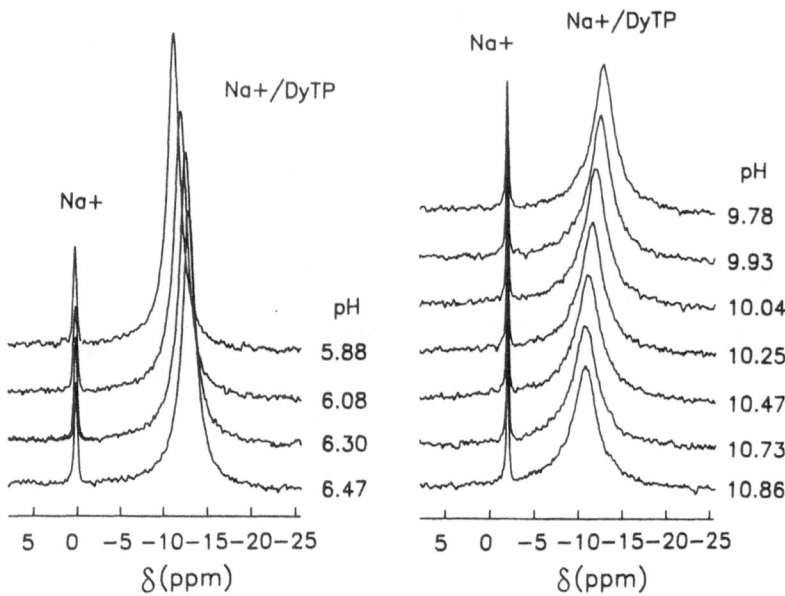

Fig. 4. Effect of pH on the sodium–23 NMR spectra of coaxial samples prepared as in Fig. 3, showing the variation of the splitting and linewidth of the DyTP-shifted signal.

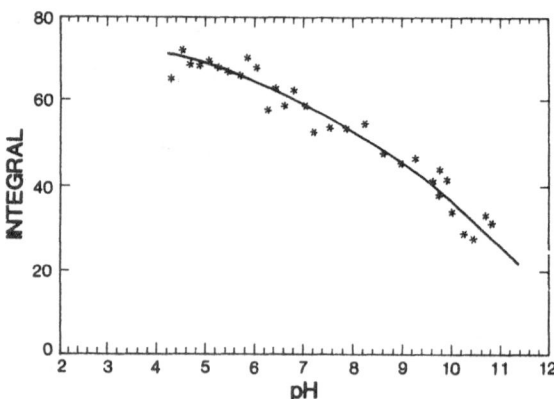

Fig. 5. Variation of the integrated intensity of fully-relaxed sodium–23 NMR signals in the presence of DyTP as a function of solution pH for data represented in Fig. 4.

spurious loss of intensity. This is what is seen for the signal of sodium bound to the DyTP as the pH is raised above about pH 6 (Figs. 4 and 5). Thus, one must be careful to control the pH of the medium during any experiments in which an accurate determination of the amount of sodium in the extracellular space is required. This is especially true for metabolising systems since they often excrete acids such as lactate or acetate into the medium during glycolysis. Adequate oxygenation must be maintained to prevent pH drift and loss of signal. Fortunately, the chemical shift difference between the two sodium signals serves as a sensitive monitor of changes in pH.

2.1   Sodium Efflux from Salt-Adapted Millet Cells

The process of adaptation of millet cells to a saline medium takes about a week for a shift to 130 mM NaCl. We examined the efflux of sodium from both adapted and non-adapted millet cells by means of Na-23 NMR and DyTP. The time dependence of the sodium resonances was measured during replacement of the external medium with an identical medium containing only half the sodium. The initial spectrum from a representative sample of NaCl-adapted cells is shown in Fig. 1A, while that for the same sample 90 min after the medium switch is shown in Fig. 1B. It is clear from the spectra in Fig. 1 that the cells lost sodium during the experiment; the kinetics of the sodium efflux are shown in Fig. 6 (open circles). The efflux curve could be fitted to the sum of two exponentials: I(t) = 23.15 exp (-t/9.15) + 76.85 exp (-t/506), which implies that 23.15% of the intracellular sodium resided

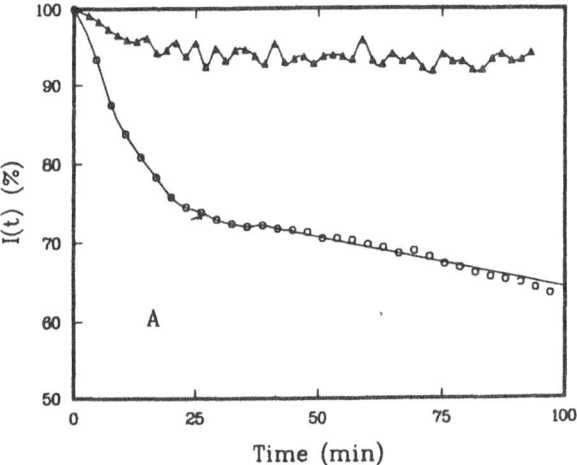

Fig. 6. Time dependence of the intracellular sodium concentration in suspensions of cultured millet cells as monitored by means of natural-abundance sodium-23 NMR. The circles represent efflux data obtained from cells adapted to growth on 130 mM NaCl, while the triangles represent data from non-adapted cells.

in a compartment which rapidly equilibrated with the medium, and that
76.85% of the intracellular sodium equilibrated at a much slower rate.
By measuring the intracellular and excluded volumes of these cells
(0.88 and 0.78 ml/g, respectively) we were able to calculate the two
fluxes as 367 and 107 nmol Na/g/min for the faster and slower
compartments, respectively at pH 6.7.

        When non-adapted millet cells were loaded with sodium for a
short time with respect to the time required for adaptation and tested
using the same experimental protocol as above, a strikingly different
pattern of sodium efflux emerged. There was very little sodium loss
during the course of the experiment (Fig. 6, triangles) compared with
the rates found for the adapted cells. In both of these cases, the
extracellular pH was constant at 6.7 over 90 min as determined from the
peak splitting. This is an indication that the DyTP was indeed not
taken up by the cells and that our oxygenation of the cells was
adequate to prevent medium acidification during the efflux period.

2.2   Sodium Influx into Millet·Cells

        The uptake of sodium by cells shifted from a medium containing
no added sodium (about 1 mM) to one containing 130 mM NaCl is shown in
Fig. 7. A linear least squares fit to the data from 6 experiments gave

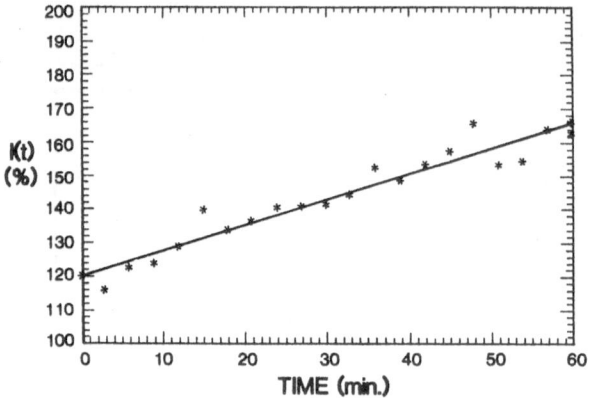

Fig. 7. Time dependence of the intracellular sodium–23 NMR signal for
millet cells grown with 1 mM NaCl shifted to a medium containing 130 mM
NaCl at time zero.

an influx of 0.757%/min. We measured the initial internal sodium
concentration as 0.93 mM or 0.82 micromol/g. The larger statistical
scatter evident in Fig. 7 arises from the smallness of the initial
internal sodium signal, and its attendant poorer signal to noise ratio.
        It is clear from the results presented above that both efflux
and influx of sodium can be measured in living cells with good time

resolution from single samples of millet cells. We have extended these
studies to include sodium transport in the roots of whole,
hydroponically-grown, plants of the salt grass Distichlis spicata.

2.3   Sodium Transport in Roots from Intact Distichlis spicata
           Plants

        The salt grass, Distichlis spicata, can grow in soil watered
by saline solutions containing up to 500 mM NaCl. It is found in the
playas of southern New Mexico, and in the salt marshes at Bodega Bay,
California. We have obtained members of both of these populations and
have grown individuals in the greenhouse using hydroponic technology in
order to control the ionic environment surrounding the roots. We have
used Na-23 NMR techniques as described above to monitor the transport
of sodium out from and into the roots of these salt-adapted plants.
The results illustrate another feature of NMR applied to living
systems; we were able to perform multiple transport experiments on the
same living plant.

2.4   Efflux of Sodium from Roots

        When the roots from Distichlis plants grown in 130 mM
NaCl-containing medium were quickly blotted and placed into an NMR tube
containing medium with no added sodium (and 5 mM DyTP) the internal
sodium moved out from the roots (Fig. 8). The kinetics of efflux are
biphasic with time constants and compartment sizes similar to those
found for the salt-adapted millet cells presented above: the equation

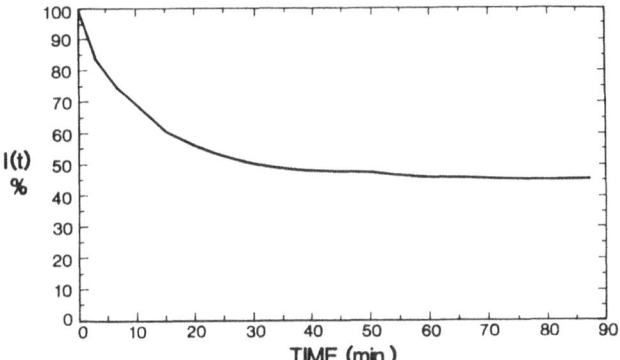

Fig. 8. Time dependence of the intracellular sodium-23 NMR signal for
Distichlis spicata. Seen here is sodium efflux from the roots of this
whole plant after the roots were placed into a medium containing 0 mM
NaCl and 5 mM DyTP. In this and the following figure, the plants were
grown hydroponicly on 130 mM NaCl and either washed extensively with
sodium-free medium for the influx experiments, or placed directly into
the NMR tube in sodium-free medium for the efflux runs.

describing the curve was found to be I(t) = 48.8 exp (-t/8.67) + 51.2 exp (-t/771). Here the fast and slow compartments contained approximately equal amounts of sodium.

2.5   Influx of Sodium into Roots

After the efflux experiment was finished, we removed the medium bathing the roots and blotted the roots to remove clinging medium. Then, the roots were placed into medium with 5 mM DyTP and 130 mM NaCl in order to measure sodium influx. The movement of sodium from the medium into these roots was faster than that found for the millet cells (Fig. 9); the influx rate was found to be 4.95%/min, with a half-time of 10.1 min. No attempts have yet been made to transform these data into fluxes since the weight of the roots is not easy to measure without sacrifice of the plant.

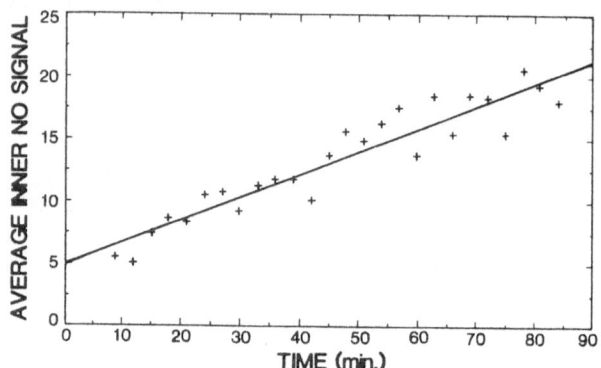

Fig. 9.   Influx of sodium into the roots of a salt-adapted whole plant, <u>Distichlis</u> <u>spicata</u>, as monitored with the aid of real-time sodium–23 NMR.

These results represent the first demonstration that Na-23 NMR can be successfully utilized to measure the parameters of sodium transport in living systems in real-time, without invasion of the tissues of interest. We have shown that the rates, and amounts of sodium efflux correlate with the ability of a plant to adapt to saline stress in the environment. Sodium-23 NMR works well for this application because plants grown in a saline environment accumulate sodium and therefore give a strong intracellular sodium NMR signal. The relatively high sensitivity of the sodium–23 nucleus translates into an ability to measure much lower sodium concentrations, such as those found in mammalian cells.

2.6 Sodium content of Human Blood Cells

Normal human blood and parenchymal cells contain sodium at a concentration that is much less than that of blood. This concentration gradient across the cell membrane is maintained at the expense of cellular ATP by means of a (Na,K)-ATPase. With the high NMR sensitivity of sodium-23 one can still measure these low intracellular amounts of sodium. An example of such a measurement is shown in Fig. 10. Normal human blood (4 ml) from a 35-year-old female volunteer was

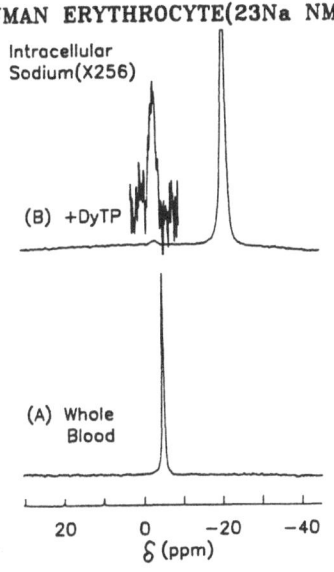

HUMAN ERYTHROCYTE(23Na NMR).

Fig. 10. Sodium-23 NMR spectra of (A) whole human blood and (B) whole human blood in the presence of DyTP showing the resolution of the sodium signal into intra- and extracellular fractions.

placed into a 10 mm NMR tube, and 0.2 ml of 100 mM DyTP was added. Spectrum A in Fig. 10 shows the sodium signal prior to the addition of the shift reagent. Atomic absorption analysis gave a sodium concentration of 138 mM for this sample. After the addition of the shift reagent (Fig. 10B) the extracellular sodium signal is shifted 17.93 ppm upfield, enabling the observation of the intracellular sodium signal. The relative integrals of these two signals were used to determine that these erythrocytes contained 5.1 mM sodium. The hematocrit for this blood sample was 52 ± 3%.

Human leukemic macrophages are another cell type to which we have applied the use of sodium-23 NMR. A sample of cells (125 million in 1.8 ml) was placed in a 10 mm NMR tube and oxygenated with a steady

HUMAN LEUKEMIC MACROPHAGES(23Na NMR).

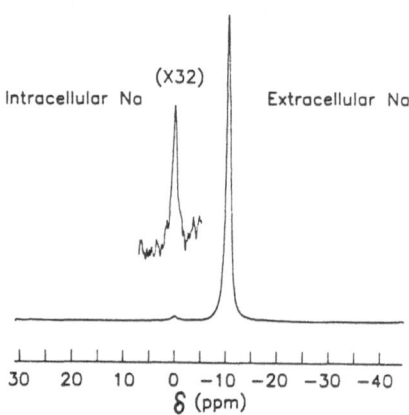

Fig. 11. Sodium-23 NMR spectrum of human leukemic macrophages in the presence of DyTP showing the intracellular sodium signal near 0 ppm.

stream of oxygen. After the addition of 5 mM DyTP the sodium spectrum (Fig. 11) shows two signals; the small signal downfield arises from the intracellular sodium, while the larger, upfield signal derives from sodium in the medium. Atomic absorption analysis gave a value of 165 mM sodium for this sample of cells suspended in phosphate-buffered saline. From the relative peak integrals we can estimate that these tumor cells contained 3.01 mM sodium or 43.2 femtomol Na/cell. These two studies demonstrate that sodium-23 NMR can be profitably used to measure the intracellular sodium concentration in living, human cells. We are now examining the transport of sodium in these human cell types.

3.0   CARBON-13 NUCLEAR MAGNETIC RESONANCE OF RAT ADIPOCYTES

Of all of the biologically important nuclides, carbon is the most interesting from the point of view of a biochemist or physiologist. Carbon forms the backbone of virtually all biomolecules; a complete description of intermediary metabolism would primarily consist of a map of the flow of carbon atoms from precursor foodstuff constituents into the product components of the cells and tissues of the organism. Indeed, there is no conclusive evidence that life itself is possible without the existence of carbon. For these and other reasons, the study of carbon biochemistry by a non-invasive, real-time technique would be of fundamental importance. Carbon-13 NMR has the needed potential to enable it to closely approach this ideal (4). The carbon-13 chemical shift range is large enough to provide superior spectral resolution compared to that of protons or phosphorus. The spectral dispersion is so great that virtually every carbon atom in a moderately complex (molecular weight around 1000) biomolecule can be resolved. This implies that the metabolic transformations of biomolecules can be studied with essentially atomic resolution, i.e., one can map the flow of single carbon atoms through a pathway. The chemical shifts of carbon nuclei are sensitive to the formation and breakage of chemical (heteronuclear and homonuclear) bonds, and to the nature of hetero-, and homo-atom substituent bonds. Although C-13 is present in nature at an abundance of only 1.1%, isotopic enrichment techniques can provide a 100-fold increase in C-13 at specific sites in a molecule so that the metabolic transformation of particular carbon atoms can be studied against a substantially reduced or absent background of natural-abundance C-13. The sensitivity of C-13 is only 1.6% that of the proton, a fact that limits the detection of C-13 to concentrations in cells or tissues to around 1 mM with modern Fourier transform spectrometers. Polarization transfer techniques will no doubt lower this by one to two orders of magnitude in the next one to two years (5). Finally, the spin-spin coupling present between two bonded, magnetic nuclei like C-13 gives NMR a unique capability to monitor the integrity of carbon-carbon bonds.

RAT EPIDIDYMAL ADIPOCYTES ^{13}C NMR

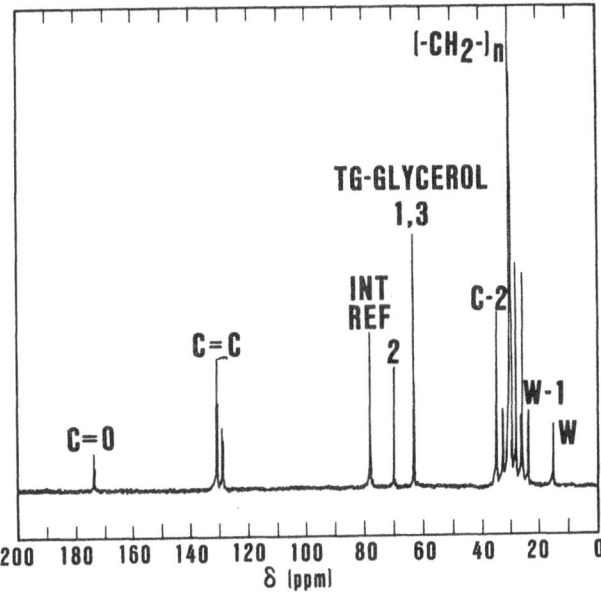

Fig. 12. A natural abundance, carbon-13 NMR spectrum of rat epididymal fat pad adipocytes. This spectrum was from 1 million cells with a signal averaging time of one minute. The excellent resolution of this spectrum provides discrete signals from almost every carbon in the triacylglycerol molecule.

3.1   Natural–Abundance C–13 NMR Spectrum of Rat Adipocytes

We have sought to use C–13 NMR to aid in the study of the
hormonal regulation of adipose tissue metabolism, since this tissue
plays an important, perhaps central, role in the etiology of diabetes
and obesity. A natural–abundance, proton–decoupled, C–13 NMR spectrum
of a suspension of rat, epididymal–fat–pad, adipocytes is shown in Fig.
12.   The spectrum can be completely assigned on the basis of published
spectra of triacylglycerols and fatty acids (6). The signals can be
assigned to 4 broad classes of carbon nuclei in differing environments
as follows: methyl and methylene (14–35 ppm), esterified glycerol
(62–70 ppm), unsaturated carbons (127–131 ppm), and carbonyls (172–174
ppm). Signals from the membranes or cytoplasm are not expected to be
seen since they constitute less than 3% of the cell mass.

Important information regarding the sites and types of
unsaturation of the fatty acyl side chains can be obtained rapidly from
the NMR spectrum. Characteristic signals from olefinic sites appear in
two places in the spectrum: near 130 ppm from the double bonded carbons
themselves and in the methylene region near 30 ppm.   The olefinic
region of the spectrum is dominated, in this case from cells from rats
given ad lib access to standard rat chow, by two signals separated by
about 1.9 ppm.   This separation arises from the magnetic inequivalence
of olefinic carbon nuclei from monoenoic and polyenoic fatty acids.
The carbon nuclei in oleic acid, for example, resonate at 130.51 and
130.76 ppm, while these same carbon nuclei in linoleate resonate at
higher (128.73, 128.91) and lower (130.96 ppm) fields. Distinct
signals from linolenate are seen at 127.84, 129.06, and 132.69 ppm;
signals from the other three olefinic carbon nuclei in linolenate
overlap those from oleate and linoleate.

The resonances from methylene carbon nuclei adjacent to
olefinic sites are shifted away from the other methylene signals due to
changes in their shielding arising from their olefinic neighbors. A
signal at 23.35 ppm comes from penultimate carbon nuclei in the fatty
acyl chain of linolenate.   The peak at 26.35 ppm is indicative of an
allylic carbon in a cis diene system; this could come from either
linoleate or linolenate.   The resonance at 27.92 ppm is characteristic
of cis allylic carbon nuclei; this could arise from either oleate or
palmitoleate.   The resonance at 32.32 ppm is uniquely assigned to the
second carbon from the methyl end of a dienoic fatty acid (6).

Certain features of these assignments have particular
relevance with respect to the usage of C–13 NMR for metabolic studies
on triacylglycerols.   Upon esterification to a fatty acid, the signals
from free glycerol (C1,3, 63.5 ppm; C2, 73.0 ppm) shift upfield
sufficiently (C1,3, –0.8 ppm; C2, –3.1 ppm) so that free and bound
glycerol can be easily resolved. This is an example of how C–13 NMR
can be used to follow the integrity of the ester bond in
triacylglycerols, and how, in a hydrolysis reaction, one could
separately follow the esterified and free glycerol simultaneously. The
chemical shift of the fatty acyl carboxyl carbon nuclei changes by –6.3
ppm upon methyl ester formation, and by another 1.3 to 2.6 ppm upfield
upon esterification with glycerol, thus offering another independent

means for determining the integrity of the ester bond by C-13 NMR.

In order to make quantitative measurements of changes in the C-13 NMR signals from the adipocytes, it is necessary to know the spin relaxation and nuclear Overhauser enhancements for each resolved resonance. We have made these measurements (7) and have used them in the analyses of the data to be presented below. An integration of the spectrum of the adipocytes can be used to provide information about the types and amounts of fatty acyl chains present in the cells in a non-disruptive, and rapid fashion. The major fatty acids are palmitic (29.9%), oleic (27.9%), linoleic (34.1%), and linolenic (2.9%). Of the unsaturated fatty acids present, 53% are oleic, 45% are linoleic, and 2.7% are linolenic. These results agree within 2% with those found using gas chromatography.

3.2   Insulin Stimulation of [1-^{13}C]glucose Incorporation

One of the classical effects of insulin on the metabolism of the adipocyte is to stimulate the incorporation of glucose into the glycerol head group of the triacylglycerol. In separate experiments (data not shown) using [ul-^{14}C]glucose in the presence of 10 mM unlabeled glucose and 10 nM insulin, we found that adipocytes synthesized triacylglycerols at a rate of 330 nmol/million cells/hr. An average adipocyte contains from 1 to 10 nmol of lipid; this rate would then correspond to a change in the NMR signal integral of from 0.3 to 3%/hr. Changes of this magnitude are easily measured given the

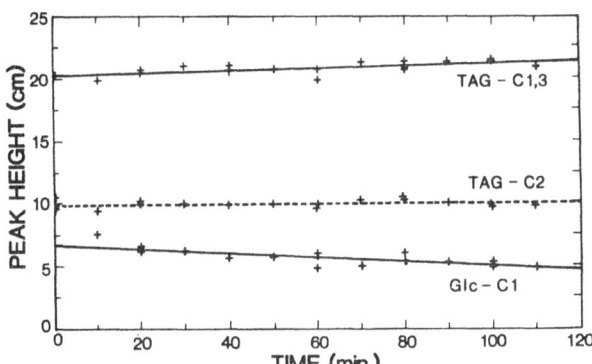

Fig. 13.   Insulin-stimulated triacylglycerol synthesis from [1-^{13}C]-glucose in rat adipocytes monitored by means of carbon-13 NMR. One notes a decrease in the glucose signal, an increase in the signal from the triacylglycerol carbon 1,3 resonance, and no change in the signal from the triacylglycerol carbon 2. These changes are to be expected on the basis of the known flow of carbon from glucose to triacylglycerols.

very high signal-to-noise ratio obtainable from suspensions of about 1 million adipocytes.

When this experiment was repeated three times, using C-13 NMR to detect the incorporation of glucose using 10 mM [1-^{13}C]glucose instead of the radioactive substrate, and 10 nM insulin, the results, at 310 K, show (Fig. 13) that the glucose was consumed by the adipocytes at a rate of 1.74 micromol/million cells/hr. The NMR signal from carbons 1 and 3 from the glycerol head group increased at a rate of 2.81%/hr, in substantial agreement with the data obtained above using C-14 glucose. The change in the total glucose signal during the course of this two-hour experiment was 1.7 times that found for the glycerol C1,3 signal. If all of the glucose was incorporated into the glycerol head group of the triacylglycerols the change in the glucose signal should have been equal to that for the glycerol signal. These data indicate that 43% of the added glucose was incorporated into other, unmeasured products including carbon dioxide and fatty acids. We have recently used sealed tubes containing hyamine to trap the evolved carbon dioxide and have found (data not shown) that there is significant labeling of the carbon dioxide. The rate of lipid synthesis shown in Fig. 3 was calculated to be about 1 micromol/million cells/hr.

The good resolution and dispersion of the C-13 NMR spectrum of adipocytes can be exploited in the present case to illustrate how certain resonances in the spectrum can be used as internal controls in order to check for systemmatic errors in the spectra from one time block to another. Labeling of carbon 2 of the glycerol moiety of the triacylglycerols will only occur if there is isotopic scrambling of the C-13, added at C1 of glucose, to C2 of glycerol-1-phosphate due to Kreb's cycle activity. There is a very minor flux through this route so that the glycerol C2 signal should be essentially constant over the course of the experiment. Any deviation from a slope of zero for the time dependence of this signal would have to arise from systemmatic effects such as floating of these very bouyant (density = 0.7) cells during the course of the experiment. The observed slope is 15.4 times smaller than that found for the glycerol C1,3 signal (0.374%/hr) providing good evidence for the absence of significant systemmatic errors in the application of this technique to the study of this process.

3.3   Isoproterenol Stimulated Lipolysis Using Natural Abundance C-13 NMR

The opposite process to that studied above is that of the breakdown of the ester bond of the triacylglycerols to form free fatty acids and glycerol. The adrenergic hormones, exemplified by epinephrine, control and promote this process. In our experiments probing the adrenergic stimulation of lipolysis, the more stable analogue, isoproterenol, was used. Incubation of adipocytes with 5 μM isoproterenol resulted (Fig. 14) in the net hydrolysis of the ester bond, with the release of free fatty acids and glycerol (Figs. 14, 15, and 16). The initial time course of the changes in the lipid glycerol C1,3 signal (Fig. 15) shows that isoproterenol stimulated lipolysis

ISOPROTERENOL STIMULATED LIPOLYSIS

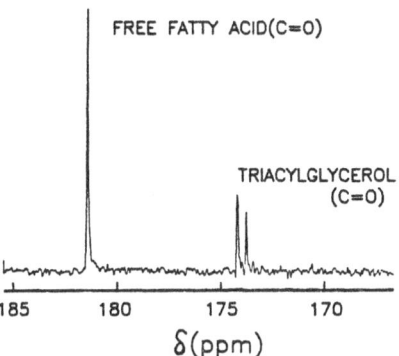

Fig. 14. Isoproterenol–stimulated lipolysis in rat adipocytes as determined by natural–abundance carbon–13 NMR. This is an example of the ability of carbon–13 NMR to provide information about the integrity of covalent bonds in biomolecules since the chemical shifts of the carbons vary according to their structure.

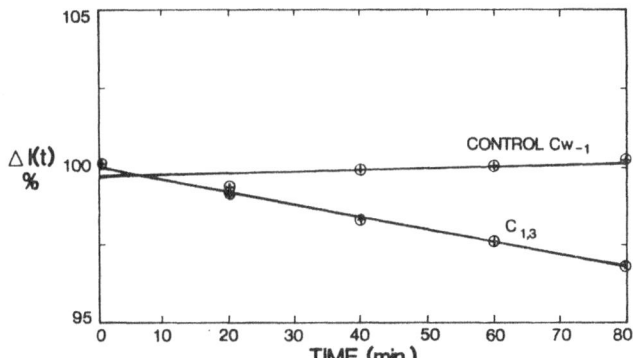

Fig. 15. Time course of isoproterenol–simulated lipolysis in rat adipocytes as monitored by natural–abundance carbon–13 NMR. The control signals were from the penultimate carbon in the fatty acyl chain of the cellular triacylglycerols. The cleavage of the glyceride bond is shown as a decrease in the signal from the covalently–bound glycerol carbon 1,3 resonance.

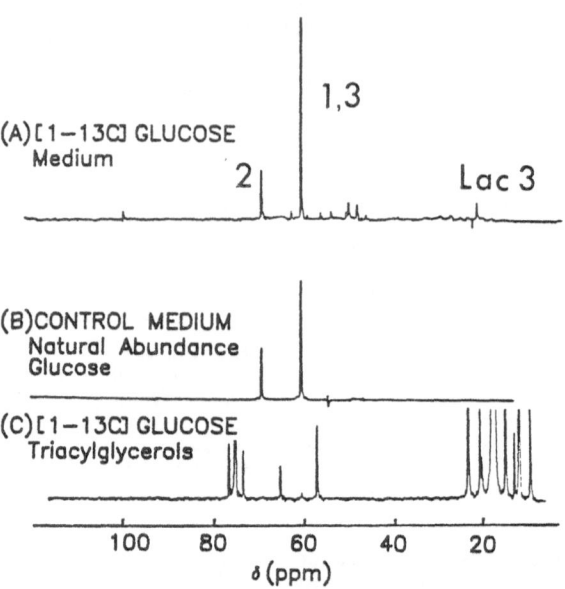

Fig. 16. Substrate cycling during lipolysis in rat adipocytes
monitored by carbon-13 NMR. Adipocytes were incubated in the presence
of 5 μM isoproterenol and either [1-^{13}C] or natural-abundance glucose.
(A) In the presence of labeled glucose the cells produced glycerol in
the medium with strong carbon-13 labeling at C1,3. (B) In the presence
of natural-abundance glucose the ratio of the glycerol C1,3 peak to
that of the C2 signal is 2:1 as expected from the random distribution
of carbon-13. (C) With labeled glucose glucose the extracted
triacylglycerols show a glyceride C1,3 to C2 signal ratio of 3.0.

stimulated lipolysis occurred at a rate of 2.4%/hr, a rate that is
close to the rate found above for the synthesis of lipids. In Fig. 15
we have used another lipid signal as an internal control; the intensity
of the resonance from the penultimate carbon in the fatty acyl chains
has virtually zero time dependence. The decrease in the glycerol
resonance intensity with time illustrates the fact that C-13 NMR can be
used to monitor the breaking of chemical bonds, since the C-13 NMR
frequency is different for the bound and free forms of glycerol. It
also points out the usefulness of natural-abundance C-13 NMR for some
purposes. It should be possible to apply these types of studies to
humans, because the C-13 NMR spectrum, at natural-abundance, of a human
arm (8) is completely dominated by signals from triacylglycerols.

3.4   Futile Cycling in Adipose Tissue

         Carbon-13 NMR is capable of resolving virutally every carbon
atom in most smaller biomolecules. Consequently, we can apply this

technique to the study of a very intriguing, and incompletely understood, facet of intermediary metabolism; a facet known as futile, or substrate, cycling. In this process, a precursor such as glucose which is labeled in a particular carbon position, is metabolized by a living system, and when the glucose pool is examined at a later time, it is found that there has been migration of the label to an initially unlabeled position. In most cases this label migration can be explained by the hypothesis that both anabolic and catabolic pathways operate simultaneously in the organism. A corollary of this hypothesis is that living systems "spin their wheels" so to speak, without doing as much useful work as the energy stored in the substrates would allow. In our work on carbohydrate metabolism in the rat liver (9) it was shown that futile cycling took place during glycogenesis at rates of from 40 to 100% of the theoretical maximum. Such high rates arose in that system because the pathways of glycogenesis and glycolysis are short and of comparable length. In the present case in the adipocyte, we sought to discover whether similar cycling took place over the longer metabolic distance from glucose to glycerol, and to measure the rates of lipogenesis during conditions favoring net lipolysis.

Adipocytes were incubated with 5 μM isoproterenol at 310 K under two conditions. For the control condition the cells were incubated with 10 mM natural abundance glucose. When all of the glucose had been consumed, the cells were separated from the medium. The triacylglycerols were extracted from the cells and dissolved in chloroform for C-13 NMR examination. C-13 NMR spectra were also taken from the medium. For the other condition, an identical aliquot of cells was incubated with the addition of 10 mM [1-^{13}C]glucose as the only differing variable. The results (Fig. 16) show several interesting features. There was substantial natural abundance glycerol release during the incubation of the control cells (Fig. 16B). Glycerol released during incubations with [1-^{13}C]glucose was labeled at C1,3 (Fig. 16A), indicating that it arose from the [1-^{13}C]glucose in the medium, rather than from lipolysis of existing triacylglycerols. The extracted triacylglycerols (Fig. 16C) showed the same labeling pattern as the glycerol (Fig. 16A). Isoproterenol stimulated glycolysis as shown by the appearance of lactate in this case and not in the control samples.

The addition of isoproterenol is classically thought to inhibit the uptake of glucose and at the same time, to stimulate lipolysis. Our results show that it does indeed stimulate lipolysis, while at the same time accelerating glycolysis. These results can be interpreted in two ways. The first is that triacylglycerols are made in the adipocyte in a first-in, first-out fashion, so that the newly made lipid molecules are the first to be hydrolyzed. This model would be appropriate for glycogen where glucosyl residues are added one at a time to precursor polymeric strands, but it is extremely unlikely for adipocytes since triacylglycerols exist as a lipid droplet without structure within the cell. The second possibility is that lipogenesis and lipolysis take place simultaneously within the adipocyte. We strongly favor this as the explanation for the labeling pattern seen for the medium glycerol in both experiments (Fig. 16 A and B) This second model is the only one which is consistent with the appearance of labeled lactate in the isoproterenol-treated cells (Fig. 16A). It may be necessary to propose new, and more significant, roles for adipose tissue in the body; that of a metabolic buffer for energy regulation, and as a significant producer of lactate and glycerol as substrates for hepatic gluconeogenesis.

4.0   POLYSACCHARIDE SYNTHESIS IN PLANT CELLS

The initiation of cell wall polysaccharide synthesis is an important obligatory first step during the process of regeneration of plant tissue from protoplasts. In order to optimize regeneration procedures a method for the monitoring of polysaccharide formation in vivo would be of considerable interest. We have used ^{13}C NMR combined with ^{13}C labeled substrates to follow the biosynthesis of cellulose and other α-glucans and glucuronoarabinoxylans in real time, in situ, within the cells of suspensions of proso millet, a monocot.

Suspensions of proso millet (Panicum miliaceum) were derived from a single callus regenerated in protoplast culture (1, 10). Exponentially growing cells (1.5 g) were harvested by filtration and suspended in a buffer of 50 mM KH_2PO_4 at a pH of 5.5 containing 50% D_2O. Proton-decoupled, ^{13}C nuclear magnetic resonance spectra were obtained with the aid of a Bruker WM300wb spectrometer operating at 75 MHz for carbon. A control natural-abundance spectrum was accumulated for 30 min from the oxygenated cell suspensions. At this time 18 mg of [1-^{13}C, 90%]-D-glucose was added and additional spectra were accumulated in 30 min blocks. For the isolation of a cellulose-enriched polysaccharide fraction other portions of cells were adapted to growth on glucose as their sole carbon source, and then cultured for 3 weeks with fresh medium containing the ^{13}C labeled substrate. During this time the cell mass tripled. Alkalai-insoluble cellulose was prepared by means of the extraction procedure of Carpita (11) and suspended in D_2O for NMR measurement.

4.1   High Resolution ^{13}C NMR Spectrum of Cellulose

In plant cells cellulose exists as a crystalline chains of β (1->4)-linked poly-D-glucose whose degree of polymerization ranges from 2,000 to 14,000 (12). From NMR studies of cello-oligosaccharides and other glucose-containing oligosaccharides (13, 14) it is expected that C1 from glucose will resonate at 103 ppm. The ^{13}C NMR spectrum (Fig. 17) of a cellulose-enriched fraction of cell wall polysaccharides isolated from millet cells grown on labeled glucose shows a major signal at 103.2 ppm which we assign to C1 of β-glucosyl residues in cellulose. This signal has a full width at half maximum of 270 ± 30 Hz which corresponds to an average mass of about 270 kD based on the dependence of T_2 and rotational correlation time on Stoke's radius and mass. This corresponds to a degree of polymerization of about 1,500 residues, a value which is at or below the lower limit estimated by

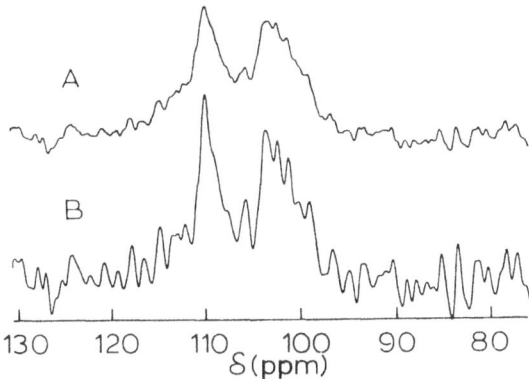

Fig. 17.   Proton-decoupled ^{13}C NMR spectrum at 75.412 MHz of cellulose purified from P. milliaceum cells grown for three weeks in 0.2 M [1-^{13}C]-D-glucose.   (A) Spectrum processed with 40 Hz digital filtration; 37,687 scans; acquisition time, 0.508 sec; pulse width, 90° (20 μs); temperature, 303K.   (B) The same data as for (A), but processed with Gaussian multiplication for resolution enhancement with -40 Hz line broadening and a peak time of 5.1 msec.   The primary signals arise from C1 of β-glucans and glucuronoarabinoxylans.

Marx-Figini (12).   Our extraction process may have degraded the chains somewhat in length.   Native cellulose should have a ^{13}C nuclear resonance width of between 370 and 2,500 Hz rendering it more difficult to observe.

The other prominent ^{13}C nuclear resonance, in the spectrum from the [1-^{13}C]-glucose fed cells, at 108.4 ppm arises from the anomeric carbon from L-α-arabinosyl residues in the glucuronoarabinoxylan which copurifies with the cellulose. We expect to find the signals from the anomeric carbon of the β(1->4)-linked xylosyl residues at a field position of about 102 ppm (14).   The signal in Fig. 17 at 103.2 ppm has a shoulder around 102.6 ppm which could be the resonance from this carbon.   Both L-α-arabinose and β-D-xylose are biosynthesized from D-glucose in millet cells, with preservation of C1 labeling.

4.2   β-glucan Synthesis from [1-^{13}C]-glucose in vivo

The natural-abundance, proton-decoupled ^{13}C NMR spectrum of millet cells (Fig. 18) shows signals from both structural and metabolic components.   The strongest signals arise from sucrose.   These cells were grown on 0.11 M sucrose, washed extensively, and resuspended in sample buffer without sucrose.   Thus it is likely that these sucrose signals originate from within the cells.   Sucrose hydrolysis takes place in these cells when transferred to a sucrose-free medium (Fig.

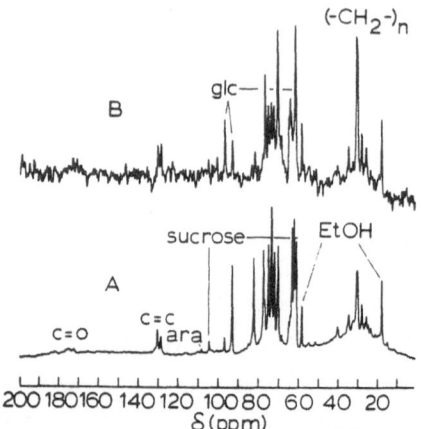

Fig. 18. Proton decoupled, natural-abundance ^{13}C NMR spectra of 1.5 g
of protoplast-derived suspension cultures of P. milliaceum cells
suspended in D_2O. (A) Cells grown in 4% sucrose, 37,349 scans with a
90° (20 μs) pulse and an acquisition time of 0.508 sec. (B) The same
sample as in (A) after 7 days growth in new, sucrose-free medium
containing 4% glucose, 826 scans in 7 minutes.

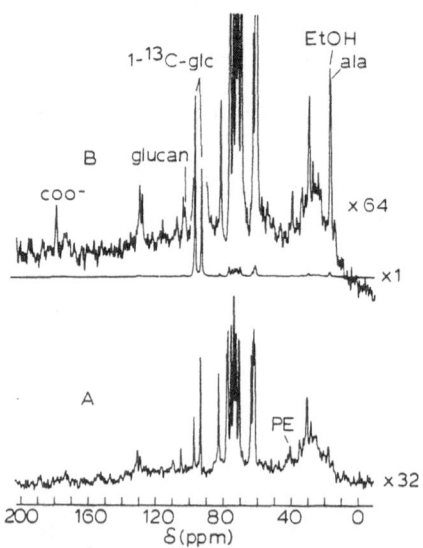

Fig. 19. (A) Natural-abundance, proton-decoupled ^{13}C NMR spectrum of
P. milliaceum cells grown for 3 weeks on natural-abundance glucose (0.2
M). This spectrum was taken as a control run for 30 min, with 12,324
scans using a 25.2° (5.6 μs) pulse. (B) ^{13}C NMR spectrum of the same
cells as in (A) 90 minutes after the addition 50 mM [1-^{13}C
(90%)]-D-glucose.

18B). When cells were incubated in this way for 7 days, about 75% of the intracellular sucrose was hydrolyzed to glucose.

In order to follow β–glucan synthesis in these cells, we adapted cells to growth on glucose by switching the carbon source from sucrose to glucose. The cells grew equally well on the glucose. Incubation of these cells with 18 mg [1–^{13}C]–glucose in the NMR tube resulted in the synthesis of a compound with a chemical shift of 103.1 ppm (Fig. 19, 20) which we identify as a β–glucan, which is most likely cellulose. The rate of increase in this signal was constant (Fig. 21); from the slope of the time course plot we can estimate that these cells made cellulose at a rate of about 0.5 μmol–glc/g–cells/hr. The width of this signal is 103 + 10 Hz, or about 2.7 times smaller than that found for the equivalent signal in the ^{13}C NMR spectrum of the cellulose–enriched fraction presented above. This difference in the linewidths probably arises from the differing positions of labeling likely to occur in the two different cases. The chronic feeding experiment would be expected to have labeled a large fraction of the total cellulose residues with ^{13}C, but the acute biosynthesis experiment would have emphasized end labeling. Terminal glucosyl residues would be expected to be much more mobile than those located closer to the center of the chains.

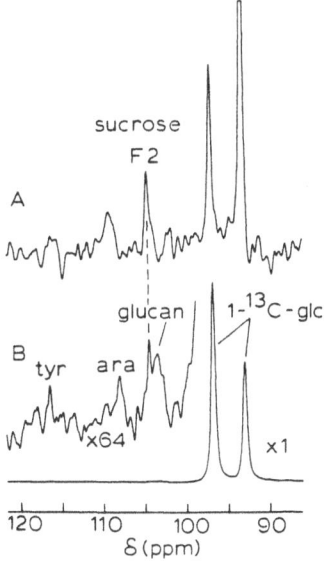

Fig. 20. An expansion of the polysaccharide anomeric carbon region of the ^{13}C NMR spectra shown in Fig. 19. (A) Control spectrum taken of the P. milliaceum cells for 30 min prior to ^{13}C–labeled substrate addition. (B) Spectrum taken 90 min after the addition of 50 mM [1–^{13}C (90%)]–D–glucose. Note the labeling of the β–glucan signal and its resolution from that of sucrose F2.

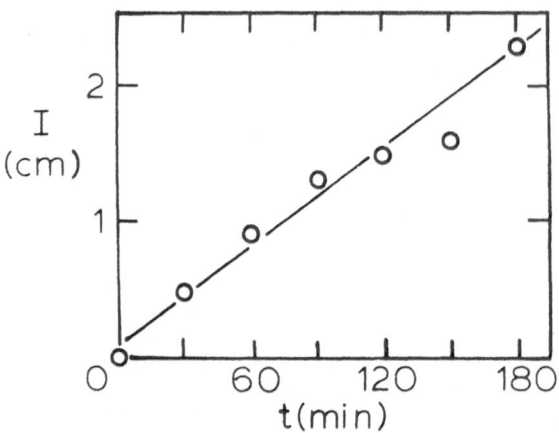

Fig. 21. Time course of β-glucan synthesis after the addition of 50 mM
[1-¹³C (90%)]-D-glucose to a suspension of protoplast-derived
suspensions of P. milliaceum cells.

        These experiments demonstrate that the synthesis of cell wall
polysaccharide material in plant cells can be monitored in situ, in
real time in the cells of moncots by means of ^{13}C NMR and ^{13}C labeling
of substrates. It will now be possible to study the regulation of this
process and its relation to the regeneration of callus tissue from
protoplasts. These studies are underway along with studies of the
structure of various alkalai-extractable cell wall fractions by means
of high resolution proton and ^{13}C NMR as well as with GC–MS.

This work was done under the auspices of the United States Department
of Energy.

5.0   REFERENCES

1. Sillerud, L. O. and Heyser, J. W. Plant Physiol. 75 (1984) 269.

2. Gupta, R. K. and Gupta, P. J. Magn. Reson. 47 (1982) 344.

3. Chu, S. C., Pike, M. M., Fossel, E. T., Smith, T. W., Balschi, J.
    A., and Springer, C. S. J. Magn. Reson. 56 (1984) 33.

4. Shulman, R. G., Brown, T. R., Ugurbil, K., Ogawa, S., Cohen, S. M.,
    and Den Hollander, J. A. Science 205 (1979) 160.

5. Sillerud, L. O., Alger, J. R., and Shulman, R. G. J. Magn. Reson. 45 (1981) 142.

6. Batchelor, J. G., Cushley, R. J., and Prestegard, J. H. J. Org. Chem. 39 (1974) 1698.

7. Sillerud, L. O., Han, C. H., Francendese, A. F., and Bitensky, M. W. J. Biol. Chem. (in press).

8. Alger, J. R., Sillerud, L. O., Behar, K. L., Gillies, R. J., Shulman, R. J., Gordon, R. E., Shaw, D., and Hanley, P. E. Science 214 (1981) 660.

9. Sillerud, L. O. and Shulman, R. G. Biochemistry 22 (1983) 1087.

10. Heyser, J. W. Z. Pflanzenphysiol. 113 (1984) 293.

11. Carpita, N. C. Plant Physiol. 72 (1983) 515.

12. Marx-Figini, M. In: Cellulose and Other Natural Polymers, R. M. Brown (Ed.) Plenum, New York (1982) 243.

13. Gast, J. C., Atalla, R. H., and McKelvey, R. D. Carbohydr. Res. 84 (1980) 137.

14. Sillerud, L. O. and Yu, R. K. Carbohydr. Res. 113 (1983) 173.

NMR MEASUREMENT OF INTRACELLULAR FREE MAGNESIUM IONS IN LIVING CELLS

Raj K. Gupta
Department of Physiology and Biophysics
Albert Einstein College of Medicine of Yeshiva University
New York, New York 10461
U.S.A.

ABSTRACT. ^{31}P NMR permits a noninvasive measurement of the extent of Mg^{2+}-complexation of ATP and the concentration of free magnesium from an accurate measurement of the Mg^{2+}-dependent chemical shift difference between the αP and βP resonances of intracellular ATP. The technique has been used to monitor intra-erythrocyte free Mg^{2+} during blood storage at $4^{\circ}C$ in standard citrate preservation media. The data indicated a marked decrease in the extent of Mg^{2+}-complexation of ATP, and in the level of intracellular free Mg^{2+}, during the shelf-life of blood stored in citrate media. Mg^{2+}-saturated and Mg^{2+}-depleted human erythrocytes exhibited the intra-erythrocyte ATP resonances at relative chemical shifts that were indistinguishable from those observed in noncellular MgATP and ATP controls, respectively. In another study, changes in intracellular free Mg^{2+} were observed in erythrocytes of patients with essential hypertension. Untreated hypertensive individuals consistently demonstrated lower levels of intra-erythrocyte free Mg^{2+} (192 ± 8 uM) than either normotensive (261 ± 10 uM) or hypertensive subjects whose blood pressure had been normalized on therapy (237 ± 8 uM). For all subjects, significant relationship existed between intra-erythrocyte free Mg^{2+} and diastolic as well as systolic blood pressure. It was concluded that significant depletion of intra-erythrocyte free Mg^{2+} is apparent in erythrocytes of subjects with essential hypertension. The observed linear relationship of free Mg^{2+} with the height of the blood pressure suggested that abnormalities of intracellular Mg^{2+} metabolism may contribute to the pathophysiology of human essential hypertension.

INTRODUCTION

Mg^{2+} is an essential component of all living cells. The intracellular concentration of free Mg^{2+} is of fundamental importance because it may regulate the activity of cellular reactions requiring this metal ion. While it is easy to measure total Mg^{2+} content of a cell by atomic absorption, a measurement of intracellular free Mg^{2+} is often more difficult. A non-invasive ^{31}P NMR method for determining free Mg^{2+} in intact cells has been described (1-3) and will be reviewed here along with some of its applications (1-11).

T. Axenrod and G. Ceccarelli (eds.), NMR in Living Systems, 335–345.
© *1986 by D. Reidel Publishing Company.*

^{31}P NMR MEASUREMENT OF INTRACELLULAR FREE MAGNESIUM

The ^{31}P NMR spectra of living cells generally show well-defined αP and βP resonances of ATP and their chemical shifts depend on the extent of Mg^{2+}-complexation by ATP. Because the level of intracellular Ca^{2+} is much lower than that of Mg^{2+}, and because Ca^{2+} resides mostly in membranes or mito-chondria, the complexation of ATP with Ca^{2+} is considered to be negligible. The chemical shift separation between the αP and βP resonances in the NMR spectrum allows a direct determination of the proportion of total intra-cellular ATP that exists as the Mg^{2+} complex. This separation is about 2.5 ppm greater for ATP than for MgATP, and for intermediate degrees of complexation the observed separation represents a weighted average, since magnesium ions exchange rapidly among ATP molecules on the NMR time scale. An accurate knowledge of the apparent dissociation constant of MgATP under simulated intracellular ionic conditions and pH would then yield free Mg^{2+} directly from the spectral data according to the following equations:

$$\phi = \frac{[ATP]_f}{[ATP]_T} = \frac{\delta_{\alpha\beta}^{cell} - \delta_{\alpha\beta}^{MgATP}}{\delta_{\alpha\beta}^{ATP} - \delta_{\alpha\beta}^{MgATP}} \qquad [1]$$

$$[Mg]_f = K_D^{MgATP} \left[\frac{1}{\phi} - 1 \right] \qquad [2]$$

where K_D^{MgATP} is the apparent dissociation constant of MgATP, $\delta_{\alpha\beta}^{cell}$ is the chemical shift separation between the αP and βP resonances of intracellu-lar ATP, $\delta_{\alpha\beta}^{ATP}$ and $\delta_{\alpha\beta}^{MgATP}$ are the values of this separation for noncellu-lar ATP and MgATP controls, respectively, $[ATP]_T$ is the concentration of total ATP, and $[ATP]_f$ is the sum of the concentrations of all ATP species not chelated to magnesium, i.e., $[KATP^{3-}]$, $[HATP^{3-}]$, and $[ATP^{4-}]$.

CHEMICAL SHIFTS OF ATP AND MgATP IN INTRACELLULAR ENVIRONMENT

An assumption implicit in the use of the NMR technique to study free Mg^{2+} in living systems is that the chemical shifts of the ^{31}P resonances of intracellular ATP respond to the presence of Mg^{2+} in a manner similar to that observed for isolated ATP. A critical part of this assumption is that, upon saturating cells with Mg^{2+}, the chemical shift separation $\delta_{\alpha\beta}^{cell}$ will decrease to that observed in isolated MgATP and that upon removal of intra-cellular Mg^{2+}, $\delta_{\alpha\beta}^{cell}$ will increase to that observed in isolated ATP. It is possible to test these assumptions using ionophore A23187 to equilibrate cytosolic free Mg^{2+} with that in the extracellular medium. Upon incubating oxygenated erythrocytes in the plasma containing divalent cation ionophore A23187 and excess Mg^{2+} which resulted in loading of erythrocytes with high internal Mg^{2+}, the observed chemical shift separation $\delta_{\alpha\beta}^{cell}$ at 22°C and 81 MHz, in a sample of stored human erythrocytes, decreased from 740 Hz to 686 Hz, a value essentially indistinguishable from that observed in extra-cellular MgATP controls under simulated intracellular ionic conditions (μ= 0.15 M) and pH (7.0) (figure 1). Incubation of the same erythrocytes in the plasma containing A23187, no added Mg^{2+} but excess EDTA to deplete most of the intracellular Mg^{2+} resulted in an increase in $\delta_{\alpha\beta}^{cell}$ to 860 Hz,

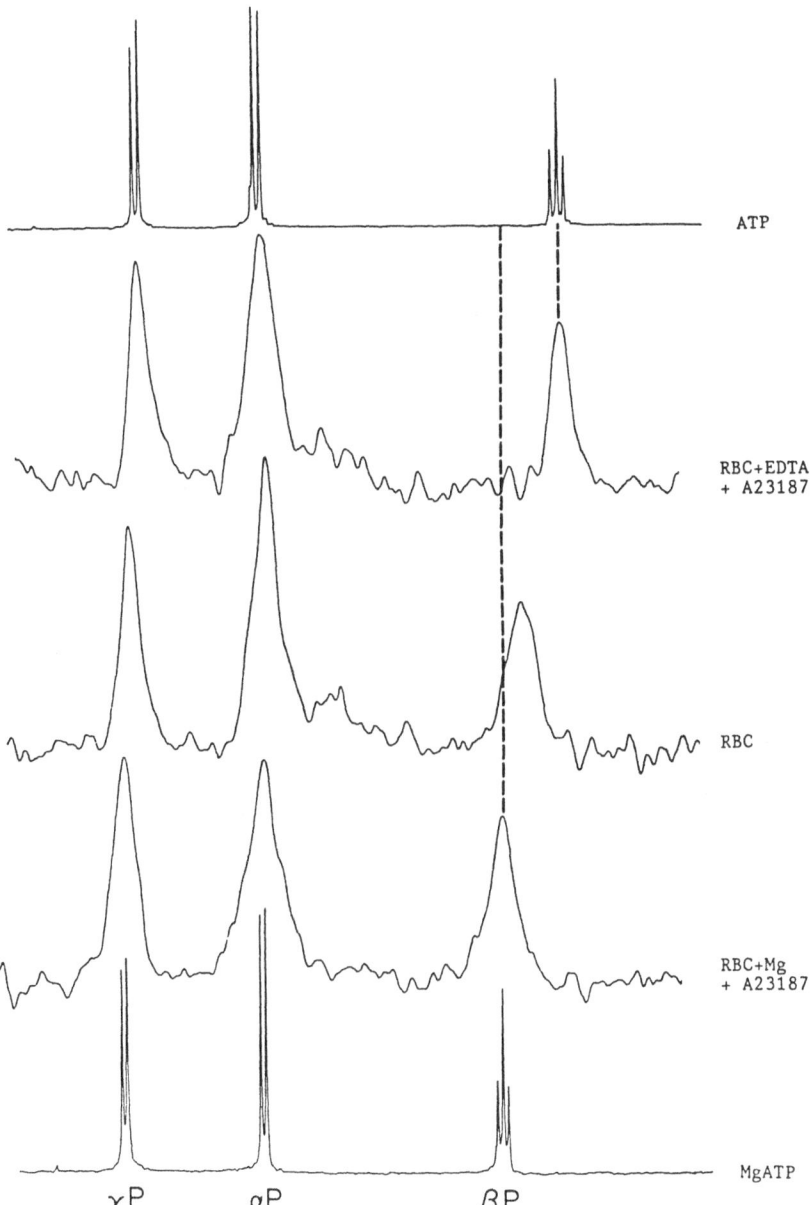

Figure 1. ^{31}P NMR spectra, at 81 MHz and 22°C, showing the effect of intracellular Mg^{2+} on the resonances of ATP in human red blood cells. Mg^{2+} and ionophore A23187 when present were at 20 mmol/l and 40 mg/l, respectively.

a value indistinguishable from that observed in extracellular ATP controls
(figure 1). The observation of similar shifts for the ATP and MgATP in
intact erythrocytes and the extracellular ATP and MgATP controls indicates
that the relative chemical shifts of the ^{31}P resonances of the red cell
ATP are determined predominantly by the normal interactions of Mg^{2+} and
ATP. The validity of the NMR method for determining free Mg^{2+} in the red
cell suggests that it is likely to be valid in other cell types as well.

DISSOCIATION CONSTANT OF MgATP

Accurate knowledge of the affinity of ATP for Mg^{2+} is crucial for calculation of free Mg^{2+} from NMR spectral data. It has recently been possible
to determine the apparent dissociation constant of MgATP by a combination
of optical and NMR techniques (5,6). An advantage of this method is that
it can be used to measure the apparent dissociation constant of MgATP at
physiological levels of the nucleotide. This may be important, since it is
possible that additional complexes form at higher concentrations of ATP.
The combination method utilizes ^{31}P NMR chemical shifts to determine the
degree of Mg^{2+}-chelation of ATP (ϕ) in a solution containing free ATP and
MgATP, and uses an indicator dye antipyrylazo III for optical measurement
of free Mg^{2+} in the same solution. Equation 2 is then used to obtain K_D^{MgATP}.
An average value of 50±10 uM has been obtained at 25°C and pH 7.2 by this
method. Other magnetic resonance methods have yielded similar values of
38±6 uM at 37°C (12), 45±8 uM at 25°C (13) and 60±10 uM at 10°C (2) for
this constant. A critical analysis of the inadequacy of various definitions of the apparent dissociation constant of MgATP and the need to avoid
mixing different definitions in data analysis has been presented (14).

APPLICATIONS OF THE ^{31}P NMR METHOD FOR FREE MAGNESIUM DETERMINATION

Measurements of intracellular free Mg^{2+} by the NMR technique have been
described in fresh human red blood cells (1), stored human erythrocytes
(10,11), erythrocytes from patients with essential hypertension (8), frog
skeletal muscle (3), Ehrlich ascites tumor cells (2), murine lymphoma
cells (15), human lymphocytes (16), dog erythrocytes (17), perfused and
ischemic heart muscle (5), rabbit urinary bladder (18), rat uterus (19),
and amphibian oocytes (9). The results consistently indicated that the
intracellular concentration of free Mg^{2+} is low, in the range 0.5±0.3 mM,
and that only a very small part of the total cell Mg^{2+} is uncomplexed in
each tissue. Low intracellular availability of Mg^{2+} supports a role for
free Mg^{2+} in the regulation of metabolic processes, e.g., the activation
and regulation of the hormone receptor-adenylate cyclase complex by
intracellular free Mg^{2+} (15,20).
    The free Mg^{2+} level in erythrocytes was found by Flatman & Lew (21)
to be low (~0.4 mM) using an ionophore A23187 method. Confirmation of NMR-
measured free Mg^{2+} levels in Ehrlich ascites tumor cells has recently been
reported by Cittadini and Scarpa, who used a null-point method with the
ionophore A23187 (22). Mg^{2+} selective microelectrodes however produced an
estimate of free magnesium in the millimolar range (3.3 mM) in intact frog
muscle (23). The use of metallochromic indicator dyes resulted in widely
different estimates of free Mg^{2+} ranging from 0.2 to 6 mM depending on the

dye used (24). It has been proposed that the most likely explanation for variability of the dye methods is that the indicator dyes behave differently inside muscle fibers than in calibrating solutions. The same may well be true for the invasive microelectrodes also. The ability to verify the applicability of ATP and MgATP ^{31}P chemical shifts in calibrating solutions to the intracellular environment in the red cell, however, indicates that the noninvasive NMR method may indeed be more reliable than the various invasive procedures in the study of living cells.

CHANGES IN INTRA-ERYTHROCYTE FREE MAGNESIUM DURING BLOOD STORAGE

The erythrocytes in liquid-stored blood undergo progressive morphologic and biochemical changes. Many of these changes are rapidly reversed after transfusion. However, an increasing number of erythrocytes suffer permanent damage during storage and are rapidly hemolyzed in-vivo. For this reason blood collected in standard preservation media has a limited shelf-life, ranging from 3 to 5 weeks in citrate-containing media which is far shorter than the 120 days life-span of erythrocytes in-vivo. The basis of this reduced survival of erythrocytes during in-vitro liquid-storage is not well understood.

Since citrate is a chelator of divalent cations, the possibility that storage in citrate media might damage cells by diminishing the intracellular concentration of free Mg^{2+} ions, which would be detrimental to cell viability, has been investigated (10,11). The ^{31}P NMR technique has been used to demonstrate a substantial decline in free Mg^{2+} during storage of blood at 4°C in standard citrate preservation media (10,11).

Changes in the ^{31}P NMR spectrum of stored erythrocytes are illustrated in figure 2 which compares the 81 MHz NMR spectra (at 22°C) of human erythrocytes immediately after collection in CPDA-1 (citrate-phosphate-dextrose-adenine) medium and after 21 days storage at 4°C. Similar changes are observed in ACD (acid-citrate-dextrose) medium. During storage the resonances arising from the 2- and 3-phosphates of 2,3-DPG diminished markedly, the P_i resonance increased and shifted downfield indicating a decrease in intracellular pH. The βP resonance of ATP became broadened and shifted upfield, the chemical shift separation between the αP and βP resonances increased indicating an increase in the fraction of total ATP not complexed to magnesium (ϕ). The $\delta_{\alpha\beta}^{MgATP}$ and $\delta_{\alpha\beta}^{ATP}$ used in the calculation of ϕ using equation 1 were obtained from measurements on model solutions with pH adjusted to match intracellular pH of stored blood which was estimated from the chemical shift separation between the P_i and the αP resonance of ATP and varied in the range 7.2 - 6.8 depending on the length of storage. A pH correction to K_D^{MgATP} which was measured at pH 7.2 was also necessary prior to use in equation 2 for estimating free Mg^{2+} at lower intracellular pH values, since protons will compete with Mg^{2+} for binding to ATP. This correction for pH changes was made assuming a pK_a for ATP^{2-} of 6.6 and that the protonated form $HATP^{3-}$ has negligible affinity for Mg^{2+}, and amounted to a correction factor of $\leqslant 1.2$ in calculating free Mg^{2+} (11).

In several blood samples stored at 4°C in ACD or CPDA-1 media, either as red cell concentrate or whole blood, the chemical shift separation $\delta_{\alpha\beta}^{cell}$ changed from an average value of 721±1.4 Hz on the day of storage to 741 ±3.4 and 774±2.8 Hz after 3-7 and 11-40 days of storage, respectively. The intracellular pH changed from 7.16±0.03 on the day of storage to 7.05±0.02 after 3-7 and 6.89±0.02 after 11-40 days of storage. The fraction of ATP not complexed to Mg^{2+}, ϕ, changed from 0.19±0.01 on the day of storage to 0.29±0.02 and 0.43±0.02 after 3-7 and 11-40 days of storage, respectively, corresponding to a decline in free Mg^{2+} from 214±7 uM on the day of storage to 138±10 uM after 3-7 days and to 81±5 uM, or about 40% of the original value, after 11-40 days of storage at 4°C. In two aliquots of blood obtained from a single donor, one of which was stored in ACD, the other in CPDA-1, the progressive increase in ϕ and decrease in free Mg^{2+} were somewhat larger for ACD than for CPDA-1 medium. The storage-induced increase in ϕ was observed for all samples examined. The rate of loss of free Mg^{2+} varied somewhat among various blood units but generally diminished after about a week of storage. Measurements, however, clearly showed that fresh units, units stored for less than a week, and units stored for more than a week were statistically distinguishable groups with respect to intra-erythrocyte free Mg^{2+}. The increase in ϕ that occurs upon storage was reversible. When stored erythrocytes with increased ϕ were incubated with plasma containing excess Mg^{2+} and A23187, the $\delta_{\alpha\beta}^{cell}$ reverted to that for isolated MgATP (figure 1). In contrast to the progressive decrease in free Mg^{2+} in citrate media, heparinized blood stored for a week exhibited decreased ATP and increased intra-erythrocyte free Mg^{2+}.

The ^{31}P NMR spectroscopy thus clearly demonstrates a substantial decrease in Mg^{2+}-complexation of ATP and in intracellular free Mg^{2+} during conventional storage of liquid blood for transfusion. The parameter $\delta_{\alpha\beta}^{cell}$ is particularly sensitive to Mg^{2+}-complexation, and the changes observed during blood storage are too large to be ascribed to any other factors. It appears likely that the observed decline in free Mg^{2+} is related to the presence of citrate in the presevation media since it is not observed in heparinized blood.

Mg^{2+} ions are essential cofactors in a number of biochemical reactions. It is the MgATP complex, rather than free ATP, that serves as a donor of high energy phosphate. Accordingly, measurements of total ATP in stored blood may be somewhat misleading as a measure of metabolic integrity since MgATP appears to decline more rapidly than total ATP. Since free Mg^{2+} even in fresh erythrocytes is probably low enough to limit the rates of certain metabolic reactions, its marked decline during storage must surely affect the physiology of the cell and may reduce the viability and life-span of liquid-stored blood. Altered intra-erythrocyte free Mg^{2+} may also affect the oxygen-transporting ability of transfused red cells and the rate at which they recover from other types of storage damage, such as 2,3-DPG depletion (11).

INTRACELLULAR FREE MAGNESIUM OF ERYTHROCYTES IN ESSENTIAL HYPERTENSION

Isolated observations over five decades suggest an association of Mg^{2+} metabolism with blood pressure regulation. Indeed, Mg^{2+} was first recommended as therapy of malignant hypertension as early as 1925 (25). Since that time, basic research has documented the ability of Mg^{2+} depletion to alter vascular smooth muscle tone, perhaps by affecting the intracellular disposition of calcium (26). In order to clarify the clinical relevance of Mg^{2+} to human hypertensive disease, ^{31}P NMR spectroscopy was utilized

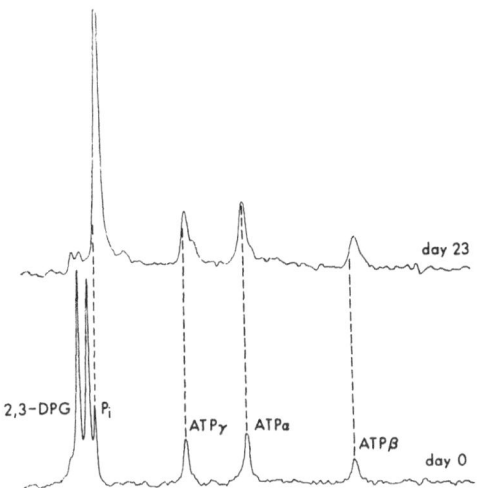

<u>Figure 2.</u> ^{31}P NMR spectra, at 81 MHz and 22°C, of blood collected in CPDA-1, on the day of collection (bottom) and after storage for 23 days at 4°C (top), showing the change in chemical shift of the ATP β resonance.

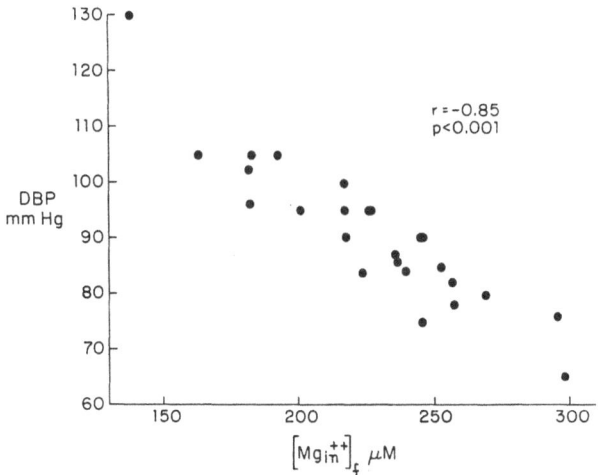

<u>Figure 3.</u> Relationship of intracellular free Mg^{2+} ($[Mg_{in}^{++}]_f$) to diastolic blood pressure (DBP) for all subjects. Regression analysis used the Pearson correlation coefficient and Student t test for level of significance (8).

to assess intra-erythrocyte levels of free Mg^{2+} ion and to relate them
to levels of blood pressure. The findings suggested consistent abnormalities of intracellular free Mg^{2+} levels in subjects with essential hypertension, which were closely linked to the height of blood pressure (8).

Hypertensive subjects, either untreated (n=11) or normotensive on
therapy (n=8), and normotensive individuals on no medical therapy (n=7)
were studied. All subjects fasted overnight, had blood pressure measured
and then, in the seated position, had peripheral venous blood drawn for
analysis of intra-erythrocyte free magnesium levels. Untreated hypertensive subjects had blood pressures (165±7/102±3 mm of Hg) significantly
higher than normotensive controls (125±8/74±3 mm of Hg) and diastolic
pressures higher than treated hypertensive subjects. Treated hypertensive
individuals had blood pressures (150±8/83±1 mm of Hg) considered to be
adequate on present medical regimens. Medical therapy in treated hypertensive subjects consisted of a variety of pharmacologic agents, including spironolactone, beta blockers, hydrochlorothiazide, nifedipine, and
prazosin. Serum levels of electrolytes did not distinguish hypertensive
subjects, either treated or untreated, from normotensive controls, and
both serum free calcium and total magnesium were within normal limits (8).

Intracellular free Mg^{2+} levels were clearly and significantly
different among the different patient groups. Normotensive controls had
intra-erythrocyte free Mg^{2+} at 261±10 uM. In comparison, untreated hypertensive subjects had intracellular free Mg^{2+} levels (192±8 uM) that were
significantly lower than those of normotensive controls. Furthermore, drug-
treated hypertensive subjects, whose blood pressures were significantly
lower than those of untreated hypertensive subjects, had intracellular
free Mg^{2+} levels (237±8 uM) significantly greater than those of the untreated hypertensive group but indistinguishable from levels in normotensive controls. Remarkable relationships were observed between intracellular free Mg^{2+} and the concurrent blood pressure for all subjects.
Systolic blood pressure correlated negatively with intracellular free Mg^{2+}
(r=-0.71, P<0.001), but diastolic blood pressure was even more strongly and
inversely linked to intracellular free Mg^{2+} (r=-0.85, P<0.001) (figure 3).

Thus individuals with essential hypertension had consistently lower
levels of intracellular free Mg^{2+} than did normotensive control subjects;
hypertensive individuals, who on therapy had achieved normalization of
their blood pressure, had levels of intracellular free magnesium that were
significantly higher than those of untreated hypertensive subjects and
indistinguishable from those of normotensive control subjects; and a continuous inverse relationship was observed between intracellular free Mg^{2+}
and the height of the blood pressure (figure 3). These findings strongly
suggest a physiologic relationship between intracellular Mg^{2+} metabolism
and blood pressure regulation and pathophysiologically suggest intracellular Mg^{2+} depletion to be common in human essential hypertension (8).

The heretofore unappreciated close quantitative relationship between
intracellular free magnesium and hypertension suggested by the NMR data is
supported by previous in-vitro and whole-animal studies and by certain
clinical observations. Altura and Altura in a series of studies have demonstrated for a variety of vascular beds in different species that Mg^{2+}
levels strongly influence vascular tone and vascular responsiveness to
pressor agents (27). Furthermore, these authors have recently shown that
dietary magnesium depletion in rats decreases levels of serum magnesium,

decreases luminal diameter of peripheral resistance vessels, and increases blood pressure (28). Similarly, it has been reported that varying dietary Mg^{2+} levels in the spontaneously hypertensive rats enhanced or retarded development of high blood pressure when animals were fed low or high Mg^{2+}-containing diets, respectively (29). Clinically, Mg^{2+} was first shown to lower blood pressure in patients with malignant hypertension as early as 1925 and by 1942 was also shown to lower pressure in some, but not all, chronic hypertensive individuals (30). The hypotensive efficacy of oral Mg^{2+} supplementation in essential hypertensive subjects on diuretic therapy has also been reported (31). Short-term Mg^{2+} therapy in essential hypertensive subjects preferentially lowered blood pressure in patients with elevated plasma renin activity (8). Significantly, these hypertensive subjects with higher renin levels had lower initial levels of serum Mg^{2+} (32).

It is of interest to speculate as to how intracellular Mg^{2+} depletion might result in the increased peripheral resistance characteristic of diverse forms of hypertensive disease. The ability of Mg^{2+} to influence blood pressure might be related to its effect on intracellular Ca^{2+} metabolism. Mg^{2+} is a weak antagonist of Ca^{2+} entry into vascular smooth muscle, and may induce vasodilatation comparable to that of calcium-channel inhibitors. Indeed, Mg^{2+} appears to potentiate verapamil-induced vasodilatation (33). The intracellular content and disposition of Ca^{2+} is also influenced by Mg^{2+}, and Ca^{2+} binding at intracellular sites may be antagonized by Mg^{2+}. Thus, magnesium shifts the force-calcium relationship of muscle contraction to the right, possibly suggestive of decreased calcium binding to myofilament regulatory sites (34). Furthermore, Mg^{2+} stimulates sarcoplasmic reticulum Ca^{2+} influx and inhibits calcium dependent-efflux. Mg^{2+} may also retard calcium efflux into the extracellular space, perhaps related to intracellular sequestration (26). Therefore, because smooth muscle tension development is directly linked to available cytosolic free Ca^{2+}, one would hypothesize that lower levels of intracellular free Mg^{2+} would be associated with higher intracellular free Ca^{2+} levels in proportion to the degree of intracellular Mg^{2+} depletion and, thus, be associated with proportionately higher blood pressures. This hypothesized reciprocal relationship between intracellular free Mg^{2+} and blood pressure is exactly what was observed (figure 3). This hypothesis is also supported by recent measurements of intracellular free calcium in normal and hypertensive human platelets (35). Regardless of hypothesized mechanisms, however, the NMR data suggest intracellular Mg^{2+} as a biochemical regulator of the physiology and pathophysiology of blood pressure control in man (8).

CONCLUSIONS

^{31}P NMR can be exploited to measure free Mg^{2+} ions in living cells and tissues. The technique has a major advantage of being noninvasive. It appears limited at present by the complexities of the cellular system, such as possible compartmentation of free Mg^{2+} in the cells. Only one set of ATP signals is, however, seen which must represent the average of nuclear and cytosolic ATP. It is likely that ATP in these areas and the mitochondria exchange rapidly. Therefore, the measurements would appear to provide a good approximation to the true level of free Mg^{2+} in intact cells.

ACKNOWLEDGEMENT

The preparation of this article and much of the research described herein
were supported by the United States National Institutes of Health Grant
AM-32030, and by National Cancer Institute Core Grant CA-13330.

REFERENCES

1. Gupta, R.K., Benovic, J.L. and Rose, Z.B. 1978, J. Biol. Chem. 253,
   pp. 6172-76.
2. Gupta, R.K. and Yushok, W.D. 1980, Proc. Natl. Acad. Sci. USA 77,
   pp. 2487-91.
3. Gupta, R.K. and Moore, R.D. 1980, J. Biol. Chem. 255, pp. 3987-93.
4. Gupta, R.K. 1980, Int. J. Quant. Chem. Quant. Biol. Symp. 7, pp. 67-73.
5. Gupta, R.K., Gupta, P., Yushok, W.D. and Rose, Z.B. 1983, Biochem.
   Biophys. Res. Commun. 117, pp. 210-216.
6. Gupta, R.K., Gupta, P., Yushok, W.D. and Rose, W.D. 1983, Physiol.
   Chem. Phys. Med. NMR 15, pp. 265-280.
7. Gupta, R.K., Gupta, P. and Moore, R.D. 1984, Annu. Rev. Biophys.
   Bioeng. 13, pp. 221-246.
8. Resnick, L.M., Gupta, R.K. and Laragh, J.H. 1984, Proc. Natl. Acad.
   Sci. USA 81, pp. 6511-6515.
9. Gupta, R.K., Kostellow, A.B. and Morrill, G.A. 1983, Biophys. J. 41,
   p. 128a.
10. Bock, J.L., Wenz, B. and Gupta, R.K. 1984, Biophys. J. 45, p. 242a.
11. Bock, J.L., Wenz, B. and Gupta, R.K. 1985, Blood, in press.
12. Gupta, R.K. and Benovic, J.L. 1978, Biochem. Biophys. Res. Commun.
    84, pp. 130-37.
13. Gupta, R.K., Benovic, J.L. and Rose, Z.B. 1978, J. Biol. Chem. 253,
    pp. 6165-71.
14. Garfinkel, L. and Garfinkel, D. 1984, Biochemistry 23, pp. 3547-3552.
15. Erdos, J.J. and Maguire, M.E. 1983, J. Physiol. (London) 337,
    pp. 351-71.
16. Rink, T.J., Tsien, R.Y. and Pozzan, T. 1982, J. Cell Biol. 95,
    pp. 189-96.
17. Wyrwicz, A.M., Schofield, J.C. and Burt, C.T. 1982, in "Probes of
    Tissue Metabolism" (J.S. Cohen, ed.), Wiley Intersci., NY, pp. 149-71.
18. Dillon, P.F., Meyer, R.A., Kushmerick, M.J. and Brown, T.R. 1983,
    Biophys. J. 41, p. 252a.
19. Degani, H., Shaer, A., Victor, T.A. and Kaye, A.M. 1984, Biochemistry
    23, pp. 2572-2577.
20. Cech, S.Y., Broadus, W.C. and Maguire, M.E. 1980, Mol. Cell. Biochem.
    33, pp. 67-92.
21. Flatman, P. and Lew, V.L. 1977, Nature 267, pp. 360-62.
22. Cittadini, L. and Scarpa, A. 1983, Arch. Biochem. Biophys. 227,
    pp. 202-208.
23. Hess, P. and Weingart, R. 1981, J. Physiol. (London) 318, pp. 14-15.
24. Baylor, S.M., Chandler, W.K. and Marshall, M.W. 1982, J. Physiol.
    (London) 331, pp. 105-37.
25. Blackfan, K.D. and Hamilton, B. 1925, Boston Med. Surg. J. 193,
    pp. 617-628.

26. Altura, B.M. and Altura, B.T. 1981, Fed. Proc. 40, pp. 2672-2679.
27. Altura, B.M. and Altura, B.T. 1978, Blood Vessels 15, pp. 5-16.
28. Altura, B.M., Altura, B.T., Gebrewold, A., Ising, H. and Gunther, T. 1984, Science 223, pp. 1315-1317.
29. Berthelot, A. and Esposito, J. 1983, J. Am. Coll. Nutr. 4, pp. 343-353.
30. Winkler, A.W., Smith, P.K. and Hoff, H.E. 1942, J. Clin. Invest. 21, pp. 207-216.
31. Dyckner, T. and Wester, P.O. 1983, Br. Med. J. 286, pp. 1847-1849.
32. Resnick, L.M., Laragh, J.H., Sealey, J.E. and Alderman, M.H. 1983, N. Engl. J. Med. 309, pp. 888-891.
33. Phillips, R.J.W. and Robinson, B.F. 1984, Clin. Sci. 66, p. 39.
34. Stephenson, W.E. 1981, Fed. Proc. 40, pp. 2662-2666.
35. Erne, P., Bolli, P., Burgissen, E., Buhler, F.R. and Bolli, P. 1983, N. Engl. J. Med. 310, pp. 1084-1088.

NMR STUDIES OF DRUG RECEPTOR COMPLEXES: ANTIFOLATE DRUGS BINDING TO
DIHYDROFOLATE REDUCTASE

J. Feeney
Physical Biochemistry Division
National Institute for Medical Research
Mill Hill, London NW7 1AA
U.K.

ABSTRACT. NMR is a useful method for studying the basis for the specificity of interactions between proteins and small ligand molecules.
We have used this method to study the binding of antifolate drugs such
as trimethoprim, methotrexate and related analogues to their target
enzyme dihydrofolate reductase. Detailed information about the conformations, ionisation states, interactions and dynamic processes within
the drug-receptor complexes has been obtained. With the data available
from X-ray and NMR studies it is possible to use molecular modelling
techniques to design inhibitors with improved binding properties.

1. INTRODUCTION

The functions of many biological systems depend, at some stage, on the
formation of non-covalent complexes between interacting molecules, and
considerable efforts are being made to understand the molecular recognition processes involved in these interactions. Typical examples are
protein-DNA, enzyme-substrate, enzyme-inhibitor, hormone-receptor and
neurotransmitter-receptor interactions. We have been using high resolution NMR spectroscopy to study the factors controlling the specificity
of such interactions in drug-receptor complexes. The aims of the work
are firstly to develop the NMR methodology for studying interactions
involving biological macromolecules in solution and secondly to provide
a basis for rational drug design. We have been studying the binding of
'antifolate' drugs such as trimethoprim (anti-bacterial) and methotrexate (anti-neoplastic) and various substrate analogues, to their target
enzyme dihydrofolate reductase (see Scheme I). This enzyme catalyses
the reduction of dihydrofolate (or folate with lower efficiency) to
tetrahydrofolate using NADPH as coenzyme.

$$\text{Folate} + \text{NADPH} + \text{H}^+ \rightarrow 7,8\text{-dihydrofolate} + \text{NADP}^+$$
$$7,8\text{-Dihydrofolate} + \text{NADPH} + \text{H}^+ \rightarrow 5,6,7,8\text{-tetrahydrofolate} + \text{NADP}^+$$

The product of the reaction, tetrahydrofolate is an important cofactor
required in the biosynthesis of purines, pyrimidines and some amino

347

T. Axenrod and G. Ceccarelli (eds.), NMR in Living Systems, 347–366.

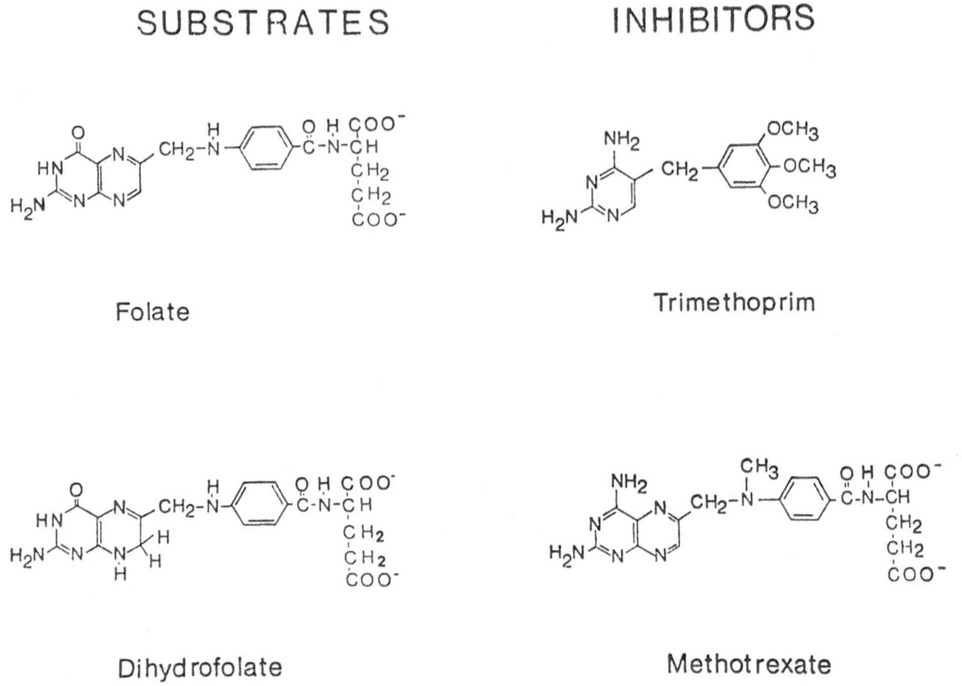

SUBSTRATES

INHIBITORS

Folate

Trimethoprim

Dihydrofolate

Methotrexate

Scheme I

acids. Thus dihydrofolate reductase is an essential enzyme in the cell and several clinically important antifolate drugs act by inhibiting this enzyme in invasive cells (1). In the case of the antibacterial drug trimethoprim, selective inhibition of the bacterial enzyme over the mammalian enzyme results from the fact that the trimethoprim binds three to four orders of magnitude more tightly to the bacterial dihydrofolate reductase. Our studies have been mainly concerned with the enzyme isolated from *Lactobacillus casei* (2) and they have been considerably aided by the availability of detailed crystallographic data on a ternary complex of the enzyme with methotrexate and NADPH(3). The enzyme has a relatively low molecular weight (17,860 Daltons) and is ideal for an NMR investigation of drug-receptor complexes.

In the present case the drug molecule D can be considered to bind to its receptor R to form a non-covalently bound complex DR

$$D + R \rightleftharpoons DR$$

The starting point in these investigations is to measure the equilibrium binding constants Ka for the complex of interest

$$Ka = \frac{[DR]}{[D][R]}$$

where [D], [R] and [DR] are the concentrations of drug, receptor and complex respectively. These measurements are usually made using fluorescence techniques (4,5,6) but NMR methods can also be used to good advantage for complexes involving weakly binding ligands (Ka < 10^3 M^{-1}) if the criteria for NMR 'fast exchange' conditions are fully satisfied (7). The Ka values allow us to estimate the binding energies (ΔG = -RTlnKa) reflecting how tightly the drugs are binding to the receptor. NMR measurements on a drug-receptor complex used in combination with the X-ray crystallographic data on related complexes often provide details of how the drug is binding in molecular terms. The NMR method can provide information about:-

  (i) *Ionisation states* in the drug-receptor complex
 (ii) *Interacting groups* in the drug and the receptor
(iii) *Conformational changes* accompanying binding and the presence of
       multiple conformational states.
 (iv) *Dynamics* of the dissociation of the complex and of molecular
       motions within the drug receptor complex (such as 'ring-flipping')

2.   ASSIGNMENT OF NMR SIGNALS IN COMPLEXES

Detailed information about the complexes can only be obtained from studying resonances which have been assigned to individual nuclei in either the bound drug molecule or the protein.

2.1 Ligand Signals

For nuclei in a very tightly bound ligand such as methotrexate (Ka > 10^{10} M^{-1}) such assignments are best made by examining isotopically labelled analogues (^2H or ^{13}C labelled) and observing the differences between spectra from the complexes of the enzyme formed with labelled and unlabelled ligands (8,9). Alternatively, assignments can be made using NOE (Nuclear Overhauser effects) measurements to connect resonances of ligand nuclei with those of assigned protein nuclei which are expected to be in close proximity from crystal structure studies. Complexes with less tightly bound ligands (Ka $\approx$ 10^6 M^{-1}) such as trimethoprim while still giving spectra showing slow exchange behaviour (separate signals being observed for bound and free species) have dissociation rate constants which allow us to use the saturation transfer method to assign the bound ligand signals. This method connects the bound signals with their corresponding free ligand signals (9-13), and also provides a direct method of measuring the dissociation rate constants (8,12,14). Complexes formed with more weakly binding ligands (Ka $\sim$ 10^3 M^{-1}) such as p-amino benzoyl-L-glutamate usually give spectra showing fast exchange behaviour where the bound and free species give a single spectrum with averaged parameters. The chemical shifts of the bound and free ligand and the equilibrium binding constant can

be calculated from analysis of binding curves where the observed averaged shift is plotted as a function of ligand concentration (15,16).
Sometimes, it is difficult to assess when conditions of true fast
exchange are present and it is possible to have a system appearing to
be in fast exchange but which has observed shifts that are not given by
the simple weighted average of the shifts in the bound and free species:
we have recently calculated the errors involved in analysing such cases
(7). We have shown that if the observed averaged shift for the ligand
can be measured at very low ligand concentrations (for example [ligand]
= 0.1 mM and [enzyme] = 1 mM] then a reliable estimate of the bound
chemical shift can usually be obtained. It is usually impossible to
see signals in the ^{1}H spectrum arising from such small amounts of ligand
in the presence of the complex spectrum from the enzyme. In collabor-
ative experiments with Kaptein we have overcome this using the photo
induced CIDNP technique (17). In the presence of a laser-excited flavin
dye, the H3',H5' proton nuclei in free p-amino benzoyl-L-glutamate are
strongly polarised and give rise to intense signals (18). This method
allows us to detect these signals in dilute solutions of the ligand
(0.1 mM) in the presence of excess enzyme (1 mM).

For complexes of the enzyme with the coenzyme, ^{31}P NMR allows us
to study the bound 2'-phosphate and pyrophosphate phosphorus nuclei
directly to obtain information about ionisation states and conformations
in the bound state (16,19-22).

2.2 Protein Signals

Using a combination of one dimensional (NOE difference spectra and spin
echo decoupling difference spectra) and two dimensional (COSY and NOESY)
experiments we have now assigned protein signals in 28 individual
residues (25). These include the aromatic protons of the five Tyr res-
isues, seven His residues, Phe 49 and several aliphatic protons in Leu,
Val, Ile and Thr residues. The assignment procedures assume that the
crystal structure of the enzyme.NADPH.methotrexate complex (3) will be
similar to its structure in solution. We have prepared and examined
selectively deuterated enzymes and these allow us to make unequivocal
assignments of signals to residue type (23-26). For example we have
compared the ^{1}H spectra of a complex formed with enzyme containing
(γ-^{2}H) labelled valine with one from a complex formed with non-labelled
valine: the difference spectrum clearly indicates the location of the
15 valine methyl signals in the spectrum (25). The detailed assignments of the high field signals from valines and 10 other residues have
been made using COSY experiments to connect nuclei which are scalar
coupled and NOESY experiments to connect nuclei in close spatial
proximity (25).

The combined use of isotopically labelled proteins with the modern
two dimensional NMR techniques now available should allow assignments
to be made for proteins as large as 40,000 Daltons.

We have also explored the potential of using ^{19}F NMR to study the
fluorine-labelled enzyme by incorporating fluorinated derivatives of
tryptophan, tyrosine or phenylalanine into the enzyme (26a,c,27,28).
The 6-fluorotryptophan labelled enzyme showed four signals two of which

showed scalar ^{19}F-^{19}F coupling (17 Hz) from a through space scalar mechanism indicating that these nuclei, from different residues, are separated by less than 4 Å (28). London and co-workers (29) have successfully incorporated γ-^{13}C Trp into dihydrofolate reductase from *S. faecium* and found evidence for two slowly interconverting states.

3. COMPLEXES WITH METHOTREXATE AND FOLATE ANALOGUES

3.1 Role of the Glutamate Moiety in Binding

From the crystal structure studies of Matthews and co-workers (3) it is known that the α-carboxylate of the methotrexate glutamate moiety forms an ion-pair with the guanidine group of the conserved Arg 57 and that the γ-carboxylate forms a second ion-pair with the imidazole ring of His 28 as shown in Figure 1. Previous NMR studies on enzyme-methotrexate complexes had shown that the latter interaction is accompanied by

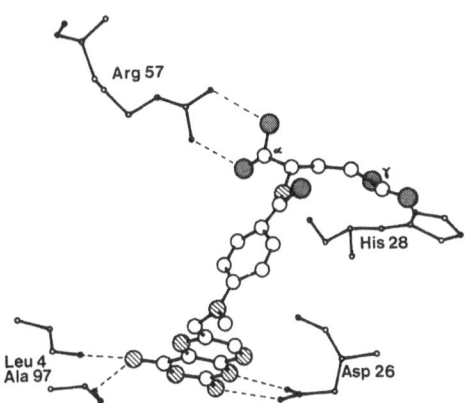

Figure 1. The conformation of methotrexate in its binding site in the ternary complex with NADPH and *L. casei* dihydrofolate reductase (From crystal data kindly supplied by D.A. Matthews (3))

an increase of one unit in the imidazole pK of His 28 as measured from the pH dependence of the histidine C2 proton resonance signals (30). NMR studies on complexes of methotrexate amides with the enzyme (31) indicate that modification of either the γ- or α-carboxylate removes this interaction with His 28 as seen from the pH titration curves of the His 28 C2 proton chemical shift shown in Figure 2. While the result was as expected for the γ-amide it was not predicted for the α-amide. Clearly the removal of the α-carboxylate-Arg 57 interaction in some way disrupts the γ-carboxylate-His 28 interaction. The removal of both interactions in the complex with the α-amide explains why modification

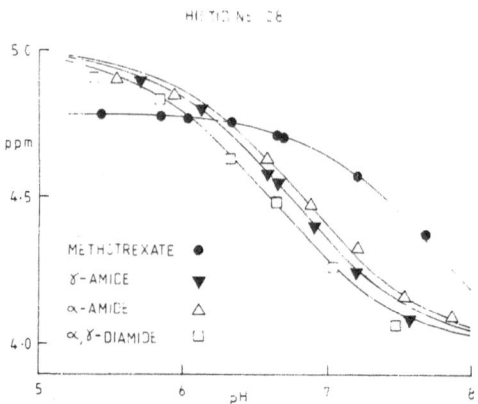

Figure 2. The titration curves resulting from plots of the C2 proton
chemical shifts of His 28 as a function of pH for complexes formed by
methotrexate and its amides with dihydrofolate reductase (31).

of the α-carboxylate has a larger effect on the binding to the enzyme
than does modification of the γ-carboxylate. Thus NMR is providing us
with a method of monitoring the ionisation state of an individual
residue in the complex and reporting on whether or not it is involved
in a strong electrostatic interaction with a nearby interacting group.
From the observed changes in binding constant in the different complexes
and knowing that both the α- and γ-interactions are broken in the
α-amide methotrexate complex we could estimate that the two interactions made similar contributions to the binding energy ($\sim$5.6 KJ mol^{-1}).
     The perturbation in the pK of His 28 is also seen in complexes of
folate and its analogues with the enzyme. In fact the p-aminobenzoyl-
L-glutamate fragment of folate also shows this effect: studies of such
weakly binding fragments can be useful in isolating which parts of the
enzyme structure are perturbed by the various parts of the complete
substrate analogue (30).

3.2 Comparison of Conformation of Folate and Methotrexate when bound
to dihydrofolate reductase

Although methotrexate has a very similar structure to folate differing
only in that it has a 4-amino substituent instead of the 4-oxy group of
folate and has a methyl group at the N10 position, this analogue binds
much more tightly to the enzyme (> 10^3 fold increase) and is not a
substrate. Such similar molecules might reasonably have been expected
to bind to the enzyme in a broadly similar manner: however a combination of X-ray crystallographic and NMR studies has shown that

methotrexate binds with its pteridine ring 'upside-down' compared to its position in the folate-enzyme complex (32-34). Using NADPH (see Scheme II) labelled with deuterium (^{2}H) at the 4-position on the nicotinamide

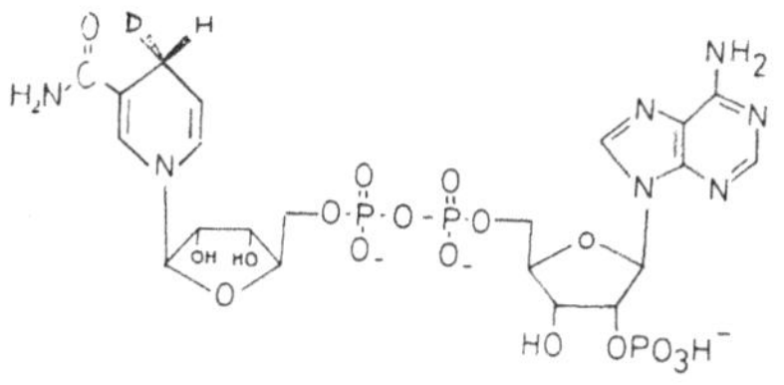

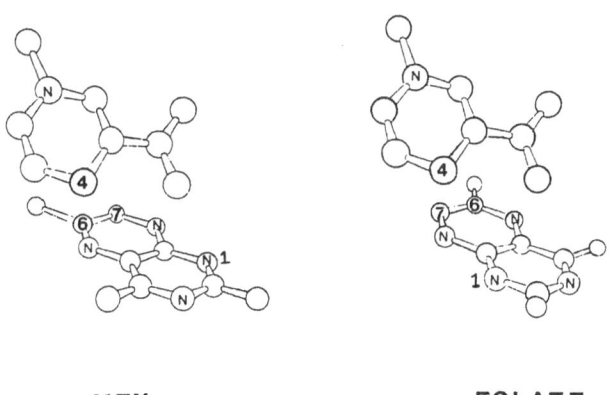

NADPH

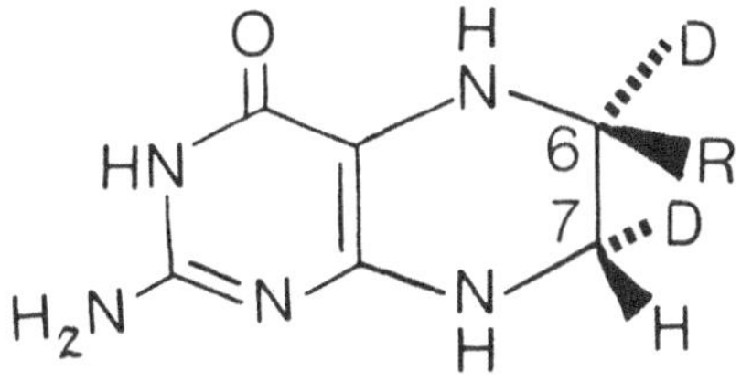

Scheme II

A-side we have reduced folate to tetrahydrofolate and shown by NMR that both transferred protons (to the 6 and 7 positions) are added to the same side of the pteridine ring. Bugg and co-workers (34) had previously determined the absolute configuration at the C-6 position of tetrahydrofolate analogues using crystallographic studies: this is as shown in Scheme II with the C-6 proton on the underside of the ring in the structure.

MTX   **FOLATE**

Figure 3. The orientation of the pteridine ring with respect to the reduced nicotinamide ring of NADPH in complexes of dihydrofolate reductase with methotrexate (left) and folate (right).

From our NMR results we now know that the proton added at C-7 is also on the underside of the ring. It is now possible to draw a complex showing how the reduced nicotinamide ring of NADPH needs to be oriented with respect to the pteridine ring of folate in order to add the two protons on the correct side of the ring: this is as shown in Figure 3. When this is compared with the crystal structure (3) of the methotrexate. NADPH.enzyme complex (Figure 3) we see that the opposite face of the pteridine ring is presented to the NADPH in this case: thus the pteridine ring of methotrexate is turned over ($\sim$ 180° about the C2-C6 axis) compared to its orientation in the folate complex. The consequence of this is that the N1 atom of methotrexate is in a completely different binding site to the N1 atom of folate. The N1 position of methotrexate has been shown to be protonated (35) and forms an electrostatic interaction with the carboxylate group of the conserved Asp 26: a similar interaction is not possible in the folate.enzyme complex and the Asp 26 is possibly acting as a proton donor in the catalytic reduction. These findings offer an explanation of why methotrexate is not a substrate for dihydrofolate reductase.

3.3 Molecular Motion and Coenzyme Induced Conformational Changes

We have used ^{19}F NMR spectroscopy to study the binding of 3',5'-difluoromethotrexate to the enzyme over the temperature range 273 to 308°. At 308°K a single resonance is observed for the two ^{19}F nuclei but as the temperature is progressively lowered the signal broadens and eventually separates into two signals of equal intensity at 273° (see Figure 4). The spectra are characteristic of nuclei undergoing exchange between two equally populated non-equivalent sites. Because of the asymmetric nature of the binding site, any fixed orientation of the benzoyl ring will lead to non-equivalence of the 3' and 5'-fluorine nuclei. The simplest exchange process leading to equivalence of the nuclei would be a 'flipping' motion about the symmetry axis of the benzoyl ring (36). Similar motions have been seen for phenylalanine and tyrosine in several proteins (37-40). Line shape analyses of the data for the 3',5'-difluoromethotrexate.enzyme complex and its ternary complexes with NADP$^+$ and NADPH indicate that the rate of ring-flipping increases in the ternary complexes even though the 3',5'-difluoromethotrexate is more tightly bound (K_{298} = 7.27 x 10^3 s^{-1}(binary); 1.88 x 10^4 s^{-1} (ternary with NADP$^+$); 2.04 x 10^4 s^{-1} (ternary with NADPH). These results clearly show that the coenzyme binding results in a conformational change which allows faster ring-flipping to take place. Examination of the crystal structure of the enzyme.methotrexate.NADPH complex reveals that steric interactions would forbid ring-flipping if the rigid binding site implied by the crystal structure were maintained: however theoretical studies (41) on the flipping of aromatic rings in proteins show that the low barriers for ring flipping can be accounted for by transient displacements of the protein atoms near the rings thus forming a relaxed protein structure where the ring-flipping is possible.

We have also seen ring-flipping behaviour for the aromatic rings in folinic acid, (5-formyltetrahydrofolate)(43,44) and trimethoprim analogues (9,42) in their complexes with the enzyme.

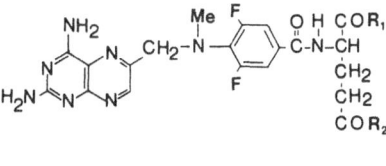

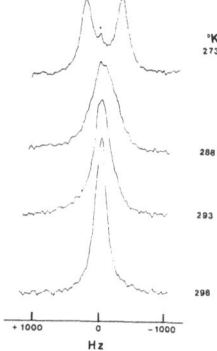

Figure 4. The ^{19}F spectra of 3',5'-difluoromethotrexate in its complex
with dihydrofolate reductase at various temperatures (36).

Direct evidence for induced conformational changes accompanying
methotrexate and coenzyme binding has also been obtained from a series
of experiments using the photo CIDNP technique to detect aromatic
residues on the surface of complexes of dihydrofolate reductase (17).
One histidine residue (probably His 22) shows an increase in accessibility when methotrexate is added to the enzyme.NADP$^+$ complex and such an
increase in accessibility could only result from a ligand induced
conformational change.

4.   COMPLEXES WITH TRIMETHOPRIM ANALOGUES

At the present time there is no published crystallographic data
available for complexes of trimethoprim with dihydrofolate reductase
from *L. casei* and we have had to use structural information from
related complexes to assist our nmr studies.

4.1 The Charged State of the Trimethoprim N1 Atom in Trimethoprim-Enzyme Complexes

We have used ^{13}C NMR spectroscopy to examine complexes of the enzyme with trimethoprim labelled with ^{13}C at the C-2 position (45). When 2 molar equivalents of [2-^{13}C]-trimethoprim are added to one equivalent of the enzyme, two ^{13}C signals are observed. One of these corresponds to free trimethoprim and its chemical shift has been titrated against pH to give a pK of 7.70 for the protonation of the N1 atom (see Figure 5). The other signal corresponds to bound trimethoprim and its chemical shift does not change with pH over the range studied indicating that

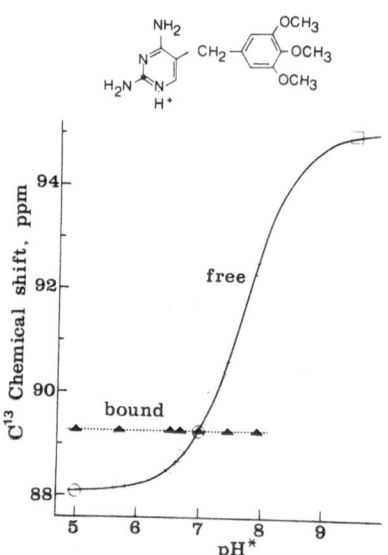

Figure 5. The pH titration curves of the ^{13}C chemical shifts of [2-^{13}C]-trimethoprim (o) free (▲) in its complex with dihydrofolate reductase (45). The solid line is calculated for a pK 7.70 and a shift difference between protonated and unprotonated forms of 7.09 ppm.

the pK of N1 protonation has increased by at least two units in binding. The ^{13}C chemical shift of the 2-carbon in bound trimethoprim is much closer to that of the protonated molecule than to the unprotonated

molecule suggesting that N1 is protonated in bound trimethoprim (45).
The difference of 1.29 ppm between the chemical shift of the bound and
protonated molecule is very similar to the corresponding difference
(1.32 ppm) observed previously by Cocco and co-workers (35) for the
corresponding carbon in bound methotrexate. This implies that the
2,4-diaminopyrimidine ring of trimethoprim is binding at the same or a
very similar binding site as that occupied by the corresponding part of
methotrexate in the enzyme-methotrexate complex.

Confirmation of the N1 protonated form of bound trimethoprim has
come from studies of complexes of the enzyme with [^{15}N - N1, N2, 2NH$_2$]
trimethoprim (46). The ^{15}N chemical shift of the N1 signal is in
excellent agreement with the value for free protonated trimethoprim.
These measurements were made using the INEPT pulse sequence which relies
on polarisation transfer being achieved via ^{15}N scalar coupling with a
directly bonded proton: observation of an intense ^{15}N signal for N1 is
thus further proof of its protonation. Finally, unequivocal confirmation of the protonation has been obtained from direct observation of
the ^{1}H signal from the N1H proton in the 500 MHz spectra of complexes
of the enzyme and trimethoprim examined in H$_2$O solution (46). The
assignment involves comparing the spectrum of the complex formed using
^{15}N labelled trimethoprim with that formed using unlabelled trimethoprim.
In the latter a ^{1}H signal observed at 14.8 ppm is a singlet whereas in
the complex with the ^{15}N labelled trimethoprim it appears as a doublet
with a splitting ($\sim$ 90 Hz) characteristic of ^{15}N-^{1}H one bond scalar
coupling: the signal is absent in spectra recorded using D$_2$O solutions.
Measurements of the line-widths of the N1H proton signals as a function
of temperature provide the rates of proton exchange with the solvent.
At 318°K the exchange rate (160 s^{-1} at 313°K) is much faster than the
dissociation rate constant for the complex (6 s^{-1} at 318°K) indicating
that the interaction involving the N1H proton and its anionic binding
site (Asp 26) can be broken without complete dissociation of the complex.
This provides some evidence for a 'zipper-type' process for the
association and dissociation of complexes (57).

4.2 The Conformation of Trimethoprim Bound to Dihydrofolate Reductase

We have used the transfer of saturation method to detect the ^{1}H signals
of bound trimethoprim in its complex with the enzyme. Initially we
attempted to observe the signals directly by using a selectively deuterated enzyme sample in which all the aromatic protons except the
2',6'-proton of the five tyrosines had been replaced by deuterium.
Figure 6 shows the low field region of the ^{1}H spectrum of the enzyme-
trimethoprim complex to which an additional molar equivalent of trimethoprim has been added (9). The five tyrosine signals from the
equivalent H2', H6' protons (rings are flipping) are clearly seen as
are the H6 and H2', H6' signals from the free trimethoprim: however
the corresponding signals from bound trimethoprim are not discernable
in the spectrum. Because there is exchange between the bound and free
trimethoprim the transfer of saturation method could be used to locate
the bound signals. Irradiation at 2.11 ppm (from dioxan) causes a
decrease in intensity of the free H2', H6' signal: thus the signal in

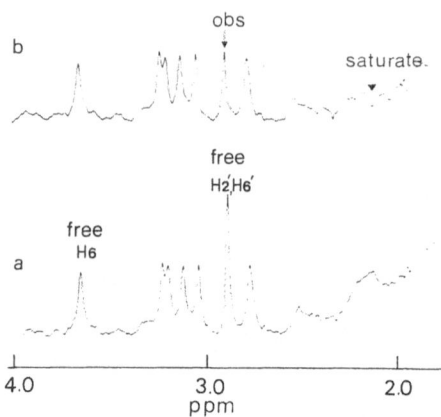

Figure 6. The aromatic region of the 270 MHz ^{1}H spectrum of selectively deuterated dihydrofolate reductase in the presence of two molar equivalents of trimethoprim (a) without irradiation (b) with selective irradiation at the frequency of the bound H2',H6' proton. The chemical shift scale is measured in ppm downfield from dioxan internal reference (9).

bound trimethoprim must be very broad (at 2.11 ppm from dioxan) probably because of slow flipping of the ring. The H6 signal was found under the high field tyrosine signal (2.76 ppm from dioxan). Selective irradiation at the frequency of the H2',H6' signal in free trimethoprim gave rise to a negative NOE effect on the H6 signal of free trimethoprim. This effect resulted from an NOE effect between the H2',H6' protons and H6 in the bound state (which would be negative) being transferred to the free ligand via the exchange between bound and free species. This was the first reported case of a transferred NOE effect involving ligands in slow exchange (9,47) and indicated that trimethoprim had a folded conformation when bound such that H6 is within 4 Å of either H2' or H6'. From a detailed analysis of the ring current effects contributing to the bound shifts of H6, H2' and H6' (assuming that the 2,4-diaminopyrimidine ring binds in a similar binding site to the corresponding part of methotrexate) we could calculate the conformation for trimethoprim when bound to dihydrofolate reductase from bacterial (E. coli and L. casei) and mammalian (SR-1) sources (9,42,47). The conformations on the bacterial enzymes are very similar and that for the L. casei-enzyme complex is shown in Figure 7. Subsequent X-ray crystallographic studies on the complex formed by trimethoprim with the E. coli enzyme gave a very similar conformation for the bound trimethoprim. In the mammalian enzyme complex, the conformation is somewhat different. Although the molecule still has a folded structure, the two aromatic rings are at less of an angle to one another than found in the bacterial enzyme complex (42).

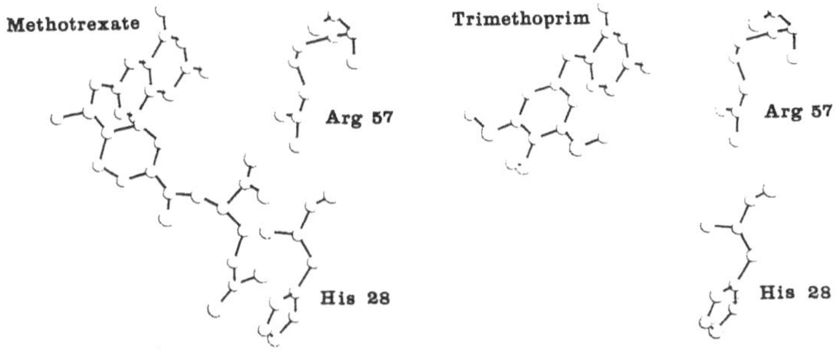

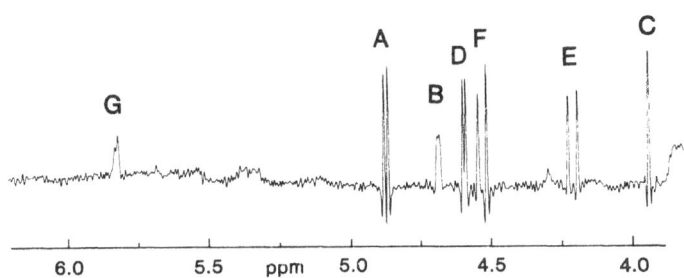

Figure 7. Conformations of methotrexate (3) and trimethoprim (9,47) in their complexes with dihydrofolate reductase: the 2,4-diaminopyrimidine fragment binds in the same binding site in each complex.

4.3 Multiple Conformations in the Ternary Complex of the Enzyme with Trimethoprim and NADP[+]

Extensive NMR studies on this complex have revealed the presence of two slowly interconverting conformations (6 s^{-1} at 304°K) which are usually in slow exchange at ambient temperatures (48-51). For example, in the ^{1}H spectrum six of the seven histidine C2 protons appear as doublets (see Figure 8) and the non-equivalence has also been detected for many

E . TMP. NADP

Figure 8. The histidine C2 proton signals in the 500 MHz spectrum of the ternary complex of trimethoprim, NADP$^+$ and dihydrofolate reductase (51) indicating the presence of two conformational states.

of the ligand nuclei using ^1H, ^{13}C, ^{15}N and ^{31}P NMR studies. Changes in structure of either the coenzyme or the trimethoprim result in changes in the relative populations of the two forms and the system appears to be a two state conformational equilibrium which can be 'switched' by the binding of ligands of different structure (50,51). Conformation I is characterised by its bound nicotinamide ring protons having very large downfield shifts (0.6 to 1.1 ppm) while those in conformation II remain virtually unchanged. Transferred NOE experiments indicate that the conformation about the glycosidic bond is different in the two conformations, conformation I being *anti-* and II being a *syn/anti* mixture similar to that seen for free NADP$^+$ in solution (51,52). It appears that the nicotinamide ring in conformation II has swung out of its binding pocket away from the enzyme surface, a process which involves changes in the conformation of the pyrophosphate moiety (detected by changes in ^{31}P chemical shifts and coupling constants) whereas in conformation I the nicotinamide remains bound to the enzyme in a manner similar to that observed in the binary complex of the enzyme with NADP$^+$. The trimethoprim conformation does not appear to change in the two conformational states of the complex although its environment is modified (51).

We have also observed multiple conformational states in other complexes such as the ternary complex of the enzyme with folate and NADP$^+$ (14,53).

5. DESIGN OF DIHYDROFOLATE REDUCTASE INHIBITORS

With the availability of detailed structural information on complexes of dihydrofolate reductase from both X-ray crystallography (3,55) and NMR spectroscopy (9,42) we have the possibility of designing trimethoprim

Methotrexate   **Brodimoprim**   **4,6-Dicarboxylate**

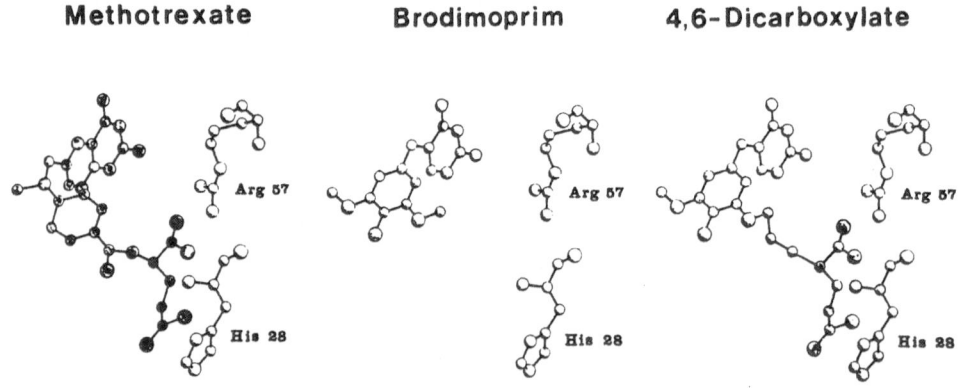

Figure 9. The conformations of (a) methotrexate(3), (b) Brodimoprim (56) (c) the 4,6-dicarboxylate analogue (III) (56) in their complexes with dihydrofolate reductase.

analogues with improved binding characteristics which could be more
selective or more active against resistant strains. In collaboration
with Dr Kompis (Hoffman la-Roche) we have been exploring this approach
using analogues of 4'-bromotrimethoprim (Brodimoprim) (56). When we
compare the bound conformations of methotrexate and 4'-bromotrimethoprim
(Figure 9a and b) it is clear that suitable modifications of the
4'-bromotrimethoprim structure in the side chain on the 3'-position
could lead to interactions with both Arg 57 and His 28. Molecular
modelling experiments indicated that the 4,6-dicarboxylate derivative
shown in Scheme III and in Figure 9c would interact with these residues.

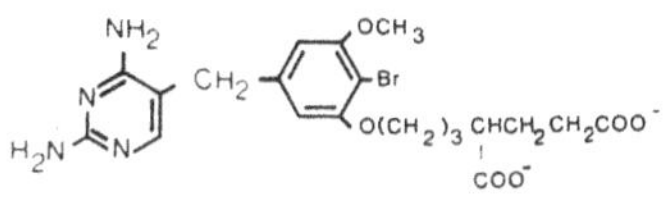

Scheme III

NMR shows that this compound binds to the enzyme in the predicted
manner, the pH dependence of the C2 proton signal of His 28 revealing
an increase of one unit in the imidazole pK in this complex. The 4,6-
dicarboxylate analogue binds 1000 fold more tightly to the enzyme than
does the parent compound while retaining its selectivity (56).

6.   CONCLUSION

The NMR method used in conjunction with X-ray crystallographic
structural data is able to provide detailed information about conformations, ionisation states, interacting groups and dynamic processes in
drug-receptor complexes. When the protein ^{1}H spectrum of *L. casei*
dihydrofolate reductase has been fully assigned, the possibilities for
characterising induced conformational changes and multiple conformational states in its complexes will be further increased.

ACKNOWLEDGEMENT

I would like to thank my colleagues at Mill Hill who have collaborated
in this work, in particular Gordon Roberts, Berry Birdsall and Arnold
Burgen.

REFERENCES

1. R.L. Blakley, 'The Biochemistry of Folic Acid and Related Pteri-
    dines'. Elsevier/North Holland, Amsterdam (1979)

2. Large scale purification and characterisation of dihydrofolate
    reductase from a methotrexate resistant strain of *Lactobacillus
    casei*. J.G. Dann, G. Ostler, R.A. Bjur, R.W. King, P. Scudder,
    P.C. Turner, G.C.K. Roberts, A.S.V. Burgen and N.G.L. Harding.
    Biochem. J. 157, 559 (1975)
3. Dihydrofolate reductase from *Lactobacillus casei* X-ray structure
    of the enzyme-methotrexate-NADPH complex. D.A. Matthews, R.A.
    Alden, J.T. Bolin, D.J. Filman, S.T. Freer, R. Hamlin, W.G.J. Hol,
    R.L. Kisliuk, E.J. Pastore, L.T. Plante, N. Xuong, and J. Kraut.
    J. Biol. Chem. 253, 6946 (1978)
4. Effects of coenzyme analogues on the binding of p-aminobenzoyl-L-
    glutamate and 2,4-diaminopyrimidine to *Lactobacillus casei*
    dihydrofolate reductase. B. Birdsall, A.S.V. Burgen and G.C.K.
    Roberts. Biochemistry 19, 3732 (1980)
5. Binding of coenzyme analogues to *Lactobacillus casei* dihydrofolate
    reductase: binary and ternary complexes. B. Birdsall, A.S.V.
    Burgen and G.C.K. Roberts. Biochemistry 19, 3723 (1980)
6. Negative cooperativity between folinic acid and coenzyme in their
    binding to *L. casei* dihydrofolate reductase. B. Birdsall, E.I.
    Hyde, A.S.V. Burgen, G.C.K. Roberts and J. Feeney, Biochemistry 20,
    7186 (1981)
7. The effect of intermediate exchange processes on the estimation of
    equilibrium constants by NMR spectroscopy. J. Feeney, J.G.
    Batchelor, J.P. Albrand and G.C.K. Roberts. J. Magn. Resonance 33,
    1 (1979)
8. ^{1}H, ^{13}C and ^{31}P NMR studies of dihydrofolate reductase-NADP$^+$-Folate
    complex: characterisation of three co-existing conformational
    states. B. Birdsall, A. Gronenborn, E.I. Hyde, G.M. Clore, G.C.K.
    Roberts, J. Feeney and A.S.V. Burgen. Biochemistry 21, 5831 (1982)
9. NMR studies of the binding of trimethoprim to dihydrofolate
    reductase. J. Cayley, J.P. Albrand, J. Feeney, G.C.K. Roberts,
    E.A. Piper and A.S.V. Burgen, Biochemistry, 18, 3886 (1979)
10. Study of moderately rapid chemical exchange reactions by means of
    nuclear magnetic double resonance. S. Forsen and R.A. Hoffman.
    J. Chem. Phys. 39, 2892 (1963)
11. Transfer of saturation NMR studies of protein-ligand complexes.
    The case of three site exchange. G.M. Clore, G.C.K. Roberts,
    A. Gronenborn, B. Birdsall and J. Feeney. J. Magn. Reson. 45, 151
    (1981)
12. ^{1}H NMR saturation transfer studies of coenzyme binding to
    Lactobacillus casei dihydrofolate reductase. E.I. Hyde, B.
    Birdsall, G.C.K. Roberts, J. Feeney and A.S.V. Burgen. Biochemistry,
    19, 3738 (1980)
13. The use of saturation transfer NMR experiments to monitor the
    conformational selection accompanying ligand-protein interactions.
    B. Birdsall, J. Feeney, G.C.K. Roberts and A.S.V. Burgen, FEBS
    Letters, 120, 107 (1980)
14. ^{13}C NMR evidence for three slowly interconverting conformations of
    the dihydrofolate reductase-NADP$^+$-Folate complex. B. Birdsall, A.
    Gronenborn, G.M. Clore, G.C.K. Roberts, J. Feeney and A.S.V.
    Burgen. Biochem. Biophys. Res. Commun. 101, 1139 (1981)

15. NMR Studies of the binding of substrate analogues and coenzyme to dihydrofolate reductase from *L. casei*. G.C.K. Roberts, J. Feeney, A.S.V. Burgen, V. Yuferov, J. Dann and R. Bjur. *Biochemistry*, 13, 5351 (1974)

16. ^{31}P NMR studies of the binding of adenosine-2'-phosphate to *L. casei* dihydrofolate reductase. B. Birdsall, G.C.K. Roberts, J. Feeney and A.S.V. Burgen. *FEBS Letters*, 80, 313 (1977)

17. Photo-CIDNP studies of the influence of ligand binding on the surface accessibility of aromatic residues in *L. casei* dihydrofolate reductase. J. Feeney, G.C.K. Roberts, R. Kaptein, B. Birdsall, A. Gronenborn and A.S.V. Burgen. *Biochemistry*, 19, (1980)

18. J. Feeney, G.C.K. Roberts, B. Birdsall and R. Kaptein. Unpublished results.

19. ^{31}P NMR studies of NADPH and NADP$^+$ binding to *L. casei* dihydrofolate reductase. J. Feeney, B. Birdsall, G.C.K. Roberts and A.S.V. Burgen. *Nature*, 257, 564 (1975)

20. ^{31}P NMR studies of complexes of NADPH and NADP$^+$ with *E. coli* dihydrofolate reductase. P.J. Cayley, J. Feeney and B.J. Kimber. *Internat. J. Biol. Macromolecules*, 2, 251 (1980)

21. Dihydrofolate reductase: interactions with the coenzyme, NADPH. J. Feeney, B. Birdsall, G.C.K. Roberts and A.S.V. Burgen, in "NMR in Biology", ed. R.A. Dwek, London, Academic Press, 111 (1977)

22. ^{31}P NMR studies of the binding of oxidised coenzymes to *Lactobacillus casei* dihydrofolate reductase. E.I. Hyde, B. Birdsall, G.C.K. Roberts, J. Feeney and A.S.V. Burgen. *Biochemistry*, 19, 3746 (1980)

23. ^{1}H Nuclear magnetic resonance studies of the tyrosine residues of selectively deuterated *Lactobacillus casei* dihydrofolate reductase. J. Feeney, G.C.K. Roberts, B. Birdsall, D.V. Griffiths, R.W. King, P. Scudder and A.S.V. Burgen. *Proc. Roy. Soc. Lond.B.* 196, 267 (1977)

24. Preparation of deuterated aromatic amino-acids for use in ^{1}H NMR studies of proteins. D.V. Griffiths, J. Feeney, G.C.K. Roberts and A.S.V. Burgen. *Biochim. Biophys. Acta*, 446, 479 (1976)

25. B. Birdsall, S.J. Hammond, M.S. Searle, J. Feeney, G.C.K. Roberts, B.J. Kimber, R.W. King and D.V. Griffiths. Unpublished results.

26a NMR studies of selectively deuterated and fluorine labelled dihydrofolate reductase. J. Feeney 'Nuclear magnetic resonance spectroscopy in molecular biology.' Proceedings of 11th Jerusalem Symposium. Edited by B. Pullman, Dordrecht, Reidel. 297 (1978)

26b ^{1}H NMR studies of the effects of ligand binding on the tryptophan residues of a selectively deuterated dihydrofolate reductase from *Lactobacillus casei*. J. Feeney, G.C.K. Roberts, J. Thomson, R.W. King, D.V. Griffiths and A.S.V. Burgen. *Biochemistry*, 19, 2316 (1980)

26c Dihydrofolate reductase: the use of fluorine-labelled and selectively deuterated enzyme to study substrate and inhibitor binding. G.C.K. Roberts, J. Feeney, B. Birdsall, B.J. Kimber, D.V. Griffiths, R.W. King and A.S.V. Burgen. In "NMR in Biology" ed. R.A. Dwek, London, Academic Press, 95 (1977)

26d. Antimetabolites: Drug Action at the Molecular Level A.S.V.
     Burgen, J. Feeney and G.C.K. Roberts, Royal Society Jubilee
     Volume 193 (1978)
27. [19]F Nuclear magnetic resonance studies of ligand binding to
     3-fluorotyrosine- and 6-fluorotryptophan-containing dihydrofolate
     reductase from *Lactobacillus casei*. B.J. Kimber, D.V. Griffiths,
     B. Birdsall, R.W. King, P. Scudder, J. Feeney, G.C.K. Roberts,
     and A.S.V. Burgen. Biochemistry, 16 (15) 3492 (1977)
28. Proximity of two tryptophan residues in dihydrofolate reductase
     determined by ^{19}F NMR. B.J. Kimber, J. Feeney, G.C.K. Roberts,
     B. Birdsall, A.S.V. Burgen and B.D. Sykes. Nature (London) 271,
     184 (1978)
29. ^{13}C NMR evidence for the slow exchange of tryptophans in
     dihydrofolate reductase between stable conformations. R.E. London,
     G.P. Groff and R.L. Blakley. Biochem. Biophys. Res. Commun. 86,
     779 (1979)
30a [1]H Nuclear magnetic resonance studies of *Lactobacillus casei*
     dihydrofolate reductase: effects of substrate and inhibitor
     binding on the histidine residues. B. Birdsall, D.V. Griffiths,
     G.C.K. Roberts, J. Feeney and A.S.V. Burgen. Proc. Roy. Soc. Lond.
     B. 196, 251 (1977)
30b The histidine residues of *L. casei* dihydrofolate reductase:
     paramagnetic relaxation and deuterium exchange studies and partial
     assignments. P. Wyeth, A. Gronenborn, B. Birdsall, G.C.K. Roberts,
     J. Feeney and A.S.V. Burgen. Biochemistry, 19, 2608 (1980)
30c The effects of coenzyme binding on the histidine residues of
     L. casei dihydrofolate reductase. A. Gronenborn, B. Birdsall, E.I.
     Hyde, G.C.K. Roberts, J. Feeney and A.S.V. Burgen. Biochemistry,
     20, 1717 (1981)
31. A ^{1}H NMR study of the role of the glutamate moiety in the binding
     of methotrexate to dihydrofolate reductase. D.J. Antonjuk,
     B. Birdsall, A.S.V. Burgen, H.T.A. Cheung, G.M. Clore, J. Feeney,
     A. Gronenborn, G.C.K. Roberts and W. Tran. Brit. J. Pharmacol.
     81, 309 (1984)
32. Stereochemistry of reduction of folic acid using dihydrofolate
     reductase. P.A. Charlton, D.W. Young, B. Birdsall, J. Feeney and
     G.C.K. Roberts. J. Chem. Soc. Chem. Commun. 922 (1979)
33. Methotrexate binding to dihydrofolate reductase. G.C.K. Roberts,
     J. Feeney, B. Birdsall, P. Charlton and D.W. Young. Nature, 286,
     309 (1980)
34. J.C. Fontecilla-Camps, C.E. Bugg, C. Temple, J. Rose, J.A.
     Montgomery and R.L. Kisliuk, 'Chemistry and Biology of Pteridines'
     Editors R.L. Kisliuk and G.M. Brown. Elsevier, North Holland, N.Y.
     235 (1979)
35. [13]C Nuclear magnetic resonance study of protonation of metho-
     trexate and aminopterin bound to dihydrofolate reductase.
     L. Cocco, J.P. Groff, C. Temple, Jr., J.A. Montgomery, R.E. London,
     N.S. Matwiyoff and R.L. Blakley Biochemistry, 20, 3926 (1981)
36. ^{19}F NMR studies of 3'5'-difluoromethotrexate binding to
     Lactobacillus casei dihydrofolate reductase. Molecular motion

and coenzyme induced conformational change. G.M. Clore, A.M. Gronenborn, B. Birdsall, J. Feeney and G.C.K. Roberts. _Biochem. J._ _217_, 659 (1984)

37. Proton magnetic resonance studies of the tyrosine residues of hen lysozyme - assignment and detection of conformational mobility. I.D. Campbell, C.M. Dobson, and R.J.P. Williams. _Proc. Roy. Soc. Lond. B._, _189_, 503 (1975)

38. Temperature dependent molecular motion of a tyrosine residue of ferrocytochrome c. I.D. Campbell, C.M. Dobson, G.R. Moore, S.J. Perkins and R.J.P. Williams. _FEBS Letters_, 70, 96 (1976)

39. Complete tyrosine assignments in the high field ^{1}H NMR spectrum of the bovine pancreatic trypsin inhibitor. G.H. Snyder, R. Rowan III, S. Karplus and B.D. Sykes, _Biochemistry_, _14_, 3765 (1975)

40. NMR investigations of the dynamics of the aromatic amino acid residues in the basic pancreatic trypsin inhibitor. K. Wüthrich and G. Wagner, _FEBS Letters_, _50_, 265 (1975)

41. The internal dynamics of globular proteins. M. Karplus and J.A. McCammon. _Crit. Rev. in Biochem._ 9 (4), 293 (1981)

42. Trimethoprim binding to bacterial and mammalian dihydrofolate reductase: a comparison by proton and carbon-13 NMR. B. Birdsall, G.C.K. Roberts, J. Feeney, J.G. Dann and A.S.V. Burgen. _Biochemistry_, _22_, 5597 (1983)

43. A ^{1}H NMR study of the complexes of the diastereoisomers of folinic acid with dihydrofolate reductase. J. Feeney, B. Birdsall, J.P. Albrand, G.C.K. Roberts, A.S.V. Burgen, P.A. Charlton and D.W. Young. _Biochemistry_, _20_, 1837 (1981)

44. Conformational studies on 5-formyl-6,7,8-tetrahydrofolic acid (folinic acid) using ^{1}H and ^{13}C NMR measurements: two interconverting conformations. J. Feeney, J.P. Albrand, C.A. Boicelli, D.W. Young and P.A. Charlton. _J. Chem. Sock. Perk. II_, 176 (1980)

45. The charge state of trimethoprim bound to _L. casei_ dihydrofolate reductase. G.C.K. Roberts, J. Feeney, A.S.V. Burgen and S. Daluge. _FEBS Letters_, _131_, 85 (1981)

46. A.W. Bevan, G.C.K. Roberts, J. Feeney and L. Kuyper. Unpublished results.

47. The use of transferred nuclear Overhauser effects in the study of the conformations of small molecules bound to proteins. J.P. Albrand, B. Birdsall, J. Feeney, G.C.K. Roberts and A.S.V. Burgen. _Internat. J. Biol. Macromolecules_, _1_, 37 (1979)

48. ^{1}H and ^{31}P NMR characterisation of two conformations of the trimethoprim-NADP[+] dihydrofolate reductase complex. A. Gronenborn, B. Birdsall, E.I. Hyde, G.C.K. Roberts, J. Feeney and A.S.V. Burgen. _Molecular Pharm._ 20, 145 (1981)

49. Direct observation by NMR of two co-existing conformations of an enzyme-ligand complex in solution. A. Gronenborn, B. Birdsall, E.I. Hyde, G.C.K. Roberts, J. Feeney and A.S.V. Burgen. _Nature_, _290_, 273 (1981)

50. A drug-receptor complex in two conformations. A.W. Bevan, B. Birdsall, A. Gronenborn, E. Potterton, G.M. Clore, G.C.K. Roberts, J. Feeney and A.S.V. Burgen. "Pteridines and Folic Acid

Derivatives" (1982)

51. Multinuclear NMR characterisation of two coexisting conformational
     states of the *Lactobacillus casei* dihydrofolate reductase trimetho-
     prim-NADP$^+$ complex. B. Birdsall, A.W. Bevan, C. Pascual, G.C.K.
     Roberts, J. Feeney, A. Gronenborn and G.M. Clore. Biochemistry,
     in press.

52. The use of transferred nuclear Overhauser effect measurements to
     compare the binding of coenzyme analogues to dihydrofolate reduct-
     ase. J. Feeney, B. Birdsall, G.C.K. Roberts and A.S.V. Burgen.
     Biochemistry, 22, 628 (1983)

53. Multiple conformations of the dihydrofolate reductase-folate-NADP$^+$
     complex. B. Birdsall, A. Gronenborn, G.M. Clore, E.I. Hyde,
     G.C.K. Roberts, J. Feeney and A.S.V. Burgen. "Pteridines and
     Folic Acid Derivatives (1982)

54. An NMR study of NADP binding to *L. casei* dihydrofolate reductase.
     J.L. Way, B. Birdsall, J. Feeney, G.C.K. Roberts and A.S.B. Burgen.
     Biochemistry, 14, 3470 (1975)

55. Crystal structures of *E. coli* and *L. casei* dihydrofolate reductase
     refined to 1.7 Å resolution. I. General features and binding of
     methotrexate. J.T. Bolin, D.J. Filman, D.A. Matthews, R.C. Hamlin
     and J. Kraut. J. Biol. Chem., 257, 13650 (1982)

56. A ^{1}H study of the interactions and conformations of rationally
     designed brodimoprim analogues in complexes with *Lactobacillus
     casei* dihydrofolate reductase. B. Birdsall, J. Feeney, C. Pascual,
     G.C.K. Roberts, I. Kompis, R.L. Then, K. Muller, and A. Kroehn.
     J. Med. Chem. (1984)

57. On the binding of Flexible Ligands to Macromolecules. A.S.V.
     Burgen, G.C.K. Roberts and J. Feeney. Nature, 253, 753 (1975)

NON-MEDICAL APPLICATIONS OF NMR-IMAGING

L.D. Hall, J. Lee, V. Rajanayagam and L. Talagala
Department of Chemistry
University of British Columbia
Vancouver, B.C.
Canada V6T 1Y6

ABSTRACT. Relatively few studies have been reported for applications of NMR-imaging methods to non-living systems. Obviously, though, many materials contain sufficient water, or fat (oil), to provide very adequate signal intensity. As a result, studies of foods, of fruits and plants, of porous media which contain water (e.g. cement), or oil (e.g. rock core samples) have been made. Unpublished work from the author's laboratory, which includes studies of hen's eggs, of wood, of oil in rock, and of ion-exchange chromatography columns, is discussed. The importance of imaging methods to evaluate the technical performance of hardware components, such as radiofrequency coils and field homogeneity is also mentioned, as is the possibility of mapping the distribution of physical and chemical properties.

Although it is understandable, indeed commendable, that the main thrust of NMR-imaging has been directed to clinical studies, this has resulted in a dearth of studies in other areas, many of which merit substantial attention in their own right. It is the purpose of this Chapter to outline a few of those studies. Right at the outset it must be emphasised that future progress in this area is critically dependent on access to suitable equipment available at an affordable price. Fortunately, several equipment manufacturers are now developing suitable devices; and, as we indicate elsewhere in this book, it is not too difficult to adapt a conventional spectrometer for imaging measurements.

Early developmental studies in NMR-imaging often involved (1) fruit, such as lemons, and it is clear that the ripening of fruit is worthy of substantial future attention. Indeed, any produce which contains a substantial component of either water, or fat, or mixtures thereof, can be imaged. The advantages of being able to study food just as it is packaged for distribution in glass, plastic, or aluminium (but not iron!) containers needs no emphasis, especially in view of the amount of food which is currently wasted due to inadequate, or uncertain storage conditions.

A logical extension of this concept is to study plants and seeds. The largest plants are trees, and the forestry industry has a variety of problems which can benefit by nmr scanning. For example, the detection of wood imperfections prior to log sawing would

T. Axenrod and G. Ceccarelli (eds.), NMR in Living Systems, 367–375.
© 1986 by D. Reidel Publishing Company.

undoubtedly increase the proportion of "clear" lumber produced. Unfortunately, the technical problems involved with imaging an entire log of 1 metre diameter and 30 metres length, and in real-time to boot, is probably beyond conceivable implementation. Nevertheless, other pertinent areas exist which are more compatible. For example, learning to optimise the heating cycle used for kiln-drying lumber could have important financial benefits. In like fashion, the well-known properties of paramagnetic species to increase the spin-lattice relaxation rate of water provides the basis for a facile method for detecting the penetration of wood preservatives which contain para-magnetic metal ions (2) (Fig 1).

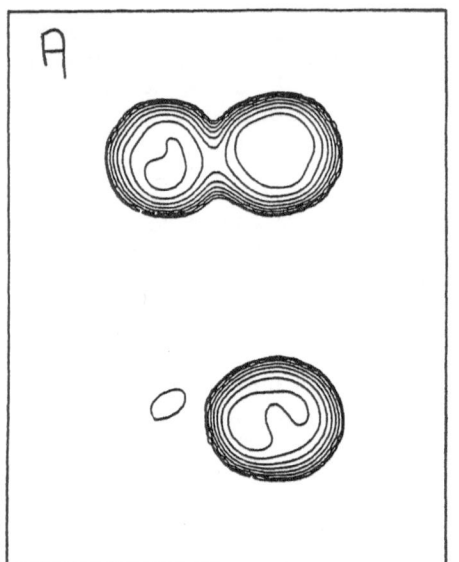 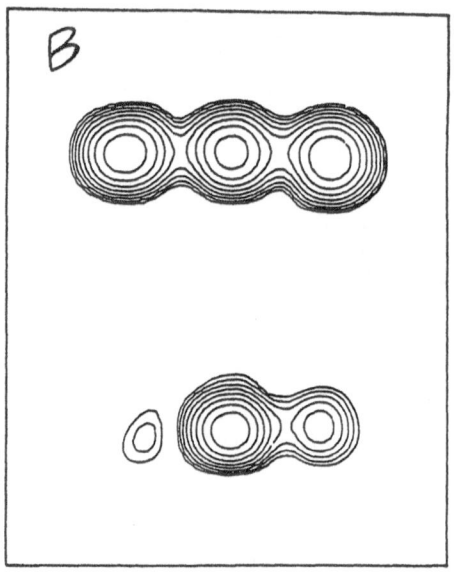

Figure 1. Cross Sectional images of branches of maple wood (Acer Rubrum) taken from a three-dimensional volume data-set, derived from the proton resonance of water. A: the upper trace shows two freshly cut pieces; the lower trace the same two samples, the one on the left having been dried for 3 hours at 110 C. B: the upper trace shows three freshly cut pieces; in the lower trace, the one in the middle is untreated, but the other two have been soaked in manganous chloride solution (1 Molar), that on the left for 3.5 hours, that on the right for 30 min. Measurements were made at 80MHz.

One area which has already received (3) substantial attention is penetration of water into porous "minerals" such as concrete, plaster, and porous rocks.

For the remainder of this chapter I will concentrate on studies which are in progress in my laboratory at U.B.C. We have two, home-built NMR devices mentioned elsewhere in this volume, but most of our

studies are made with the 80 MHz system, for which we have probes
which can accept samples up to 12 cm diameter.

Our own studies of living systems have emphasised proton-
imaging, of rats, (4) of seeds (5), and of eggs (5). The long-term
objective of the latter area is to follow sequentially the
development of a chick embryo. However, we have already studied the
effects of storage on eggs, and also the effects of heating. For a
fresh egg, the proton-image shows the four separate types(5) of
albumin, and some fine structure can also be seen in the yolk. Even
after hard-boiling, the seemingly homogeneous white of the egg still
shows separate domains.

With regards to non-living systems we have chosen several areas
which have substantial commercial importance. One of these involves
(6) the detection of hydrocarbons distributed in porous media such
as that of oil-bearing strata. The difficulty is that many such
rocks contain a sufficiently high level of paramagnetic species to
broaden the oil resonances beyond detectability. Nevertheless, the
potential use of this approach as an aid to the investigation of
enhanced oil recovery warrants substantial efforts. Our preliminary
experiments (Fig 2) have involved oil, trapped in porous glass

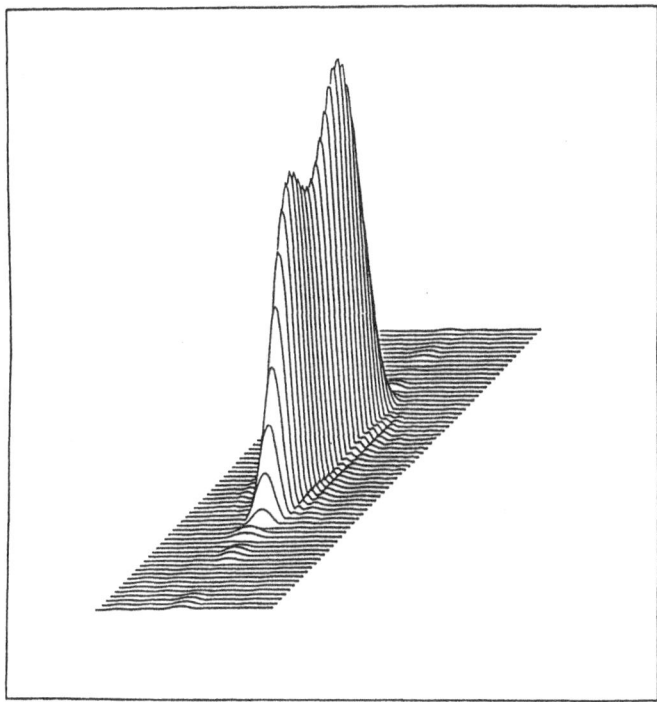

Figure 2. Projection - image of oil in a sintered glass frit showing
the distribution along a plane.

blocks, in limestone and sand blocks, and in rock core samples.
Dectection of the oil itself is trivial; however, it is more
difficult to make the measurement in the presence of the aqueous
solutions used for polymer flooding and this is where our major
efforts are being directed at present.

Given, that in industry, many chemical and biochemical,
processes are performed in columns, we have chosen to develop probes
and sample holders suitable for such studies (6). One example will
suffice to illustrate this area. An ion-exchange column packed in a
glass tube was developed with aqueous copper sulphate. The water on
the column was then imaged (8) using the inversion recovery pulse
sequence incorporated into a three-dimensional volume-imaging
measurement. The vertical slice along the length of the column
obtained with a long value of the time between the 180° pulse and the
imaging-pulse showed the outline of the total shape of the column
(Fig 3A). It was then possible to choose appropriate values for that

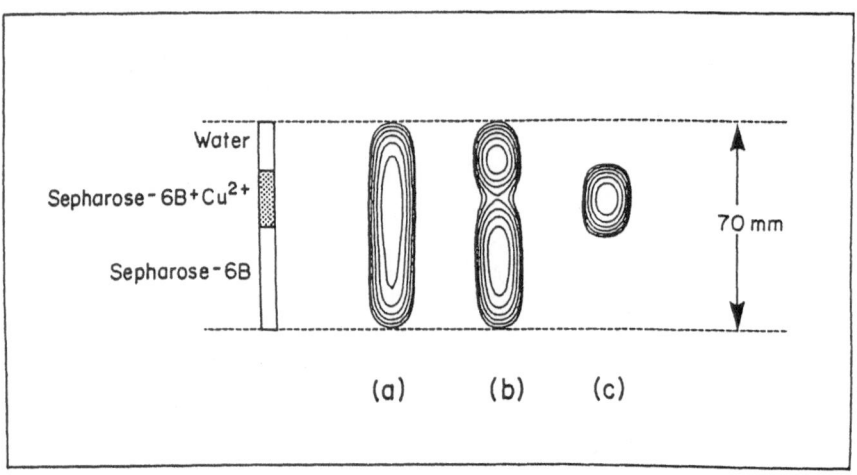

Figure 3. Data from a chromotography column containing ca 10^{-5} moles
copper (II) adsorbed on a column of "chelating sepharose-6B". The
images shown in (a), (b) and (c) are single slices drawn from a 3D
volume data set based on four scans 16 x 16 x 512 digital increments,
using an inversion-recovery pulse sequence (180 - t - 90), and with
the t-delay interval set at 3sec, 10msec, and 300ms respectively.

delay period to make images in which the water in the vicinity of the
copper ions can be distinguished from that of the column packing.
This rather simple example is pertinent to several areas of NMR-
imaging. Most importantly, it demonstrates the concept of

"molecular amplification", which can serve to overcome the ultimate limitation of NMR, namely low signal-to-noise sensitivity. In this case, it would be impossible by NMR to detect directly the ca 20 x 10^{-6} grams of copper ions on the column. However, because each copper ion influences either directly, or indirectly, a large number of water molecules, those can jointly act as a composite reporter group showing the location of the copper ions. In this case the molecular amplification factor is estimated to be ca 10^5. It seems that similar approaches to this will be mandatory if NMR is to be used to study biological events which take place at micromolar concentrations.

For studies of chemical transformations which occur on columns containing immobilised-enzymes, or -cells, isotopic enrichment will confer the same advantages as those already demonstrated for homogeneous systems; particularly, carbon-13 will be widely used.

So far in this article we have been concerned with studies of objects. It is important to note, however, that many interesting phenomena can be studied by imaging methods. Technical evaluation of imaging-hardware and -procedures constitutes a major non-medical use for imaging. Obvious examples are studies of suitably designed phantoms. For example, the image of a regular grid of tubes containing aqueous media can be used (9) to evaluate the linearity of the overall image produced; in much the same way phantoms consisting of "line pairs" can be used to define the detected resolution. And the image of a homogeneous volume of liquid provides compelling insight concerning the homogeneity of the B_1-field distribution within the probe. Although this information is important to volume-imaging probes, the more spectacular use (10) is in the evaluation of radiofrequency penetration from a surface-coil. It will be recalled that the early studies involving surface-coils made the tacit assumption that the penetration depth was equal to the coil-radius. More recent theoretical studies have demonstrated (11) the limits of this assumption. Furthermore, a number of laboratories have developed methods whereby the effective penetration depth can be varied (12). We have used three dimensional volume imaging to evaluate these and other aspects of surface coils. In practice, a large beaker containing, for example, dilute aqueous copper sulphate is placed on top of the coil and is then "imaged" in the usual way (10). Given that the sample is homogeneous, variations in the resultant image intensity reflect the spatial distribution of the B_1-field (Fig 4). Insight gained in this way is invaluable in its own right.

It also suggests a number of procedures whereby improved spatial localisation can be achieved. Consider, for example, a spectroscopic measurement using a surface coil and a spectrometer with facilities capable of producing a linear field-gradient perpendicular to the surface of the coil, and a frequency selective pulse. With the gradient on, the latter can be used (10,13) to excite into resonance any "slice" of defined thickness, and depth. The spectrum of the corresponding volume, which has the form of a hockey puck (using a

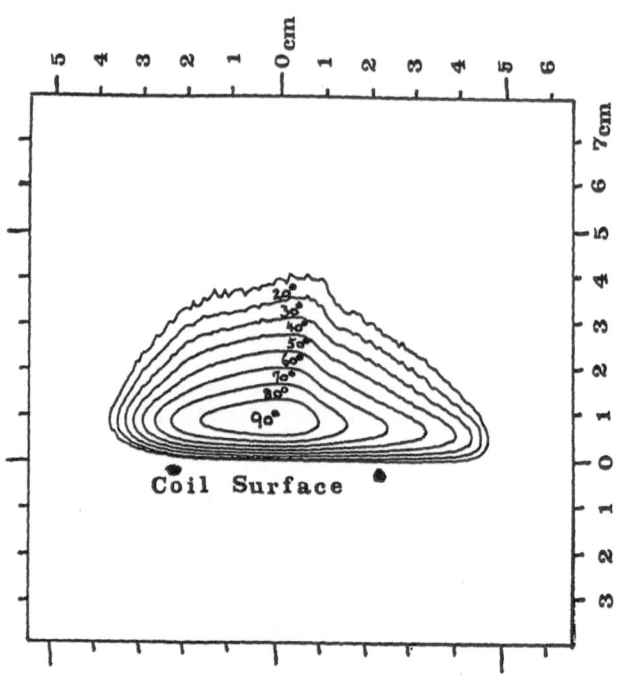

Figure 4.   Experimentally determined slice-image derived from a 3D volume data set of a beaker of water placed on top of a circular surface coil; the simple slice shown, is perpendicular to the surface of the coil.

Canadianism!), is then acquired with the gradient off. Slices at various depths can be measured, either by varying the frequency, or, if many slices parallel to the surface are required, by inspection of slices taken from a three dimensional volume data set obtained using a non-selective pulse.

    A question which has to be answered is whether, or not, the results obtained from studies such as those summarised here really justify the capital investments involved. Is it worthwhile using a $400,000 instrument to image an egg, when a 5 cent candle does a splendid job? Clearly this criticism can only be answered by data and examples, and those are not being produced very rapidly at present because of the paucity of suitable equipment. Although the number of instruments is likely to increase rapidly starting in 1985, so much remains to be done that there will be ample room for many new research groups. Specific industries which could well benefit from an active involvement in this area include the food industry, those involved in oil recovery, especially enhanced oil recovery and recovery from oil shales, industries concerned with the development of new concrete composites such as those reinforced with organic polymer fibres, industries involved with insulation, or composite materials, which are exposed to water under the influence of pressure, or heat, or both.

Phenomena which can be studied by imaging methods include the characterisation of the distribution and physical status of individual chemical constituents and mapping of their variations. Distribution studies are best followed by chemical shift resolved tomography. Physical characterisation involves measurement of the spin-lattice and spin-spin relaxation rates of the individual chemical species. The intrinsic variations of these parameters can be used qualitatively to heighten the contrast of slice images. For example, when studying the distribution of oil-water mixtures in porous media advantage can be taken of the differential between the relaxation rates to suppress the signals from either the oil or the water, and hence selectively eliminate their contribution from the final image. This can be a useful alternative to a chemical shift resolved imaging measurement. The quantitative measurement of relaxation rates by "imaging" is extremely difficult even for a single species characterised by a simple relaxation rate. Thus studies of systems which have multiple exponential relaxation have to be regarded as being no more than barely feasible; certainly they require substantial time and dedication. A third parameter, well used (14) for studies of small samples, is the self-diffusion coefficient. It is now technically feasible (15) to measure this parameter by imaging methods, which raises a number of exciting possibilities.

The advent of chemical shift resolved tomography means that it is now possible to map the spatial distribution of any property, chemical, or physical, which can influence the chemical shift of any resonance signal, whether it be of an endogenous species or of an exogenous species deliberately added as a "probe". Two examples, of many, will suffice to make this point. It is well known that the chemical shifts of the protons of imadazole (16) and of the ^{31}P resonance of inorganic phosphate (17) are dependent on pH. Thus these can be used (18) to map pH distribution. In like fashion, temperature distributions can be measured (18) using known variations of shift and relaxation parameters.

Although the emphasis in this Chapter has been on mapping the overall distribution of substances or properties, it is worth noting in conclusion that access to an NMR device capable of holding an object which is 7 - 50 cm in diameter automatically makes feasible a wide variety of simple, point-specific measurements. Thus, for studies of materials which, although complex in chemical composition, are otherwise homogeneous in distribution, it is only necessary to make a measurement on the total volume, or even a part thereof. For example, assay of an unopened bottle of vintage wine is now feasible. Furthermore, even when the material itself has an inhomogeneous distribution, volume-specific methods can be used to characterise just a local region. If that region is near the surface of the object then a surface-coil (10) can be used to provide a crude spatial localisation. Even when the region of interest is deep inside the sample, point spectra can be obtained using a combination of frequency-selective radiofrequency pulses and field-gradients. The main advantage of these approaches is that they are faster than chemical shift imaging, which is important when sample throughput has to be high, or when the low effective concentration of the nuclear species of interest necessitates extensive time averaging to obtain and adequate signal-to-noise ratio.

Acknowledgements

It is a pleasure to thank the other members of the U.B.C group whose efforts have made feasible the unpublished results reported here; especial mention must be made to Dr. S. Sukumar and to Tom Marcus and Cedric Neale. This work was supported by generous grants from the Presidents of the Natural Science and Engineering Research Council of Canada, and of the Medical Research Council of Canada, to whom we are indebted.

References

1. W.S. Hinshaw, P.A. Bottomley and G.N. Holland, Nature 270 722 (1977); E.R. Andrew, P.A. Bottomley, W.S. Hinshaw, G.N. Holland, W.S. Moore, C. Simaroj and B.S. Worthington, Proc. Congr. Ampere, 20th, Tallinn, U.S.S.R. p. 53 (1978); P.C. Lauterbur, in NMR in Biology (R.A. Dwek, I.D. Campbell, R.E. Richards and R.J.P. Williams, eds) pp 323-335, Academic Press, New York, 1977; P. Mansfield and I.L. Pykett J. Magn. Reson. 29 355 (1978); W.S. Hinshaw, J. Appl. Phys. 47 3709 (1976); R.J. Ordidge, R.R. Rzedian and P. Mansfield, Bull. Magn. Reson. 2 432 (1980); P.C. Lauterbur, Pure Appl. Chem 40 149 (1974).

2. L.D. Hall and V. Rajanayagam, to be published.

3. R.J. Gummerson, C. Hall, W.D. Hoff, R. Hawkes, G.N. Holland and W.S. Moore, Nature 281 56 (1979).

4. L.D. Hall, J. Schachter and L. Talagala, to be published.

5. L.D. Hall and J. Lee; L.D. Hall, S.L. Luck and V. Rajanayagam, to be published.

6. L.D. Hall and V. Rahanayagam, to be published

7. L.D. Hall, T. Marcus, C. Neale, B. Powell, J. Sallow and S. L. Talagala, J. Magn. Reson., in press.

8. L.D. Hall and V. Rajanayagam, J.C.S. Chem. Commun., 499, (1985)

9. L.D. Hall, V. Rajanayagam and S. Sukumar, J. Magn. Reson., 60 199 (1984).

10. L.D. Hall and J. Lee, to be published.

11. J.L. Evelhoch, M.G. Crowley and J.J.H. Ackerman, J. Magn. Reson. **56** 110 (1984).

12. M.R. Bendall and R.E. Gordon, J. Magn. Reson. **53** 365 (1983); D.I. Hoult, Prog. NMR. Spec. **12** 41 (1978); A.J. Shaka and R. Freeman, J. Magn. Reson. **59** 169 (1984).

13. P.A. Bottomley, T.B. Foster and R.D. Darrow, J. Magn. Reson., **59** 338 (1984).

14.   E.O. Stejskal and J.E. Tanner, J. Chem. Phys. **42** 288 (1965) E.D. Finch, in <u>The Aqueous</u> Cytoplasm, ed. A.D. Keith, p. 64-89, Marcel Dekker, Inc., New York 1979; P.T. Callaghan, K.W. Jolley and R.S. Humphrey, J. Coll, Interface Sci., **93** 521 (1983).

15. L.D. Hall and S.L. Luck, to be published.

16. D. L. Rubenstein, and A.A. Isab, Anal. Biochem., **121** 423 (1982).

17. R.B. Moon and J. H. Richards, J. Bio. Chem. **248** 7276 (1973).

18. L.D. Hall and L. Talagala, to be published.

OTHER METHODS FOR IMAGING THE INTACT HUMAN BODY

L.D. Hall
Department of Chemistry
University of British Columbia
Vancouver, B.C.
Canada V6T 1W5

ABSTRACT. A brief overview is given of other methods which are available for producing an image from the intact human body. These fall into three main groups. First, methods which use X-rays (X-ray photography and CT scanning). Second, nuclear medicine methods involving gamma-emitting radionuclides (gamma photography and SPECT); and another which uses positron emitting radionuclides (PET). Finally, ultrasound methods. These are compared, and then a more detailed overview given of the PET technique.

Given that the major thrusts of most new developments in both magnetic resonance "imaging" and "spectroscopy" have been directed to clinical studies of man, it is important that one should be aware of alternative techniques which are already available with which the nmr methods must compete. This chapter will briefly survey four such methods, two which produce an anatomical image (X-ray and ultrasound) and two which can be used to map in-vivo metabolism [Positron Emission Tomography (PET) and Single Photon Emission Computed Tomography (SPECT)]. As will be seen, in some instances these methods can be complimentary with NMR, in others NMR will eventually displace them, whereas NMR cannot hope to compete with some others.

At the outset it must be recognised that any "imaging" (or spectroscopic) measurement of necessity involves the interaction between some form of "radiation" and some component of the object which is to be studied. For example, in the case of "sight", the electromagnetic energy lies in the visible region of the frequency spectrum, and it interacts with the electrons of the molecules on the outer surface of the object. For medical imaging, where the interest mainly involves the internal structures of the intact body, it is obvious that the radiation must be able to penetrate through the body tissues in order that it may first interact, and second exit from the body carrying with it the information which is of interest. It so happens that only a limited number of "frequency windows" exist which are suitable. Radiofrequencies up to at least 100 MHz can penetrate through tissues without undue attenuation; this makes possible the NMR studies which are discussed elsewhere in this book.

T. Axenrod and G. Ceccarelli (eds.), NMR in Living Systems, 377–383.

X-rays, gamma rays, and high frequency sound waves, are also suitable and lead to the methods discussed in this chapter.

1. X-RAY METHODS

The discovery by Roentgen that X-rays could pass through human tissues, yet were selectively attenuated by bone, led with remarkable rapidity to transmission X-ray photography, which continues to be the most widely used of the imaging methods. A divergent beam of X-rays is beamed towards the appropriate part of the patient's body, behind which is located a sheet of X-ray-sensitive photographic film. Preferential absorption of the X-rays proportional to the electron density of the tissue, produces the well known "shadowgraph" in which the outline of the bones is displayed with remarkably high resolution.

This method has many advantages, including low capital cost and ease of use. Its principle disadvantage is that because it produces a two-dimensional display of a three-dimensional object, it sacrifices structural information. This is not a serious problem for studies of teeth, for example, but can be for studies of the whole head.

Recognition of this limitation, prompted Hounsfield to develop Computed Axial Tomography. In this method, a colimated beam of X-rays is used to form a slice image of the region of interest. Many different procedures are now used; however, in essence they all involve the same principle. The beam of X-rays is passed through the body from a number of different directions and the intensity of the transmitted beam measured for each of them. The resultant sets of data are then combined mathematically using the well known "back-projection" algorithm to reconstruct the image of the slice defined by the X-ray beam. Modern CT scanners can directly produce high resolution images of any region of the body. Since the image contrast depends principally on the very small differences between the electron density of the different tissues it is remarkable that this method gives the amount of contrast which it does. When the intrinsic contrast is insufficient, external contrast agents are frequently used; for example, barium sulphate for studies of the gastrointestinal tract, and various iodinated organic substances for imaging the vascular system (as in angiography).

The principle disadvantages of this method include the fact that the physical structure of the gantry upon which the X-ray transmitter and receiver are mounted, limits the method to the production of transverse sections. And although such slices through the upper skull have revolutionised the diagnosis of head pathology, studies of the lower part (the posterior fossa) are complicated by the image artifacts produced by the very dense bone structure at the base of the skull. Nevertheless, in terms of "picture taking", this is the bench mark against which proton NMR tomography must compete (vide-infra).

2. ULTRASOUND

Of all the competitive methods, only ultrasound is sufficiently non-invasive to make it well suited to serial studies, or to studies in gynaecology. The method depends on the reflection of very high frequency sound waves (2-15 MHz) at the interface between different organs. Several different methods are available which produce images in real time. This method is probably capable of substantial further development. Certainly it has the dual merits of low capital cost, and of portability.

3. TECHNIQUES IN NUCLEAR MEDICINE

In contrast to the methods of the first section where the source of the radiation is external to the body, all techniques in nuclear medicine use gamma rays generated within the patient's body by a suitable radiolabelled substance. In two of the methods the gamma rays come directly from the administered radionuclide; however, for positron emission tomography the gamma rays are actually generated in the tissue by positron annihilation.

In clinical practice, nuclear medicine methods are generally used to provide a "map" of the physiological function. The spatial resolution is relatively poor (of the order of a cubic centimetre). However, the signal-to-noise sensitivity is extremely high and in that regard this method has substantial advantages over NMR spectroscopy.

These methods require the administration to the patient of a radioactive nuclide which has been incorporated into a suitable "carrier". This can take the form of a physical dispersion of an atomic species; or, for biochemical studies the nuclide can be chemically part of a complex organic substance (as in the case of 2-deoxy-2-^{18}F-fluoro-$\underline{D}$-glucose).

Again, the simplest detection method involves the projection, onto a two-dimensional plane, of the total distribution of radioactivity in the region of interest. For many purposes, the resultant loss of spatial information is of no concern, as, for example, in the evaluation of thyroid activity.

Nevertheless, the advantages of information displayed as tomographic slices is sufficiently compelling that here too, methods have been developed which enable slice selection to be performed. The difficulty in extending the conventional gamma camera methods to this end arise from the variable extent to which the gamma rays interact with the body tissues. Nevertheless, the technique of Single Photon Emission Computed Tomography (SPECT), merits a substantial investment of effort.

4. POSITRON EMISSION TOMOGRAPHY

The most sophisticated (and expensive!) of the nuclear medicine methods is Positron Emission Tomography. The method depends on the fact that certain radionuclides emit positrons; in tissue, these travel distances of the order of millimetres before they are annihilated by an electron. That annihilation event produces instantaneously a pair of gamma rays, each of 511 KEV energy, which travel in opposite directions (angle <u>ca</u> 180°). The region of interest is surrounded by a ring of many separate gamma ray detectors, interconnected for "coincidence counting"; that is the system only records an "event" when two detectors simultaneously register the arrival of a gamma ray. Knowledge of which pair of detectors is triggered, physically defines the axis along which the original positron annihilation occurred. Once sufficient of these pair-wise events have been counted, the intensity information for the individual detectors can be combined using the well known back-projection algorithm, to provide a slice image which displays the distribution of the positron annihilation events in that physical plane, and hence the distribution of the original radiolabelled substance. In turn, that distribution can be interpreted in terms of the particular biochemical or physiological function under investigation.

This brief summary has glossed over several important facts. First, all the positron emitting nuclides have short half lives; the longest of the commonly used radionuclides, ^{18}F, is 110 minutes; those of other species are:- ^{11}C, 20 min; ^{13}N, 10 min; ^{15}O, 2 min; ^{75}Br, 1.6 hr; ^{122}I, 4min. The shortness of these half lives has two important implications. From the standpoint of the patient it means that the radionuclide remains in circulation through the body for a relatively short time, which reduces the radiation dose experienced by the tissues; clearly this is a substantial benefit. From the purely technical viewpoint, the shortness of these half lives has several, draconian disadvantages. It is a general perception that the <u>total</u> time available for a PET measurement should be less than the equivalent of five, half-life times. It follows then, that in general it is not possible to ship positron emitting radionuclides over any great distance; hence, each PET group requires access to a dedicated cyclotron. The same time-limitation has equally dramatic implications for the chemical syntheses used, which have to be not only efficient in terms of yields (both chemical and radiochemical), but also extremely fast. We return to this point later.

The final point of this introduction is that the technical demands of the PET method are so varied and extreme, that it is necessary to have a large, interdisciplinary team. Coupled with the very high capital costs involved, this also means that each patient study is extremely expensive.

I shall now explore, step by step, the sequence of a typical PET measurement in order to provide the reader with some feeling for the magnitude of this undertaking. The key intellectual feature is the decision as to which chemical species can be used to probe the phenomenon of interest. This necessitates considerable insight as to the <u>in-vivo</u> biochemistry involved. Some prior knowledge of the kinetics of the biochemical and physiological changes is also mandatory because of the shortness of the half lives of the radionuclide used.

Thus, at the outset, one has to define which phenomenon should be studied and which is the most appropriate substrate to follow it; the choice of radionuclide depends on the life time of the phenomenon itself, and also on the available chemistry.

The next two stages are both technical. First and most expensive, is access to a suitable cyclotron, and appropriate targets, to produce the appropriate radionuclides. This involves a substantial team of cyclotron-engineers and physicists, plus a nuclear chemist to ensure that the nuclear chemical reactions are induced as planned, that the product has appropriate radiopurity, and in adequate quantities. It is appropriate to mention, en passant, that generator-produced PET-radionuclides may eventually become available.

The next stage is to develop a suitable chemical synthesis; this must be rapid (remember that the whole process, from cyclotron to acquisition of clinical data, must be completed within 3-5 half lives), and high yielding. The intellectual philosophy which is to be followed is very different from that of any conventional organic synthesis. The cost of the starting material is completely irrelevant since only microgrammes of products will be produced! Likewise the complexity of the chemistry which precedes the labelling stage is unimportant, the clock does not start ticking until the radiolabelling step. However, thereafter time is everything, and all processes, not just the reaction itself, have to be simple and fast. Thus, it is useless to use a fast reaction if the subsequent deblocking, or purification, steps take too long. This represents a series of substantial intellectual and technical challenges.

Once a basic synthesis has been developed using cold materials, it is checked using the appropriate radionuclide. Frequently, this involves a reduction in quantities of several orders of magnitude, occasionally with disasterous results as surface adsorption on the apparatus takes it toll on the product yields!

Then the radio-pharmacist enters the scene, charged with responsibility for checking the material for its chemical, radioisotope and pharmaceutical purity. The latter has to be done by checking the long term validity of the procedure, the product from an individual synthesis being administered to the patient long before the check for the presence of pathogens has been completed.

Finally, the problem comes of getting the entire technical team to synchronise their efforts to the study of patients; this involves two additional requirements. First, that the team be able to guarantee to produce a labelled substance ready for the arrival of the patient who, with the attendant doctors will tak a dim view of being kept waiting too long. The second is that, if it is successful, the examination will have to be repeated with different patients over a period of several years; this requirement has some important implications for staffing the project, since most highly skilled Ph.D. chemists such as those required to pioneer the above syntheses, are generally not attracted to the prospect of repeating a synthesis several times each week for an extended period of time.

In general, the complete procedure involving the administration of the substance to man, will first be evaluated using a healthy volunteer. In that and the subsequent examinations, the examination is under the supervision of the clinical coworker, who administers the material to the patient who has already been positioned in the tomograph. Then the data are acquired and subjected to data processing to produce the spatial maps which show the distribution of the substance, or its metabolites which had been labelled with the positron-emitter. The quantitative data from those images then forms the base for the calculations to produce the diagnostic result.

Although the latter processes all sound straightforward, this is a gross oversimplification. The tomograph itself represents yet another major investment, probably mainly financial, although it is also necessary to have a trained staff, even when a turn-key system has been purchased.

The amount of data produced, even from a single study is immense and if several patient studies are made in a single day, then it is mandatory to have a substantial computer, along with trained operators, to process the data. In this context it is not obvious to the uninitiated, that for many PET procedures the clinically useful data do not come directly from the image itself, but, rather from fitting to a mathematical model. The development of those models can in itself be a massive undertaking, involving extensive studies in animals and a detailed insight into the biochemistry and physiology of the tissues which are under study, and to the resultant mathematical model. That all this is frequently taken for granted, probably stems from the fact that the use of 2-deoxy-2-fluoro-D-glucose was itself established so rapidly only because of the previous extensive studies of 2-deoxy-D-glucose.

Given the magnitude both of the capital expenditures involved, as well as the size of the team, it is clear that PET cannot become a widely used routine tool as it stands. Indeed, there are some who take the jaundiced view that it is not a clinically viable tool because it does not allow detailed repeated studies of a single patient. Others suggest that NMR-spectroscopy will anyway displace it.

My own views are as follows. First, that at present it is the only feasible method for mapping the spatial distribution of some biological transformations in man; this is especially so for events in the brain which occur at micro-molar concentrations, or lower. Second, that it is already feasible to contemplate many procedures which include at least some of the desirable features of PET, but which do not necessitate such expensive capital equipment. For example, use of nuclides which emit single gamma rays as the basis for "Single Photon Emission Computed Tomography" (SPECT) has already begun in some centres. This can use relatively inexpensive gamma ray equipment, and nuclides with somewhat longer half lives, thus avoiding the need for an on site cyclotron.

Three features of the PET method could undergo substantial changes in the near future. First, use of PET nuclides generated as "daughter products" from a radionuclide which has a substantially longer half life could lead to "generator isotopes", again reducing the dependence on a cyclotron. However, even that could become less of a problem if less expensive, simpler, cyclotron designs could be established. This is potentially the most important opportunity since none of the nuclides which are available from generators for PET, or SPECT, are those which are isotopes of the fundamental building blocks of biochemical substances, namely carbon, nitrogen, oxygen nor, even, as close as fluorine. Finally, attention should be drawn to the fact that new designs for gamma counting equipment could be adapted to PET measurements. Besides reducing substantially the cost for a head scanner, this could open up the whole area of body studies, with particular emphasis on the metabolic status of the heart.

Given the central role of diseases of the brain and heart and also of cancer, in the current spectrum of mortality and disability to which man is at present subject in the developed nations, it is clear that there is an ongoing need for methods which can be used to follow in-vivo the biochemical transformations of normal and diseased tissues. The ideal technique would be one which is capable of detecting at the most micro-molar quantities; which is non-invasive and hence can be used for serial studies; which is sufficiently inexpensive that it can be used widely in medical research centres and in hospitals, and which is flexible in the sense that new questions can be posed and answered without the need for many man-years of preliminary experimentations.

The reader of this chapter will have concluded that no single method currently available is even remotely satisfactory in more than one of the above categories. Clearly this provides an alluring challenge both to "industry" and to "academe" to develop the necessary intellectual and technical resources, and to the "clinical" and "biochemical" practitioners to identify those biochemical substances whose measurement would lead to clinically important diagnostic procedures. That this can only happen if there is close collaboration between the diverse array of different disciplines in turn poses a substantial opportunity for "university administrators", and the "Government funding agencies" to develop new organisation procedures which cut across the present departmental structures, many of which have performed admirably in the past, but which are now too inflexible to cope with contemporary opportunities, let alone those of the future.

HOW TO COPE WITH THE LITERATURE OF NMR OF LIVING SYSTEMS

L.D. Hall and W.A. Stewart
Department of Chemistry
University of British Columbia
Vancouver, B.C.
Canada V6T 1W5

ABSTRACT. Studies pertinent to this area cover such a wide range of topics and are published in so many different journals, that it is impossible to keep track using conventional methods. Fortunately, both the medical imaging industry, and the medical profession itself, have both responded with the development of computer-based surveys, which help alleviate the problem.

That the literature concerning NMR studies of living systems is expanding at an ever increasing rate, is an encouraging indication of the widespread acceptance which the method is receiving. The major drawback is that it faces those involved in this area with the daunting task of attempting to keep up with what others have done. Although this same situation applies to many other scientific and medical areas, in the case of NMR the problem is compounded by the diversity of interests which have converged on this subject. These range from the expected aspects of science, technology and computing, through the range of areas of application such as the life- and medical- sciences, to the legislative and financial aspects of the health-care delivery authorities. Although few practitioners will have to have a comprehensive survey of all of these areas, most will need at least some knowledge of each. This is a formidable task.

In what follows, we shall attempt to analyse this problem and discuss some strategies which we have found to be useful within the context of our own research group. Although others will almost certainly wish to choose their own balance between computer-searches and direct perusal of the journals themselves, it seems highly probable that everyone will use at least some measure of each approach.

Initially, any newcomer to this area will be more interested in a general survey than an in-depth compilation. Such surveys are most efficiently obtained from the numerous textbooks which have already been published on this topic. A summary of some of the titles of journals available up to 1984 are listed in references 1 to 15. A beginning reseacher may choose to invest in the one monograph which is exclusively dedicated to the literature (10). This book includes a number of interesting cross indexes, including those based on the direct literature, and on patent literature, and includes summaries of the names of persons who are active in the field. Although not

385

T. Axenrod and G. Ceccarelli (eds.), NMR in Living Systems, 385–390.

stimulating reading as such, this is an invaluable compilation since it includes not only magnetic resonance imaging but also appropriate references to NMR spectroscopy.

In this same context however we draw attention to the fact that many of the magnetic resonance imaging companies have themselves produced brochures which are extremely helpful; in particular, the quality of the diagrams included in those brochures are of extremely high quality.

Once a satisfactory level of general expertise and knowledge is available, the researcher will then need access to the literature pertinent to their own areas of future research. The same textbooks will provide a direct entree to the early literature and in particular will identify some of the "classical" references. So too, will a perusal of the professional journals which are directly pertinent to the researcher's other interests; the reference lists included in those publications also have the merit of including references which have been judged by others at least to be worthy of citation, will include most, if not all, of the "classical" references.

Eventually, most researchers will wish to have the security associated with a comprehensive bibliography of all of the pertinent references, and it is at this stage that it is mandatory to make use of a computer-aided literature search. The key feature of such searches is of course the prior development of an optimised set of "key words" which will ensure that, in addition to culling all of the pertinent references, the computer programme minimises the number of extraneous ones; this is not an easy task. The same computer-based method will also be invaluable when a researcher wishes to evaluate the possibilities of moving into a new area.

Our own experience in this area has been influenced substantially by the excellent co-operation which we have received from members of the various libraries of the University of British Columbia and the following discussions rest heavily on the advice which we have received from them; indeed it includes in some instances direct quotations.

What can be searched on a database?

Words (or phrases) are searched, primarily from the title, abstracts (if there is one), added indexing terms, or names from the author's area. Some databases also have codes to express particular concepts.

What is computer searching logic?

The logic involves the use of the Boolean logical operators AND, OR NOT. The OR operator broadens a search (example: cats OR dogs). The AND narrows (example: articles with cats AND dogs). The NOT operator eliminates articles with a particular concept (example: cats NOT dogs).

A search involves the creation of groups of citations (called sets), each group generally representing a particular concept. The sets are then combined in such a way so as to give the desired combination, and thus give the pertinent articles.

Since Boolean logic does not reflect complex human logic, many unwanted articles, which have the correct concepts but incorrect inter-relationships, may appear. Several database suppliers have helped to overcome this problem by use of "word adjacency" techniques (one more reason for a precise sentence describing what is wanted).

I shall now summarise some of the databases which we have accessed ourselves in the course of our own research studies.
1. Medline Database: this is produced by the U.S. National Library of Medicine (NLM) and provides journal articles with emphasis on medicine. It can be accessed in three different ways which are as follows. 1, NLM or MEDLARS; this is the cheapest way but also the least capable. It costs approximately 57 cents per minute before 2 p.m. and 44 cents per minute after 2 p.m. 2, BRS: this is more expensive than the above, but also more capable. It costs U.S. $19 per hour plus 4 cents for each citation. 3, DIALOG: this is the most capable but also more expensive than either of the above. It costs U.S. $44 per hour plus costs for other services.

All three of the above methods for accessing the Medline database are fairly sophisticated, and although they can be accessed directly we have found it more convenient to make use of the UBC library service. However there are two other routes which are less sophisticated and which can be used by an individual researcher. These are entitled: 1. BRS after-dark: this is expensive but unsophisticated. 2. DIALOG's knowledge index.

ATOMINDEX

This is produced by the International Atomic Energy Agency and provides access to the journal articles, monographs, conference proceedings and technical reports. This contains information not found in other bases.

CHEM.ABS

This database can be accessed in a variety of ways including BRS, DIALOG, and in Canada, a system referred to as CAN/OLE. If access to abstracts of papers are required then it is necessary to use the system CAS which is operated by the Chemical Abstract Service.

INSPEC:

This is produced by the Institute of Electrical Engineers of the United Kingdom. Its emphasis is on physics, electrical engineering, computing, and other technological aspects. It can be accessed through various of the larger systems such as BRS, DIALOG, CAN/OLE etc. and is relatively expensive.

NTIS:

This is the National Technical Information System and its emphasis is on technical reports generated by federally funded research in the United States. It can be accessed through BRS, DIALOG, CAN/OLE etc.

The databases summarised as numbers 1 and 2 above are probably the most widely used. Chemical abstracts is particularly good for studies which involve science, but it tends to be rather expensive.

Although the above computer-aided literature searches are necessary if a systematic coverage of the literature is required, they are certainly not a substitute for direct perusal of current journals. For any individual researcher with a broad range of interests this then remains a substantial task. In our laboratory at UBC we have attempted to share this task as follows. Each research worker is assigned several specific journals and is charged with responsibility for leafing through the entire contents of each issue. A photocopy is then made of the title page including the abstract, of each article which appears to be relevant to the interests not only of that researcher but of the entire group. Those copies are then placed in a binder which is circulated through all of the membership of the research group, so that the individual researcher has a reasonable chance of deciding which of the papers is worthy of more detailed study. An automatic bonus of this approach is that it encourages the membership of the research group to share the broader ranges of interest of the entire group.

We do not feel it appropriate to give more detailed advice concerning literature searches, because individual research groups will have to tailor their needs to the resources which they have available. One thing only is obvious, namely that the size and scope of nuclear magnetic resonance is going to increase at a progressively more rapid rate both in terms of technical developments, and in terms of the variety and number of applications. Although we can anticipate that this expansion of interest will be accompanied by the development of more specific databases and search profiles, and also by the development of publications which specialise exclusively in the area of NMR, it is inconceivable that the number of publications in which NMR reports are published will ever diminish. The only bright spot on the horizon is for the person who is interested in fundamental developments, who will find that these represent a small fraction of the total number of papers being published; those "classics" will of course be mandatory reading.

ACKNOWLEDGEMENTS. It is a great pleasure to acknowledge the excellent help which we have received from the staff of the libraries of the University of British Columbia as we have ourselves struggled with these immense problems. In particular, we wish to thank Jim Henderson, Computer Search Services Coordinator, Woodward Library, U.B.C. and Susan Chan, Computer Programmer, Health Service Research and Development.

ADDRESSES

1. NLM or MEDLARS: Medlars Management Section
   Bibliographic Services Division
   National Library of Medicine
   8600 Rockville Pike
   Bethesda, Maryland 20014
   Phone: (301) 496-6193
   In Canada: Medline Coordinator
   Health Science Resource Center
   Canadian Institute for Scientific and
     Technical Information
   Ottawa, Ontario K1A OS2
   Phone: (613) 993-1604

2. BRS: Bibliographic Retrieval Service, Inc.
   1200 Route 7
   Latham, New York 12110
   Phone: (518) 783-1161, or 800-345-4BRS

3. DIALOG: Dialog Information Services, Inc.
   3460 Hillview Avenue
   Palo Alto, California
   Phone: (415) 858-2700
   Telex: 334499
   Customer Services: (415) 858-3810

In Canada: Micromedia Ltd/DIALOG
   144 Front Street West
   Toronto, Ontario M5J 2L7
   Phone: 112-800-387-2689
   or (416) 593-5211

4. CAN/OLE: Canada Online Enquiry
   Client Services CAN/OLE & CAN/SDI
   Canadian Institute for Scientific and Technical
     Information
   National Research Council of Canada
   Ottawa, Ontario K1A OS2
   Phone: (613) 993-1210

5. CAS: Chemical Abstracts Service
   Customer Service Representative
   P.O. Box 3012
   Columbus, Ohio 43210
   Phone: (614) 421-6940

REFERENCES

1. NMR of Intact Biological Systems. Eds. R.J.P. Williams, E.R. Andrew, G.K. Radda, Phil. Trans. Roy. Soc., **289**, 379 (1980).

2. NMR-Imaging.   Eds. R.L. Witcosky, N. Karstaedt, C.L. Partain, Bowman Grey School Med., Winston-Salem (1981).

3. NMR in Medicine. Ed. R. Damadian, Springer-Verlag (1981).

4. NMR-Imaging in Medicine. Eds. L. Kaufman, L.E. Crookes, A.R. Margulis, Igaku-Shoin, Tokyo (1981).

5. NMR and Its Applications to Living Systems, D.G. Gadian, Oxford-Clarendon Press, Oxford (1982).

6. NMR Imaging. P. Mansfield and P.G. Morris, Ed. J.S. Waugh, Academic Press, London (1982).

7. NMR-Tomography, NMR-Scanner Techniques and the Theory of Image Reconstruction, V. Bangert, V.D.I.-Verlag, Dusseldorf (1982).

8. Nuclear Magnetic Resonance Imaging. Eds. C.L. Partain, T.L. James, Rollo and R.R. Price, Saunders Co., Philadelphia (1981).

9. Medical Imaging Systems, A. Macousky, Prentice Hall, Englewood Cliffs (1983).

10. NMR Imaging - A Comprehensive Bibliography, J. Jaklovsky, Addison-Wesley Pub. Co., Reading (1983).

11. NMR Imaging - Basic Principles. S.W. Young, Raven Press, New York (1984).

12. Clinical Magnetic Resonance Imaging. Eds. A.R. Margulis, C.B. Higgins, L. Kaufman and L.E. Crooks, Rad. Res. Ed. Fndtn., San Francisco (1983).

13. Nuclear Magnetic Resonance - NMR Imaging. C.L. Partain, Saunders Co., Philadelphia (1983).

14. Magnetic Resonance in Medicine and Biology, M.A. Foster, Ed. R. Anstey, Pergammon Press, Oxford (1984).

15 Biomedical Magnetic Resonance. Eds. T.L. James, A.R. Margulis, Rad. Res. Ed. Fndtn., San Francisco (1984).

LIST OF PARTICIPANTS

AIELLO, F.
Via Giovanni Bonanno, 59
90100 Palermo
Italy

ALBRAND, J. P.
C. E.N.G. - D.R.E.
Laboratoire de Chemie, 85X
38041 Grenoble Cedex
France

ALGER, J.
Department of Molecular Biophysics and
Biochemistry
P.O. Box 6666
Yale University
New Haven, Connecticut 06511
USA

ARNOLD, W.
Department of Biochemistry
Medical Center
University of Kansas
Kansas City, Kansas 66103
USA

AXENROD, T.
Department of Chemistry
The City College of the City University of New York
New York, N.Y. 10031
USA

BALDASSARI, A.M.
Istituto Anatomia Umana Normale
dell'Universita' di Bologna
Via Irnerio, 48
48100 Bologna
Italy

BARR, R.
Apartment 301
12000 Fairhill Avenue
Cleveland, Ohio 44120
USA

BAX, A.
Building 2, Room 109
National Institutes of Health
Bethesda, Maryland 20205
USA

BAZZO, R.
Via Campano, 14
28100 Novara
Italy

BECKER, E.D.

Building 1, Room 118
National Institutes of Health
Bethesda, Maryland 20205
USA

BEDINI, L.

Istituto di Elaborazione dell'Informazione
Via S. Maria, 46
56100 Pisa
Italy

BELL, J.

Department of Chemistry
Birbeck College
University of London
London WC1E 7HX
United Kingdom

BELLITTO, L.

Istituto Fisiologia Clinica
Via Savi, 8
56100 Pisa
Italy

BERTOLINI, L.

Dpartimento di Fisica
Universita' di Pavia
Via Bassi, 6
27100 Pavia
Italy

BIANUCCI, A.M.

Istituto di Chimica Farmaceutica
Universita' di Pisa
Via Bonanno, 6
56100 Pisa
Italy

BOICELLI, A.

National Research Council
Institute of Anatomy
University of Bologna
Via Irnerio, 48
40126 Bologna
Italy

BONADONNA, F.

Via Villafranca, 38
90100 Palermo
Italy

BORASI, G.

Servizio di Fisica Sanitaria
Ospedale Niguarda
Piazza Ospedale Maggiore, 3
20162 Milano
Italy

BORSETTO, C.

Centro Studi Biochimici sul Morbo di Cooley
Via Luigi Borsari, 46
44100 Ferrara
Italy

BORST, C.

Laboratorium-Experimentele Cardiologie
Catharijnesingel, 101
3511 GV Utrecht
The Netherlands

BOTTINI, S.

Istituto di Elaborazione dell'Informazione
Via S. Maria, 46
56100 Pisa
Italy

BRADAMANTE, S.

Universita' di Milano
Via C. Golgi 19
20133 Milano
Italy

BRAI, M.

Istituto di Fisica
Universita' di Palermo
Via Archirafi, 36
90123 Palermo
Italy

BRUNNER, P.

Spectrospin AG
Industriestr., 26
8117 Fallanden
Switzerland

CAIRI, M.

Department of Chemistry
University of Ioannina
45332 Ioannina
Greece

CALVANI, P.

Dipartimento di Fisica
Universita' di Roma
Piazzale Aldo Moro, 2
00185 Roma
Italy

CARPINELLI, G.

Istituto Superiore di Sanita
Laboratorio di Biologia Cellulare
Viale Regina Elena, 299
00161 Roma
Italy

CASIERI, C.

Dipartimento di Fisica
Universita' di Roma
Piazzale Aldo Moro, 2
00185 Roma
Italy

CAVAGNA, F.

Analyt. Labor G865
Hoechst AG
6230 Frankfurt/M, 80
FRG

CECCARELLI, G.

Istituto di Chimica Fisica
Universita' di Pisa
Via Risorgimento, 35
56100 Pisa
Italy

CIRAOLA, L.

Viale E. Cialdini, 3
Firenze
Italy

CONTI, F.

Istituto di Chimica Fisica
Universita' di Roma
Piazzale Aldo Moro, 5
00185 Roma
Italy

COUTINHO, I. B.

Universidade Nova de Lisboa
Quinta da Torre
2825 Monte da Caparica
Portugal

DALLAND, M.

Department of Chemistry
University of Bergen
Allegt. 41
N-5000 Bergen
Norway

DE BIE, M.

Laboratory for Organic Chemistry
State University of Utrecht
Croesestraat, 79
3522 AD Utrecht
The Netherlands

DE JONG, J.W.

Cardiochemical Laboratory- Thoraxcenter
Erasmus University
P.O. Box 1738
3000 DR Rotterdam
The Netherlands

DE LUCA, F.

Dipartimento di Fisica
Universita' di Roma
Piazzale Aldo Moro, 2
00185 Roma
Italy

DE SIMONE, B.C.

Dipartimento di Fisica
Universita' di Roma
Piazzale Aldo Moro, 2
00185 Roma
Italy

EAGAN, W.

Food and Drug Administration
Building 29, Room 430
8800 Rockville Pike
Bethesda, Maryland 20205
USA

FEENEY, J.

National Institute for Medical Research
The Ridgeway, Mill Hill
London, NW7 1AA
United Kingdom

FINOCCHIARO, P.

Facolta di Ingegneria
Viale Andrea, 6
95125 Catania
Italy

FRANCOIS, A

Vaste Stof-Fysica en Magnetisme
Katholieke Universiteit Leuven
Celestijnenlaan 200D
B-3030 Leuven
Belgium

FROELICH, T.

Universitats-Kinderklinik
Im Neuenheimerfeld, 150
D-6900 Heidelberg
FRG

GANSSEN, A.

Siemens Aktiengesellschaft
Bereich Medizinische Technik
Postfach 3260
Henkestrasse, 127
8520 Erlangen
FRG

GENDEL, E.

420 East 55th Street
New York, N.Y. 10022
USA

GEROTHANASSIS, I.   Department of Chemistry
                      University of Ioannina
                      45332 Ioannina
                      Greece

GIULIANI, A.M.   Area Della Ricerca Del C.N.R.
                      C.P. 10
                      00016 Monterotondo Stazione
                      Roma
                      Italy

GOBETTO, R.   Istituto di Chimica Generale
                      ed Inorganica dell'Universita
                      Corso Massimo D'Azeglio
                      410125 Torino
                      Italy

GRASSINI, S.   Istituto di Chimica Fisica
                      Universita' di Pisa
                      Via Risorgimento, 35
                      56100 Pisa
                      Italy

GRILLO-RUGGIERI, F.   Istituto di Radiologia
                      Universita' di Genova
                      Viale Benedetto XV, 10
                      16132 Genova
                      Italy

GUPTA, R.   Department of Physiology and Biophysics
                      Albert Einstein School of Medicine
                      Bronx, N.Y. 10461
                      USA

HALL, L.   Department of Chemistry
                      University of British Columbia
                      2036 Main Mall
                      Vancouver, B.C. V6T 1Y6
                      Canada

HINTON, J.   Department of Chemistry
                      University of Arkansas
                      Fayetteville, Arkansas 72701
                      USA

HOULT, D.I.   Building 13, Room 3W13
                      National Institutes of Health
                      Bethesda, Maryland 20205
                      USA

KIEFER, B.
Institut fur Biophysik
University of Giessen
Leihgestener Weg, 217
D-6300 Giessen
FRG

LANDONI, L.
Via Grigna, 3
20025 Legnano
Italy

LAVANCHY, N.
Laboratoire de Physiologie Animale
Universite de Grenoble
B.P. 68
38402 St-Martin-D'Heres Cedex
France

LO ZITO, A.
Via Mezzini, 15
Raffadali
Agrigento
Italy

MACLEAN, C.
Chemistry Laboratory
Free University of Amsterdam
De Boelelaan, 1083
1081 HV Amsterdam
The Netherlands

MACRI, M.A.
Via Cassioli, 150
00169 Roma
Italy

MAIER, M.
Charing Cross Medical School
The Reynold's Building
St. Dunstan's Road
London W6 8RP
United Kingdom

MANGIARACINA, P.
161A Maspeth Avenue
Brooklyn, N.Y. 11211
USA

MARAVIGLIA, B.
Dipartimento di Fisica
Universita' di Roma
Piazzale Aldo Moro, 2
00185 Roma
Italy

MASON, R.P.   Department of Organic Chemistry
                               University of Cambridge
                               Lensfield Road
                               Cambridge CB2 1EW
                               United Kingdom

MINGUZZI-RANZI, A.   Department of Physics
                               University of Bologna
                               Via Irnerio, 46
                               40126 Bologna
                               Italy

MOR, P.   Via Manzoni, 9
                               25127 Brescia
                               Italy

MUSTARELLI, P.   Dipartimento di Fisica
                               Universita' di Pavia
                               Via Bassi, 6
                               27100 Pavia
                               Italy

NALBANTOGLU, M.   TBTAK Marmara Research Institute
                               P.K. 21
                               Gebeze-Kocaeli
                               Turkey

NARBAD, A.   Department of Microbiology
                               University College-Cardiff
                               Newport Road
                               Cardiff CF2 1TA
                               United Kingdom

NUCCETELLI, C.   Dipartimento di Fisica
                               Universita' di Roma
                               Piazzale Aldo Moro, 2
                               00185 Roma
                               Italy

PAVONI, P.   Viale Cortina d'Ampezzo, 179
                               00135 Roma
                               Italy

PUPI, A.   Istituto di Medicina Nucleare
                               Universita' di Firenze
                               Viale Morgagni, 85
                               50134 Firenze
                               Italy

RANDALL, E.W.   Department of Chemistry
Queen Mary College
Mile End Road
London E1 4NS
United Kingdom

REMY, C.   L.M.C.E.C.
Departement de Biophysique
UER de Medecine
38700 La Tronche,
France

RESCIGNO, A.   Section of Neurological Surgery
School of Medicine
Yale University
New Haven, Connecticut 06510
USA

ROTOLO, E.   Vicolo della Banca, 4
33100 Udine
Italy

SANTOS, H.   Centro de Quimica Estrutural
Instituto Superior Tecnico
Av. Rovisco Pais
1096 Lisboa Codex
Portugal

SCANDURRA, G.   Via Trieste, 28
S. Venerina
Catania
Italy

SEPIACCI, G.   Vicolo della Banca, 4
33100 Udine
Italy

SHAW, D.   General Electric Company
260 Bath Road
Slough, Berks. SL1 4ER
United Kingdom

SILLERUD, L.   Los Alamos National Laboratory
MS M886
P.O. Box 1663
Los Alamos, New Mexico 87545
USA

STALMANS, W.L.R.

Katholieke Universiteit
School of Medicine
Afdeling Biochemie
Campus Gasthuisberg
Herestraat, 49
B-3000 Leuven
Belgium

TAVERNI, N.

Via Panciatichi, 37
50127 Firenze
Italy

TURAN, B.

Department of Physiology
Faculty of Medicine
University of Ankara
Sihhiye-Ankara
Turkey

TURNER, D.

Department of Chemistry
The University
Southampton SO 9 5NH
United Kingdom

TURNER, N

Dyson Perrins Laboratory
Oxford University
South Parks Road
Oxford OX1 3QY
United Kingdom

TURNER, R

Department of Physics
University of Nottingham
University Park
Nottingham NG7 2RD
United Kingdom

VAN CRAEN, J.

Woluwelaan, 100
1920 Diegem
Belgium

VALENZA, G.

Via G. Cosentino, 20
90145 Palermo
Italy

VALENZA, M.

Istituto di Fisica
Universita' di Palermo
Via Archirafi, 36
90123 Palermo
Italy

VEIL, E.

Hauptstrasse,44
7441 Schlaitdorf
FRG

VELLUCCI, F.

Ansaldo Biomedicale
Via Pierino Pesce, 5
16151 Sampierdarena
Genova
Italy

VIORA, E.

Cattedra di Patologia Ostetrica e Ginocologia
Via Ventimiglia, 3
10126 Torino
Italy

VITTADINI, G.

Via Follo, 50
20134 Milano
Italy

WEBB, G.A.

Department of Chemistry
University of Surrey
Guildford, Surrey GU2 5XH
United Kingdom

WILLEM, R.

Vrije Universiteit Brussel
T.W./ AOSC
Pleinlaan, 2
B-1050 Brussels
Belgium

YILMAZ, A.

P.K. 36
Diyarbakir
Turkey

ZIESSOW, D.

Institute for Physical and Theoretical Chemistry
Technical University of Berlin
Strasse des 17, Juni, 112
D-1000 Berlin
Germany

ZOLLE, I.

Allgemeines Krankenhaus der Stadt
Abteilung fur Nuclearmedizin der Med. Univ. Klinik
Garnisongasse, 13
1090 Wien
Austria